Drug Information for Teens

TEEN HEALTH SERIES

First Edition

Drug Information for Teens

Health Tips about the Physical and Mental Effects of Substance Abuse

Including Facts about Alcohol, Anabolic Steroids, Club Drugs, Cocaine, Depressants, Hallucinogens, Herbal Products, Inhalants, Marijuana, Narcotics, Stimulants, Tobacco, and More

Edited by Karen Bellenir

Omnigraphics

615 Griswold Street • Detroit, MI 48226

Bibliographic Note

Because this page cannot legibly accommodate all the copyright notices, the Bibliographic Note portion of the Preface constitutes an extension of the copyright notice.

Edited by Karen Bellenir

Teen Health Series

Karen Bellenir, *Managing Editor*
David A. Cooke, MD, *Medical Consultant*
Elizabeth Barbour, *Permissions Associate*
Dawn Matthews, *Verification Assistant*
Carol Munson, *Permissions Assistant*
Laura Pleva Nielsen, *Index Editor*
EdIndex, Services for Publishers, *Indexers*

* * *

Omnigraphics, Inc.

Matthew P. Barbour, *Senior Vice President*
Kay Gill, *Vice President—Directories*
Kevin Hayes, *Operations Manager*
David P. Bianco, *Marketing Consultant*

* * *

Peter E. Ruffner, *President and Publisher*

Frederick G. Ruffner, Jr., *Chairman*

ISBN 0-7808-0444-9

Library of Congress Cataloging-in-Publication Data

Drug information for teens : health tips about the physical and mental effects of substance abuse / edited by Karen Bellenir.-- 1st ed.
p. cm. -- (Teen health series)
"Including facts about alcohol, anabolic steroids, club drugs, cocaine, depressants, hallucinogens, herbal products, inhalants, marijuana, narcotics, stimulants, tobacco, and more."
Includes bibliographical references and index.
ISBN 0-7808-0444-9
1. Teenagers--Drug use--United States. 2. Teenagers--Alcohol use--United States. 3. Teenagers--Health and hygiene--United States. 4. Drugs--United States--Physiological effect. 5. Drug abuse--United States--Prevention. 6. Alcoholism--United States--Prevention. I. Bellenir, Karen. II. Series.
HV5824.Y68 D774 2002
362.29--dc21
2002074858

Printed in the United States

Table of Contents

Part IV: Other Abused Drugs And Chemicals

Part V: Other Drug-Related Health Concerns

Part VI: Treatment For Substance Abusers

Part VII: Drug Statistics And Policy Controversies

Part VIII: Resources For Help And Additional Information

Preface

About This Book

Teens live in a world marked by transition. As adolescents leave childhood behind and prepare to enter adulthood, they begin to explore new ideas and take more risks. This inclination can lead to experimentation with alcohol, tobacco, and other drugs. Some may try a substance—just once... or twice.

"Every drug user starts out as an occasional user," says Alan Leshner, Director of the National Institute on Drug Abuse. "To be sure, no one ever starts out using drugs intending to become a drug addict."

Drug use, however, creates changes in the way the brain functions. At some point, which varies among individuals and is affected by the characteristics of different substances, the brain becomes altered. An occasional, voluntary drug user becomes a compulsive, addicted user.

According to recent surveys, more than half of American young people have tried an illicit drug by the time they finish high school; 62% of high school seniors say they have been drunk at least once. More than four million kids between the ages of 12 and 17 are current smokers, and approximately 14 million teens are considered at moderate or high risk of substance abuse.

Drug Information for Teens provides adolescents with facts about drug use, abuse, and addiction. It describes the physical and mental effects of alcohol, tobacco, marijuana, ecstasy, inhalants, and many other drugs and chemicals that are often abused. It includes information about the process that leads from casual use to addiction and offers suggestions for resisting peer pressure and helping friends stay drug free. A section on drug statistics and policy controversies offers facts about drug trends and current issues such as the medical use of marijuana and drug legalization. Resource directories provide contact information for national organizations, hotlines and helplines, and other sources of support.

How To Use This Book

This book is divided into parts and chapters. Parts focus on broad areas of interest. Chapters are devoted to single topics within a part.

Part I: Understanding Substance Use, Abuse, And Addiction begins with a quiz on drug-related knowledge. It provides information about the brain processes that are affected by drug use and describes how addictions develop. Tips on drug prevention efforts and facts about peer pressure are also included.

Part II: Alcohol presents facts about alcohol use, abuse, and addiction in teens, their friends, and family members. It includes suggestions for avoiding situations in which alcohol may be offered, reviews the risks associated with binge drinking, summarizes treatment options for people with alcohol-related problems, and offers tips for helping friends who may be reluctant to seek help on their own.

Part III: Tobacco provides information about cigarettes and other nicotine products, such as chewing tobacco, cigars, and pipes. Health risks associated with second-hand smoke are also discussed.

Part IV: Other Abused Drugs And Chemicals offers basic information about some of the most commonly abused substances, including anabolic steroids, cocaine, ecstasy, LSD, heroin, inhalants, and marijuana. Also included are facts about legally available substances of concern, such as caffeine, herbal products, and medications.

Part V: Other Drug-Related Health Concerns covers some important topics that are associated with drug use but not necessarily related to the direct effects of the substances themselves. These include drug-facilitated rape and other issues surrounding sex under the influence of intoxicating substances; the spread of infectious diseases that can be transmitted via drug paraphernalia; impaired driving; violence; learning disabilities; emotional and behavioral problems; and the relationship between drugs and suicide.

Part VI: Treatment For Substance Abusers presents information about the various methods and medications that are used in substance abuse treatment. It offers encouragement to seek help before problems become overwhelming and provides tips for helping friends and family members who may be reluctant to seek treatment.

Part VII: Drug Statistics And Policy Controversies summarizes observed trends in substance use among middle- and high-school students. It explains the Controlled Substances Act and offers information about some controversial drug-policy issues, including the medical use of marijuana, and drug legalization.

Part VIII: Resources For Help And Additional Information includes a directory of national organizations able to provide drug-related information and a directory of places able to provide support services, including hotline and helpline phone numbers and organizations that sponsor support groups. A state-by-state list of referral services will help readers find local information, and a chapter of additional reading presents lists of books, magazines and journals, and web pages that can be used as a starting point for further research.

Bibliographic Note

This volume contains documents and excerpts from publications issued by the following government agencies: Center for Substance Abuse Prevention (CSAP); Centers for Disease Control and Prevention (CDC); Drug Enforcement Administration (DEA); National Clearinghouse for Alcohol and Drug Information (NCADI); National Institute of Drug Abuse (NIDA); National Institute of Justice; National Institute on Alcohol Abuse and Alcoholism (NIAAA); Substance Abuse and Mental Health Services Administration (SAMHSA); U.S. Department of Health and Human Services

(DHHS); U.S. Department of Justice (DoJ); and the U.S. Food and Drug Administration (FDA).

In addition, this volume contains copyrighted documents and articles produced by the following organizations: A.A. World Services, Inc./A.A. Grapevine, Inc.; American Academy of Family Physicians; American Civil Liberties Union; American Psychiatric Association; Australian Nutrition Foundation, Inc. (Nutrition Australia); California Dental Association; Connecticut Clearinghouse; Do It Now Foundation; Focus Adolescent Services; Harvard School of Public Health; Hazleden Foundation; Indiana Prevention Resource Center; National Alliance for the Mentally Ill; National Association for Children of Alcoholics; National Center on Addiction and Substance Abuse at Columbia University (CASA); Pennsylvania Liquor Control Board; Project Inform; Reuters Health; and Youth Media Network.

Full citation information is provided on the first page of each chapter. Every effort has been made to secure all necessary rights to reprint the copyrighted material. If any omissions have been made, please contact Omnigraphics to make corrections for future editions.

Acknowledgements

In addition to the organizations listed above, special thanks are due to verification assistant Dawn Matthews, permission specialist Liz Barbour, and editorial assistant Buffy Bellenir.

Note From The Editor

This book is part of Omnigraphics' *Teen Health Series*. The series provides basic information about a broad range of medical concerns. It is not intended to serve as a tool for diagnosing illness, in prescribing treatments, or as a substitute for the physician/patient relationship. All persons concerned about medical symptoms or the possibility of disease are encouraged to seek professional care from an appropriate health care provider.

At the request of librarians serving today's young adults, the *Teen Health Series* was developed as a specially focused set of volumes within

Omnigraphics' *Health Reference Series*. Each volume deals comprehensively with a topic selected according to the needs and interests of people in middle school and high school. If there is a topic you would like to see addressed in a future volume of the *Teen Health Series*, please write to:

Editor
Teen Health Series
Omnigraphics, Inc.
615 Griswold Street
Detroit, MI 48226
E-mail: editorial@omnigraphics.com

Our Advisory Board

The *Teen Health Series* is reviewed by an Advisory Board comprised of librarians from public, academic, and medical libraries. We would like to thank the following board members for providing guidance to the development of this series:

Dr. Lynda Baker, Associate Professor of Library and Information Science, Wayne State University, Detroit, MI

Nancy Bulgarelli, William Beaumont Hospital Library, Royal Oak, MI

Karen Imarisio, Bloomfield Township Public Library, Bloomfield Township, MI

Karen Morgan, Mardigian Library, University of Michigan-Dearborn, Dearborn, MI

Rosemary Orlando, St. Clair Shores Public Library, St. Clair Shores, MI

Medical Consultant

Medical consultation services are provided to the *Teen Health Series* editors by David A. Cooke, MD. Dr. Cooke is a graduate of Brandeis University, and he received his MD degree from the University of Michigan. He completed residency training at the University of Wisconsin Hospital and Clinics. He is board-certified in Internal Medicine. Dr. Cooke currently works as part of the University of Michigan Health System and practices in

Brighton, MI. In his free time, he enjoys writing, science fiction, and spending time with his family.

Part 1

Understanding Substance Use, Abuse, And Addiction

Chapter 1

Are You Drug Smart?

Eggs-Istential Questions

If drug information were money, we'd all be zillionaires by now.

Think about it. Sometimes, it almost seems like it's everywhere you look today—on TV, at school, in magazines, in ads zooming past on buses, and looming down from billboards.

"This is a frying pan. This is an egg. This is an egg in a frying pan. Drugs are like this, only different. Any questions?"

It's usually well-intentioned. And most of it's true (in one way or another), but a lot of it's just dumb. And what isn't dumb, can be eggs-cruciatingly boring the 5,000th time around.

That's why we put together this quiz: to let you sort out what you really know from what you only might think you know about drugs and alcohol.

So be like an egg in a non-teflon frying pan: Stick around. Because sometimes, there's a world of difference between the two. And the difference can add up to something a lot more precious to all of us than money.

About This Chapter: Text in this chapter is from "Are You Drug Smart? Test Your Chemical IQ," by Jim Parker, Do It Now Foundation, Catalog No. 103, © January 2001; reprinted with permission.

Questions

1. "Special K" is a PCP-like drug that can cause users to believe they've been contacted by extraterrestrials.

a. true b. false

2. Hash oil is derived from hashish and rarely contains other drugs.

a. true b. false

3. Which can increase the risk of HIV infection?

a. alcohol
b. cocaine
c. heroin or other IV drug use
d. all of the above

> ✤ **It's A Fact!!**
>
> This quiz is from a pamphlet that is one in a series of publications on drugs, behavior, and health published by Do It Now Foundation. You can call or write for a complete list of available titles, or check them out online at http://www.doitnow.org.
>
> Do It Now Foundation
> P. O. Box 27568
> Tempe, AZ 85285
> Phone: 480-736-0599

4. Which of the following drugs is most often linked to incidents of date rape?

a. Rohypnol c. alcohol
b. cocaine

5. The main active ingredient in most forms of "herbal ecstasy" is:

a. St. John's wort
b. ephedrine
c. a user's own imagination
d. something else

6. "Ecstasy" is:

a. an amphetamine-based hallucinogen
b. a powerful barbiturate
c. an orange powder with purple "flavor crystals"

7. What's the best treatment for heroin overdose?

a. mouth-to-mouth resuscitation
b. induce vomiting

8. Does cocaine produce dependence?

a. yes b. no

9. Which is used in Native American religious ceremonies?

a. bhang c. peyote
b. guarana

10. Which class doesn't cause physical dependence?

a. opiates
b. hallucinogens
c. barbiturates

11. "Designer drugs" are:

a. safe and effective when taken as directed
b. copycat chemicals designed to mimic illegal drugs
c. made in Third World sweatshops by child chemists

12. Alcohol contains about how many calories per ounce?

a. 75
b. 125
c. 200
d. 350

13. The most potent form of marijuana or cannabis is:

a. hashish
b. kif
c. ganja
d. mojo

14. Which is most likely to trigger overdose with alcohol?

a. marijuana
b. amphetamine
c. barbiturates

15. What side effects are linked to long-term use of anabolic steroids?

a. heart disease
b. impotence
c. severe acne
d. all of the above

16. Which drug causes the most proven birth defects?

a. LSD
b. marijuana
c. alcohol
d. heroin

17. The most-widely used tranquilizer in America is:

a. Xanax®
b. Darvon®
c. Valium®
d. C-SPAN

18. A cheap, smokable form of cocaine is known as:

a. snap
b. crack
c. pop
d. rock
e. b and d

19. On the street, PCP is sold as:

a. angel dust
b. tic
c. wac
d. all of the above

20. "Ice" is a smokable form of which drug?

a. methamphetamine
b. barbiturate
c. cocaine
d. LSD

✔ Quick Tip

Add It Up

Are you broke again? Don't know where your money is going? Take a look at what you're spending your money on. Chances are, if you're supporting bad habits such as smoking cigarettes, drinking alcohol, or using marijuana or other illicit substances, you're spending quite a chunk of change. If you don't believe it, try out this expense calculator and see how much money you could be spending on something else!

Cigarette Use			
Packs of cigarettes smoked in a week.	Times Price per pack.	=	Average Monthly Subtotal
Alcohol Use			
Average number of drinks drank in one setting.	Times Price per drink.	Times a week you drink =	Average Monthly Subtotal
Substance Use			
Drug: Cocaine Heroin Methamphetamines Marijuana	Price you pay	Times units used per month =	Average Monthly Subtotal
Totals			
Add it up		=	Average Monthly Total
		Times 12 =	Yearly Expenditures

From "Drug Calculator," The National Clearinghouse for Alcohol and Drug Information, an interactive undated web calculator available at http://www.health.org/features/interact/calc/; cited 11.19.01.

Answers

1. *(a) strange, but true.* Various users of the dissociative anesthetic ketamine (AKA "K" or "Special K")—including early researcher Dr. John Lilly—have reported that they felt in telepathic contact with extraterrestrials while under K's influence. None has produced autopsy photos or other forms of proof, though, despite the fact that Fox would probably pay a fortune for the TV rights.

2. *(a) true.* In nearly all cases, hash oil really is just that, a concentrate of hashish in an alcohol solution.

3. *(d) all of the above.* Although only heroin and other injectable drugs are linked directly to transmission of the AIDS virus (through the sharing of contaminated needles), alcohol, cocaine, and other drugs can lead to high-risk sex, which can increase risk of infection.

4. *(c) alcohol.* Although the sleeping pill Rohypnol® was labeled the date-rape drug by the media in the mid-'90s (since it could be slipped undetected into an unsuspecting woman's drink and caused full or partial amnesia in victims), all the drugs listed (and perhaps all drugs period) have been linked to date rape. Still, alcohol figures into more reports of date rape and sexual assault than any other drug.

5. *(b) ephedrine.* The main ingredient in most forms of herbal ecstasy is the natural bronchodilator ephedrine, with other natural stimulants (including caffeine) thrown in to impress the gullible. The natural antidepressant St. John's wort hasn't turned up in herbal "E" yet, but that doesn't mean it won't, given the tight new controls the U.S. Food and Drug Administration has imposed on over-the-counter sale of ephedrine. (If you guessed (c) you're right, too—maybe even more right. Give yourself full credit.)

6. *(a) an amphetamine-based hallucinogen.* "Ecstasy" is known pharmacologically as MDMA. Its chemical structure is similar to both mescaline and amphetamine.

7. *(a) mouth-to-mouth resuscitation.* Making the victim of a heroin overdose throw up not only doesn't help, it can even make things worse. Since most heroin users inject the drug, there's no good reason to induce vomiting.

8. *(a) yes.* Like other potent stimulant drugs, cocaine can cause serious dependence.

9. *(c) peyote.* The peyote cactus, which grows in the southwestern U.S. and Mexico, is still used in ceremonies of the Native American Church. Religious use of peyote dates back thousands of years.

10. *(b) hallucinogens.* While hallucinogens do not cause addiction or withdrawal, all opiates and barbiturates do.

11. *(b) copycat chemicals designed to mimic illegal drugs.* Designer drugs are designed to simulate such controlled drugs as heroin and amphetamine. Since they're usually untested, they can pose serious risks to unwitting human guinea pigs.

12. *(c) 200.* Beverage alcohol contains about 200 calories per ounce. Add mixer, a pineapple slice, and a little straw umbrella, and you come up with lots of calories—but no nutrition. (Unless you eat the pineapple or the umbrella.)

13. *(a) hashish.* Ganja and kif are common names for marijuana in India and the Middle East.

14. *(c) barbiturates.* In combination, alcohol and other depressant drugs can produce a deadly synergism, with effects more multiplicative than additive. Translation? Mix alcohol and downers, and 3 + 3 doesn't add up to 6, but something more like 9. And for some people, it can add up to a lot more than that.

15. *(d) all of the above.* Synthetic versions of the male sex hormone testosterone, steroids can cause a number of side effects, including heart disease, acne, and impotence. Need any other reasons to leave them alone?

16. *(c) alcohol.* The No. 1 cause of birth defects in America is alcohol. Babies born to women who drink during pregnancy can suffer permanent defects known as Fetal Alcohol Syndrome. Even occasional drinking can cause problems, and may increase chances of stillbirth, growth retardation, and miscarriage.

17. *(a) Xanax.* Although Valium held the top spot for years (and, for a while, was the most widely-prescribed drug of all), Xanax rules the roost today. Both are members of the drug family known as benzodiazepines.

18. *(e) b and d.* Both "crack" and "rock" are the same thing—a form of cocaine sold in small chunks, which are smoked by users. But no matter what you call it, crack has made a name for itself as the king of street drugs—and as one mother of an addiction.

19. *(d) all of the above.* Even though PCP is used medically only as an animal tranquilizer, that hasn't stopped people from wolfing it down. The reason it often travels under aliases is that it's so unpredictable and so often unpleasant that users don't exactly clamor for it or ask it for it by name. Large doses can cause hallucinations, delusions, amnesia, and overdose.

20. *(a) methamphetamine.* A concentrated form of crystal methamphetamine, "ice" is smoked, just like crack cocaine. It carries all the risks of traditional amphetamine use, and then some, due to the rapid onset of its effects and the intensity of its high, plus the unknown hazards of direct exposure of lung tissue to meth vapors.

Scoring Guide

19-20 right. Drug eggs-pert! Congratulations, ace. You're at the head of the class, drug information-wise. Still, you did mess up the grading curve for everyone else.

16-18 right. Over easy! Eggs-cellent score, dude/dudette! If drug information really was money, you'd be rolling in it. Keep up the good work!

☞ Remember!!

What you don't know can hurt you, and that's especially true when what you don't know about is drugs and alcohol.

Take care. And be careful of what you take.

13-15 right. Slightly runny. Not bad, but your drug info quotient is slightly soft-boiled, and could stand a little improvement. Just don't try to catch up by experimenting on yourself.

10-12 right. You must be yolking! Take two drug education pamphlets and call us in the morning, lest you eggs-acerbate a bad situation.

Less than 10. Egg-gads! Consider yourself among the world's great chemical illiterates, but don't get egg-ocentric about it. Run—don't walk—to the nearest computer and visit Do It Now at http://www.doitnow.org/pages/nowhome2.html, or check out some of the other resources listed in the last section of this book.

Chapter 2

Teenagers And Drugs

Teenagers may be involved with legal or illegal drugs in various ways. Experimentation with drugs during adolescence is common. Unfortunately, teenagers often don't see the link between their actions today and the consequences tomorrow. They also have a tendency to feel indestructible and immune to the problems that others experience.

Using alcohol and tobacco at a young age increases the risk of using other drugs later. Some teens will experiment and stop, or continue to use occasionally, without significant problems. Others will develop a dependency, moving on to more dangerous drugs and causing significant harm to themselves and possibly others.

Adolescence is a time for trying new things. Teens use drugs for many reasons, including curiosity, because it feels good, to reduce stress, to feel grown up or to fit in. It is difficult to know which teens will experiment and stop and which will develop serious problems.

About This Chapter: Information in this Chapter is from "Drugs and Teen Substance Abuse," Copyright © 2000 Focus Adolescent Services, Salisbury, MD. Information provided by the American Academy of Child and Adolescent Psychiatry (AACAP) and the National Institute of Drug Abuse. Reprinted with permission. The full text and other information can be found on the Focus Adolescent Services website at http://www.focusas.com.

Substances That Are Abused

Teenagers abuse a variety of drugs, legal and illegal.

- **Alcohol**
- **Tobacco:** Teens who smoke are three times more likely than nonsmokers to use alcohol, eight times more likely to use marijuana, and 22 times more likely to use cocaine. Smoking is associated with a host of other risky behaviors, such as fighting and engaging in unprotected sex.
- **Prescribed medications** (such as Ritalin and OxyContin)
- **Inhalants:** Known by such street names as huffing, sniffing, and wanging, the dangerous habit of getting high by inhaling the fumes of common household products is estimated to claim the lives of more than a thousand children each year. Many other young people, including some first-time users, are left with serious respiratory problems and permanent brain damage.
- **Over-the-counter** cough, cold, sleep, and diet medications (such as Coricidin)
- **Marijuana:** About one half of the people in the United States have used marijuana, many are currently using it and some will require treatment for marijuana abuse and dependence.
- **Stimulants:** The possible long-term effects include tolerance and dependence, violence and aggression, malnutrition due to suppression of appetite. Crack, a powerfully addictive stimulant, is the term used for a smokeable form of cocaine. In 1997, an estimated 1.5 million Americans, age 12 and older, were chronic cocaine users.

✤ It's A Fact!!
Who Is At Risk?

Teenagers at risk for developing serious alcohol and drug problems include those:

- with a family history of substance abuse
- who are depressed
- who have low self-esteem, and
- who feel like they don't fit in or are out of the mainstream

- **Club drugs:** This term refers to drugs being used by teens and young adults at all-night dance parties such as "raves" or "trances," dance clubs, and bars. MDMA (Ecstasy), GHB, Rohypnol (Rophies), ketamine, methamphetamine, and LSD are some of the club or party drugs gaining popularity. Because some club drugs are colorless, tasteless, and odorless, they can be added unobtrusively to beverages by individuals who want to intoxicate or sedate others. In recent years, there has been an increase in reports of club drugs used to commit sexual assaults.
- **Depressants:** These are drugs used medicinally to relieve anxiety, irritability, tension. There is a high potential for abuse and, combined with alcohol, effects are heightened and risks are multiplied.
- **Heroin:** Several sources indicate an increase in new, young users across the country who are being lured by inexpensive, high-purity heroin that can be sniffed or smoked instead of injected. Heroin has also been appearing in more affluent communities.
- **Steroids:** Anabolic steroids are a group of powerful compounds closely related to the male sex hormone testosterone. From 1998 to 1999, there was a significant increase in anabolic steroid abuse among middle-schoolers.

The use of illegal drugs is increasing, especially among young teens. The average age of first marijuana use is 14, and alcohol use can start before age 12. The use of marijuana and alcohol in high school has become common.

Drug use is associated with a variety of negative consequences, including increased risk of serious drug use later in life, school failure, and poor judgment which may put teens at risk for accidents, violence, unplanned and unsafe sex, and suicide.

Warning Signs Of Teen Substance Abuse

- **Physical:** Fatigue, repeated health complaints, red and glazed eyes, and a lasting cough.
- **Emotional:** Personality change, sudden mood changes, irritability, irresponsible behavior, low self-esteem, poor judgment, depression, and a general lack of interest.

- **Family:** Starting arguments, breaking rules, or withdrawing from the family.
- **School:** Decreased interest, negative attitude, drop in grades, many absences, truancy, and discipline problems.
- **Social problems:** New friends who are less interested in standard home and school activities, problems with the law, and changes to less conventional styles in dress and music.

✔ Quick Tip

Your Parents May Need To Know About Treatment Issues

Parents can help through early education about drugs, open communication, good role modeling, and early recognition if problems are developing. If there is any suspicion that there is a problem, parents must find the most appropriate intervention for their child.

The decision to get treatment for a child or adolescent is serious. Parents are encouraged to seek consultation from a psychiatrist or mental health professional when making decisions about substance abuse treatment for children or adolescents.

- Parents and families must be informed consumers and should be involved in their child's recovery.
- No single treatment is appropriate for all teens.
- It is important to match treatment settings, interventions, and services to each individual's particular problems and needs. This is critical to his or her ultimate success in returning to healthy functioning in the family, school, and society.
- Effective treatment must attend to the multiple needs of the individual—not just the drug use.
- Any associated medical, psychological, social, and cognitive problem must be addressed.
- Remaining in treatment for an adequate period of time is critical for treatment effectiveness and positive change.
- Each person is different and the amount of time in treatment will depend on his or her problems and needs. Research shows that for most individuals, the beginning of improvement begins at about 3 months

Some of the warning signs listed above can also be signs of other problems. Parents may recognize signs of trouble but should not be expected to make the diagnosis.

Consulting a physician to rule out physical causes of the warning signs is a good first step. This should often be followed or accompanied by a comprehensive evaluation by a psychiatrist or mental health professional.

into treatment. After this time, there is usually further progress toward recovery.

- Counseling (individual and/or group) and other behavioral therapies are critical components of effective treatment.
- In therapy, teens look at issues of motivation, build skills to resist drug use, replace drug-using activities with constructive and rewarding behaviors, and improve problem-solving skills. Behavioral therapy also facilitates interpersonal relationships and the teen's ability to function in the home and community.
- Addicted or drug-abusing individuals with coexisting mental disorders should have both disorders treated in an integrated way.
- Because addictive disorders and mental disorders often occur in the same individual, individuals should be assessed and treated for the co-occurrence of the other type of disorder.
- Medical detoxification is only the first stage of addiction treatment and by itself does little to change long-term drug use.
- Medical detoxification safely manages the acute physical symptoms of withdrawal associated with stopping drug use. While detoxification alone is rarely sufficient to help addicts achieve long-term abstinence, for some individuals it is a strongly indicated precursor to effective drug addiction treatment.
- Treatment does not need to be voluntary to be effective.
- Strong motivation can facilitate the treatment process. Sanctions or enticements in the family, school setting, or juvenile justice system can increase significantly both treatment entry and retention rates and the success of drug treatment interventions.
- Recovery from addiction can be a long-term process and frequently requires multiple episodes of treatment.

☞ Remember!!

As with other chronic illnesses, relapses to drug use can occur during or after successful treatment episodes. Addicted individuals may require prolonged treatment and multiple episodes of treatment to achieve long-term abstinence and fully restored functioning. Participation in self-help support programs during and following treatment often is helpful in maintaining abstinence. You and your parents should ask what aftercare treatment services are available for continued or future treatment.

Chapter 3

Oops: How Casual Drug Use Leads To Addiction

It is an all-too-common scenario: A person experiments with an addictive drug like cocaine. Perhaps he intends to try it just once, for "the experience" of it. It turns out, though, that he enjoys the drug's euphoric effect so much that in ensuing weeks and months he uses it again—and again. But in due time, he decides he really should quit. He knows that despite the incomparable short-term high he gets from using cocaine, the long-term consequences of its use are perilous. So he vows to stop using it.

His brain, however, has a different agenda. It now demands cocaine. While his rational mind knows full well that he shouldn't use it again, his brain overrides such warnings. Unbeknown to him, repeated use of cocaine has brought about dramatic changes in both the structure and function of his brain. In fact, if he'd known the danger signs for which to be on the lookout, he would have realized that the euphoric effect derived from cocaine use is itself a sure sign that the drug is inducing a change in the brain—just as he would have known that as time passes, and the drug is used with increasing regularity, this change becomes more pronounced, and resistant to being changed, until finally his brain has become addicted to the drug.

About This Chapter: Text in this chapter is from "Oops: How Casual Drug Use Leads to Addiction," by Alan I. Leshner, Ph.D., Director, National Institute of Drug Abuse, National Institutes of Health, January 2001; available online at http://www.nida.nih.gov/Published_Articles/Oops.html.

And so, despite his heartfelt vow never again to use cocaine, he continues using it. Again and again.

His drug use is now beyond his control. It is compulsive. He is addicted.

While this turn of events is a shock to the drug user, it is no surprise at all to researchers who study the effects of addictive drugs. To them, it is a predictable outcome.

> ✎ **Weird Words**
>
> Biochemistry: The chemistry of living organisms and of the chemical, molecular, and physical changes occurring therein. (Biochemical is a word that refers to biochemistry.)
>
> Euphoria: A feeling of well-being, commonly exaggerated and not necessarily well founded.
>
> Source: From *Stedman's Medical Dictionary, 27th Edition*, Copyright © 2000 Lippincott Williams & Wilkins. All rights reserved.

Unintended Consequences

To be sure, no one ever starts out using drugs intending to become a drug addict. All drug users are just trying it—once or a few times. Every drug user starts out as an occasional user, and that initial use is a voluntary and controllable decision. But as time passes and drug use continues, a person goes from being a voluntary to a compulsive drug user. This change occurs because over time, use of addictive drugs changes the brain—at times in big dramatic toxic ways, at others in more subtle ways, but always in destructive ways that can result in compulsive and even uncontrollable drug use.

The fact is, drug addiction is a brain disease. While every type of drug of abuse has its own individual "trigger" for affecting or transforming the brain, many of the results of the transformation are strikingly similar regardless of the addictive drug that is used—and of course in each instance the result is compulsive use. The brain changes range from fundamental and long-lasting changes in the biochemical makeup of the brain, to mood changes, to changes in memory processes and motor skills. And these changes have a tremendous impact on all aspects of a person's behavior. In fact, in addiction the drug becomes the single most powerful motivator in the life of the drug user. He will do virtually anything for the drug.

Table 3.1. Addictive Potential Of Narcotics. (From "Drugs with Addictive Potential," Copyright © Connecticut Clearinghouse, a program of Wheeler Clinic, Inc.; reprinted with permission.)

Drug	Pharmaceutical & Street Names	Physical Dependence	Withdrawal Symptoms	Tolerance	Duration Of High (hrs)	Method Of Use	Short & Long Term Effects	Effects of Overdose
NARCOTICS								
Heroin	Diacetylmorphine, Horse, Smack	High	Watery eyes Runny nose Yawning Loss of appetite Gooseflesh Irritability Tremors Panic Cramps Diarrhea Nausea Chills & sweating	Yes	3-6	Injected, Sniffed, Smoked	Euphoria Drowsiness Respiratory depression Constricted pupils Nausea Constipation Pulmonary edema	Slow & shallow breathing Clammy skin Pinpoint pupils Convulsions Respiratory failure Coma Possible death
Morphine	Duramorph, MS-Contin, Roxanol, Oramorph SR	High		Yes	3-6	Oral, Smoked, Injected		
Codeine	Tylenol w/codeine, Empirin w/codeine, Robitussin A-C, Fiorinal w/codeine, APAP w/codeine	Moderate		Yes	3-6	Oral, Injected		
Hydrocodone	Tussionex, Lorcet, Vicodin, Hycodan	High		Yes	3-6	Oral		
Hydromorphone	Dilaudid	High		Yes	3-6	Oral, Injected		
Oxycodone	Percodan, Percocet, Tylox, Roxicet, Roxicodone	High		Yes	4-5	Oral		
Methadone & LAAM	Dolophine, Methadose, Levo-alpha-acetylmethadol, Levomethadyl acetate	High		Yes	12-72	Oral, Injected		
Fentanyl & Analogs	Innovar, Sublimaze, Alfenta, Sufenta, Duragesic	High		Yes	0.1-72	Injected, Transdermal Patch		
Other Narcotics	Percodan, Tylox Percocet, Opium, Darvon, Talwin, Buprenorphine, Meperidine (Peth-idine), Demerol	Low To High		Yes	Varies	Oral, Injected		

Table 3.2. Addictive Potential Of Depressants. (From "Drugs with Addictive Potential," Copyright © Connecticut Clearinghouse, a program of Wheeler Clinic, Inc.; reprinted with permission.)

Drug	Pharmaceutical & Street Names	Physical Dependence	Withdrawal Symptoms	Tolerance	Duration Of High (hrs)	Method Of Use	Short & Long Term Effects	Effects of Overdose
DEPRESSANTS								
Chloral Hydrate	Noctec, Somnos, Felsules	Moderate	Anxiety Insomnia Tremors Delirium Convulsions Possible death	Yes	5-8	Oral	Slurred speech Disorientation Drunken behavior Slow reflexes Impaired memory, judgement & coordination	Shallow respiration Clammy skin Dilated pupils Weak/rapid pulse Coma Possible death
Barbiturates	Amytal, Florinal, Nembutal, Tuinal, Seconal, Phenobarbital, Pentobarbital, Barbs	Moderate to High		Yes	1-16	Oral, Injected		
Benzodiazepines	Ativan, Dalmane, Diazepam, Xanax, Librium, Serax, Valium, Tranxene, Verstran, Versed, Halcion, Paxipam, Restoril, Rohypnol, Roofies	Low		Yes	4-8	Oral, Injected		
Glutethimide	Doriden	High		Yes	4-8	Oral		
Alcohol/Ethanol	Beer, Wine, Liquor	High		Yes	Varies	Oral		
Other Depressants	Equanil, Miltown, Noludar, Placidyl, Valmid, Methaqualone, GHB	Moderate		Yes	4-8	Oral		

Table 3.3. Addictive Potential Of Stimulants. (From "Drugs with Addictive Potential," Copyright © Connecticut Clearinghouse, a program of Wheeler Clinic, Inc.; reprinted with permission.)

Drug	Pharmaceutical & Street Names	Physical Dependence	Withdrawal Symptoms	Tolerance	Duration Of High (hrs)	Method Of Use	Short & Long Term Effects	Effects of Overdose
STIMULANTS								
Cocaine	Coke, Flake, Snow, Crack	Possible	Apathy Long periods of sleep Irritability Depression Disorientation	Yes	1-2	Sniffed, Smoked, Injected	Increased alertness Excitation Euphoria Increased pulse rate & blood pressure Insomnia Loss of appetite Psychosis Heart attack or stroke	Agitation Increased body temperature Hallucinations Convulsions Possible death
Amphetamine/ Methamphetamine	Biphetamine, Desoxyn, Dexedrine, Obetrol, Ice	Possible		Yes	2-4	Oral, Injected, Smoked		
Methylphenidate	Ritalin	Possible		Yes	2-4	Oral, Injected, Inhaled		
Other Stimulants	Adipex, Didrex, Ionamin, Melfiat, Plegine, Captagon, Sanorex, Tenuate, Tepanil, Prelu-2, Preludin, Methcathinone, Khat	Possible		Yes	2-4	Oral, Injected		
Nicotine	Cigarettes, Cigars, Chewing Tobacco, Dip, Snuff	High		Yes	0.2-0.4	Smoked, Chewed, Transdermal Patch		

Table 3.4. Addictive Potential Of Cannabis. (From "Drugs with Addictive Potential," Copyright © Connecticut Clearinghouse, a program of Wheeler Clinic, Inc.; reprinted with permission.)

Drug	Pharmaceutical & Street Names	Physical Dependence	Withdrawal Symptoms	Tolerance	Duration Of High (hrs)	Method Of Use	Short & Long Term Effects	Effects of Overdose
CANNABIS (THC)								
Marijuana	Pot, Acapulco Gold, Grass, Reefer, Sinsemilla, Thai Sticks, Weed, Blunts	Unknown	Reports of insomnia Hyperactivity Decreased appetite Irritability	Yes	2-4	Smoked, Oral	Euphoria Relaxed inhibitions Increased appetite Disorientation	Fatigue Paranoia Possible psychosis Disorientation
Tetrahydro-cannabinol	THC, Marinol	Unknown		Yes	2-4	Smoked, Oral		
Hashish & Hashish Oil	Hash, Hash oil	Unknown		Yes	2-4	Smoked, Oral		

Table 3.5. Addictive Potential Of Hallucinogens. (From "Drugs with Addictive Potential," Copyright © Connecticut Clearinghouse, a program of Wheeler Clinic, Inc.; reprinted with permission.)

Drug	Pharmaceutical & Street Names	Physical Dependence	Withdrawal Symptoms	Tolerance	Duration Of High (hrs)	Method Of Use	Short & Long Term Effects	Effects of Overdose
HALLUCINOGENS								
LSD	Acid, Microdot	None	Unknown	Yes	8-12	Oral	Illusions & hallucinations Altered perceptions of time/distance	Longer, more intense "trip" episodes Psychosis Possible death
Mescaline & Peyote	Mescal, Buttons, Cactus	None		Yes	8-12	Oral		
Amphetamine Variants	2, 5-DMA, STP, MDA, MDMA, Ecstasy, DOM, DOB	Unknown		Yes	Varies	Oral, Injected		
Phencyclidine & Analogs	PCE, PCPy, TCP,PCP, Hog, Loveboat, Angel Dust	Unknown		Yes	Days	Oral, Smoked		
Other Hallucinogens	Bufotenine, Ibogaine, DMT, DET, Psilocybin, Psilocyn, 'shrooms	None		Possible	Varies	Smoked, Oral, Injected, Sniffed		

Table 3.6. Addictive Potential Of Inhalants. (From "Drugs with Addictive Potential," Copyright © Connecticut Clearinghouse, a program of Wheeler Clinic, Inc.; reprinted with permission.)

Drug	Pharmaceutical & Street Names	Physical Dependence	Withdrawal Symptoms	Tolerance	Duration Of High (hrs)	Method Of Use	Short & Long Term Effects	Effects of Overdose
INHALANTS								
Organic Solvents	Gasoline, Lighter fluid, Spray paint, Paint thinners, Hair spray, Nail polish remover, Degreasers, Cleaning fluid	Low	Unknown	Yes	0.1-1.0	Inhaled	Poor motor coordination Impaired vision & memory Lightheaded-ness Drunken behavior	Sudden death Brain, liver & kidney damage Glaucoma
Nitrites	Amyl nitrite (poppers, snappers) Butylnitrite (air freshener)	Unknown		Yes				
Nitrous Oxide	Laughing gas, Whipped cream propellant	Unknown		Unknown				

This unexpected consequence of drug use is what I have come to call the oops phenomenon. Why oops? Because the harmful outcome is in no way intentional. Just as no one starts out to have lung cancer when they smoke, or no one starts out to have clogged arteries (which in turn cause heart attacks) when they eat fried foods, no one starts out to become a drug addict when they use drugs. But in each case, though no one meant to behave in a way that would lead to tragic health consequences, that is what happened just the same, because of the undetected, destructive biochemical processes at work.

While we haven't yet pinpointed precisely all the triggers for the changes in the brain's structure and function that produce the "oops" phenomenon, a vast body of hard evidence shows that it is virtually inevitable that prolonged drug use will lead to addiction. From this we can soundly conclude that drug addiction is indeed a brain disease.

I realize that this flies in the face of the notion that drug addiction boils down to a serious character flaw—that those addicted to drugs are just too weak-willed to quit drug use on their own. But the moral weakness notion itself flies in the face of all scientific evidence, and so it should be discarded.

Biological And Behavioral Factors

It should be stressed, however, that to assert that drug addiction is a brain disease is by no means the same thing as saying that those addicted to drugs are not accountable for their actions, or that they are just unwitting, hapless victims of the harmful effects that use of addictive drugs has on their brains, and in every facet of their lives.

Just as their behavior at the outset was the turning point that put them on a collision course with compulsive drug use, their behavior after becoming addicted is just as critical if they are to be effectively treated and to recover.

At minimum, they have to adhere to their drug treatment regimen. But this can pose an enormous challenge. The changes in their brain that turned them into compulsive users make it a challenging task to control their actions and complete treatment. Making it even more difficult is the fact that their craving becomes more heightened and irresistible whenever they are exposed to any situation that triggers a memory of the euphoric experience of drug use. Little wonder, then, that most compulsive drug users can't quit on their own, even if they want to (for instance, at most only 7 percent of those who try in any one year to quit smoking cigarettes on their own actually succeed). This is why it is essential that they enter a drug treatment program, even if they don't want to at the outset.

Clearly, a host of biological and behavioral factors conspires to trigger the oops phenomenon in drug addiction. So the widely held sentiment that drug addiction has to be explained from either the standpoint of biology or the standpoint of behavior, and never the twain shall meet, is terribly flawed. Biological and behavioral explanations of drug abuse must be given equal weight and integrated with each other if we are to gain an in-depth understanding of the root causes of drug addiction and then develop more effective treatments. Modern science has shown us that we reduce one explanation to the other—the behavioral to the biological, or vice versa—at our own peril. We have to recognize that brain disease stemming from drug use cannot and should not be artificially isolated from its behavioral components, as well as its larger social components. They all are critical pieces of the puzzle that interact with and impact on one another at every turn.

A wealth of scientific evidence, by the way, makes it clear that rarely if ever are any forms of brain disease only biological in nature. To the contrary, such brain diseases as stroke, Alzheimer's, Parkinson's, schizophrenia, and clinical depression all have their behavioral and social dimensions. What is unique about the type of brain disease that results from drug abuse is that it starts out as voluntary behavior. But once continued use of an addictive drug brings about structural and functional changes in the brain that cause compulsive use, the disease-ravaged brain of a drug user closely resembles that of people with other kinds of brain diseases.

Treatment For Addiction

It's also important to bear in mind that we now see addiction as a chronic, virtually life-long illness for many people. And relapse is a common phenomenon in all forms of chronic illness—from asthma and diabetes, to high blood pressure and addiction. The goals of successive treatments, as with other chronic illnesses, are to manage the illness and increase the intervals between relapses, until there are no more.

An increasing body of scientific evidence makes the compelling case that the most effective treatment programs for overcoming drug addiction incorporate an array of approaches—from medications, to behavior therapies, to social services and rehabilitation. The National Institute on Drug Abuse published *Principles of Effective Drug Addiction Treatment*, which features many of the most promising drug treatment programs to date. As this booklet explains, the programs with the most successful track records treat the whole individual. Their treatment strategies place just as much emphasis on the unique social and behavioral aspects of drug addiction treatment and recovery as on the biological aspects. By doing so, they better enable those who have abused drugs to overcome the unexpected consequences of drug use and once again lead fruitful lives.

Chapter 4

Brain Function And Drug Abuse

Brain Anatomy

The brain consists of several large regions, each responsible for some of the activities vital for living. These include the brainstem, cerebellum, limbic system, diencephalon, and cerebral cortex (Figure 4.1).

The brainstem is the part of the brain that connects the brain and the spinal cord. It controls many basic functions, such as heart rate, breathing, eating, and sleeping. The brainstem accomplishes this by directing the spinal cord, other parts of the brain, and the body to do what is necessary to maintain these basic functions.

The cerebellum, which represents only one-eighth of the total weight of the brain, coordinates the brain's instructions for skilled repetitive movements and for maintaining balance and posture. It is a prominent structure located above the brainstem.

On top of the brainstem and buried under the cortex, there is a set of more evolutionarily primitive brain structures called the limbic system (Figure 4.2). The limbic system structures are involved in many of our emotions

About This Chapter: Text in this chapter is excerpted from *Mind Over Matter: Teacher's Guide*, National Institute on Drug Abuse, NIH Pub. No. 98-3592. To obtain a copy of this publication, call the National Clearinghouse for Alcohol and Drug Abuse Information at 800-729-6686.

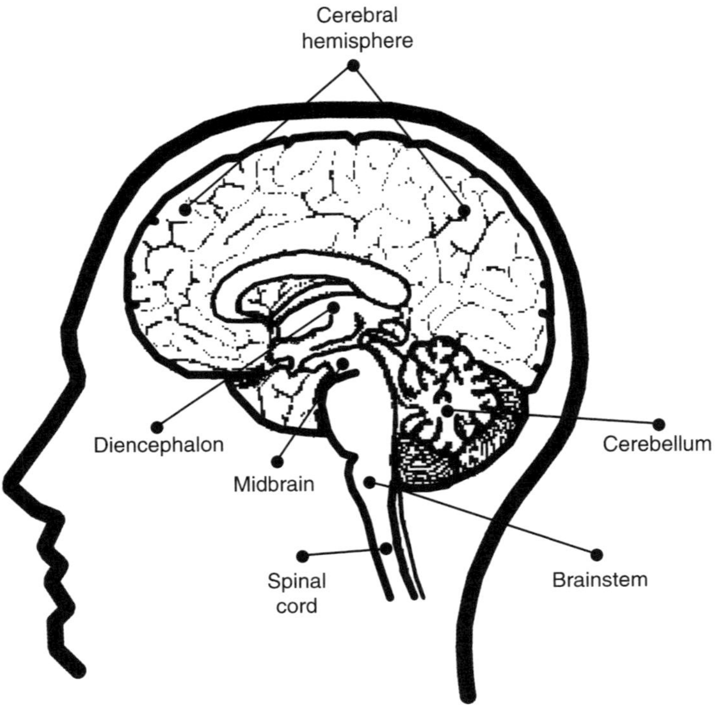

Figure 4.1. This drawing of a brain cut in half demonstrates some of the major regions of the brain.

✎ Weird Words

Neurotransmission: A process by which one cell releases a specific chemical agent (a neurotransmitter) to cross a synapse to stimulate or inhibit another cell.

Synapse: The functional membrane-to-membrane contact of the nerve cell with another nerve cell, an effector (muscle, gland) cell, or a sensory receptor cell.

Source: From *Stedman's Medical Dictionary, 27th Edition*,

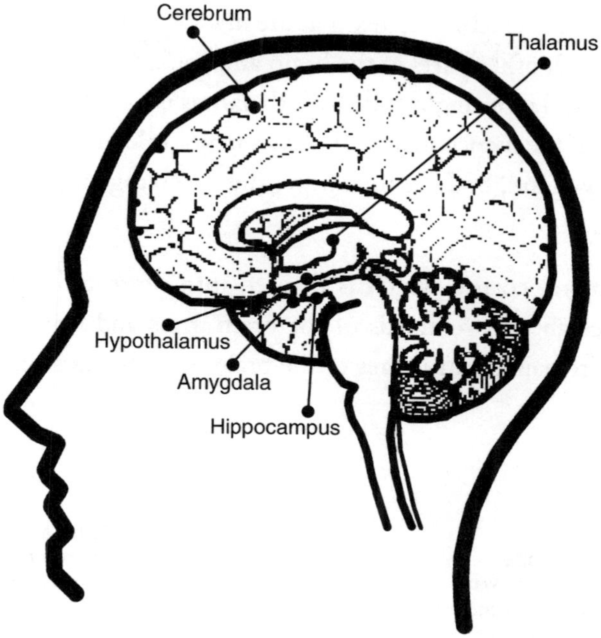

Figure 4.2. This drawing of a brain cut in half demonstrates some of the brain's internal structures. The amygdala and hippocampus are actually located deep within the brain, but are shown as an overlay in the approximate areas that they are located.

and motivations, particularly those that are related to survival, such as fear, anger, and emotions related to sexual behavior. The limbic system is also involved in feelings of pleasure that are related to our survival, such as those experienced from eating and sex. Two large limbic system structures called the amygdala and hippocampus are also involved in memory. One of the reasons that drugs of abuse can exert such powerful control over our behavior is that they act directly on the more evolutionarily primitive brain-stem and limbic structures, which can override the cortex in controlling our behavior. In effect, they eliminate the most human part of our brain from its role in controlling our behavior.

The diencephalon, which is also located beneath the cerebral hemispheres, contains the thalamus and hypothalamus (Figure 4.2). The thalamus is involved in sensory perception and regulation of motor functions (movement). It connects areas of the cerebral cortex that are involved in sensory perception and movement with other parts of the brain and spinal cord that also have a role in sensation and movement. The hypothalamus is a very small but important component of the diencephalon. It plays a major role in regulating hormones, the pituitary gland, body temperature, the adrenal glands, and many other vital activities.

The cerebral cortex, which is divided into right and left hemispheres, encompasses about two-thirds of the brain mass and lies over and around most of the remaining structures of the brain. It is the most highly developed

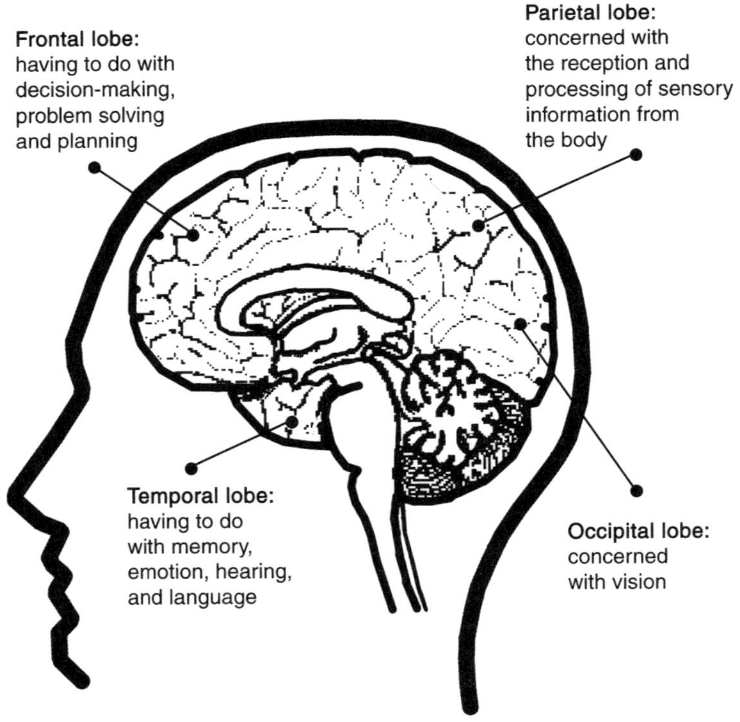

Figure 4.3. This drawing of a brain cut in half demonstrates the lobes of the cerebral cortex and their functions.

part of the human brain and is responsible for thinking, perceiving, and producing and understanding language. It is also the most recent structure in the history of brain evolution. The cerebral cortex can be divided into areas that each have a specific function (Figure 4.3). For example, there are specific areas involved in vision, hearing, touch, movement, and smell. Other areas are critical for thinking and reasoning. Although many functions, such as touch, are found in both the right and left cerebral hemispheres, some functions are found in only one cerebral hemisphere. For example, in most people, language abilities are found in the left hemisphere.

Nerve Cells And Neurotransmission

The brain is made up of billions of nerve cells. Typically, a neuron contains three important parts (Figure 4.4): a central cell body that directs all activities of the neuron; dendrites, short fibers that receive messages from other neurons and relay them to the cell body; and an axon, a long single fiber that transmits messages from the cell body to the dendrites of other neurons or to body tissues, such as muscles. Although most neurons contain all of the three parts, there is a wide range of diversity in the shapes and sizes of neurons as well as their axons and dendrites.

The transfer of a message from the axon of one nerve cell to the dendrites of another is known as neurotransmission. Although axons and dendrites are located extremely close to each other, the transmission of a message from an axon to a dendrite does not occur through direct contact. Instead, communication between nerve cells occurs mainly through the release of chemical substances into the space between the axon and dendrites (Figure 4.5). This space is known as the synapse. When neurons communicate, a message, traveling as an electrical impulse, moves down an axon and toward the synapse. There it triggers the release of molecules called neurotransmitters from the axon into the synapse. The neurotransmitters then diffuse across the synapse and bind to special molecules, called receptors, that are located within the cell membranes of the dendrites of the adjacent nerve cell. This, in turn, stimulates or inhibits an electrical response in the receiving neuron's dendrites. Thus, the neurotransmitters act as chemical messengers, carrying information from one neuron to another.

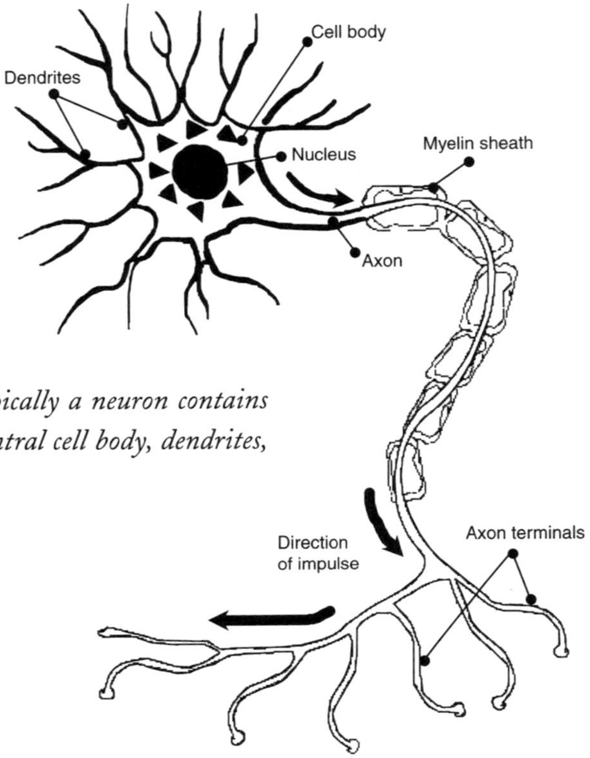

Figure 4.4. A Neuron. Typically a neuron contains three important parts: a central cell body, dendrites, and an axon.

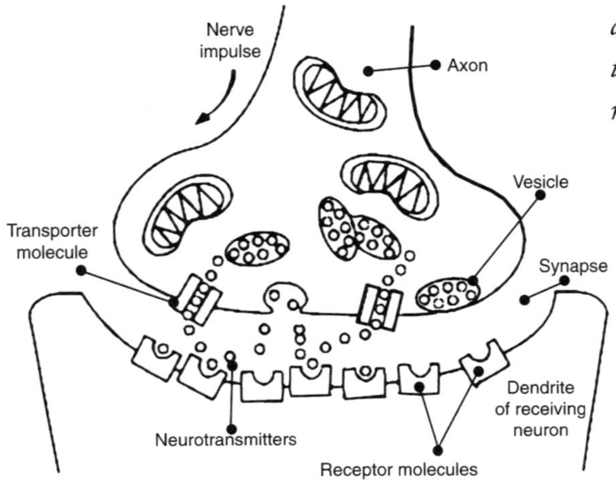

Figure 4.5. Re-uptake. Re-absorption of an enzyme by transporter molecules is called re-uptake.

There are many different types of neurotransmitters, each of which has a precise role to play in the functioning of the brain. Generally, each neurotransmitter can only bind to a very specific matching receptor. Therefore, when a neurotransmitter couples to a receptor, it is like fitting a key into a lock. This coupling then starts a whole cascade of events at both the surface of the dendrite of the receiving nerve cell and inside the cell. In this manner, the message carried by the neurotransmitter is received and processed by the receiving nerve cell. Once this has occurred, the neurotransmitter is inactivated in one of two ways. It is either broken down by an enzyme or reabsorbed back into the nerve cell that released it. The reabsorption (also known as re-uptake) is accomplished by what are known as transporter molecules (Figure 4.5). Transporter molecules reside in the cell membranes of the axons that release the neurotransmitters. They pick up specific neurotransmitters from the synapse and carry them back across the cell membrane and into the axon. The neurotransmitters are then available for reuse at a later time.

As noted above, messages that are received by dendrites are relayed to the cell body and then to the axon. The axons then transmit the messages, which

✤ It's A Fact!!

Myth: Drug addiction is voluntary behavior.

Fact: A person starts out as an occasional drug user, and that is a voluntary decision. But as times passes, something happens, and that person goes from being a voluntary drug user to being a compulsive drug user. Why? Because over time, continued use of addictive drugs changes your brain—at times in dramatic, toxic ways, at others in more subtle ways, but virtually always in ways that result in compulsive and even uncontrollable drug use.

From "Exploring Myths about Drug Abuse," by Alan I. Leshner, Ph.D., Director, National Institute on Drug Abuse, January 25,2001.

are in the form of electrical impulses, to other neurons or body tissues. The axons of many neurons are covered in a fatty substance known as myelin. Myelin has several functions. One of its most important is to increase the rate at which nerve impulses travel along the axon. The rate of conduction of a nerve impulse along a heavily myelinated axon can be as fast as 120 meters/second. In contrast, a nerve impulse can travel no faster than about 2 meters/second along an axon without myelin. The thickness of the myelin covering on an axon is closely linked to the function of that axon. For example, axons that travel a long distance, such as those that extend from the spinal cord to the foot, generally contain a thick myelin covering to facilitate faster transmission of the nerve impulse. (Note: The axons that transmit messages from the brain or spinal cord to muscles and other body tissues are what make up the nerves of the human body. Most of these axons contain a thick covering of myelin, which accounts for the whitish appearance of nerves.)

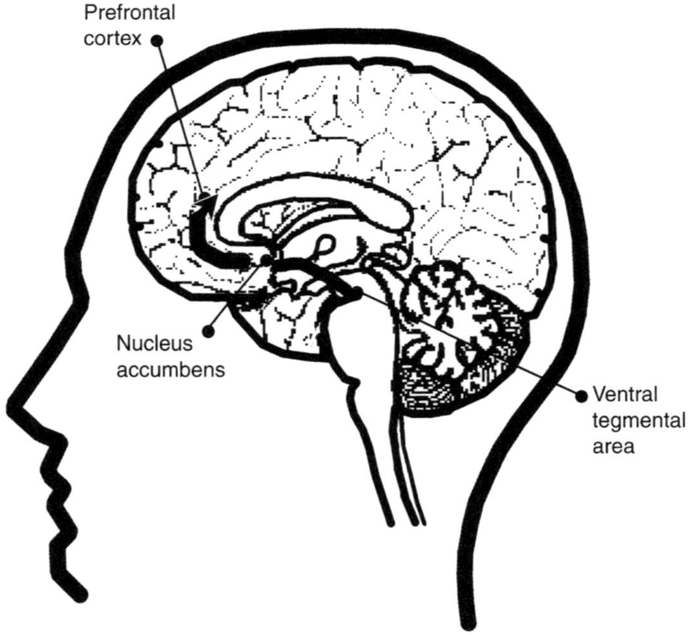

Figure 4.6. This drawing of a brain cut in half demonstrates the brain areas and pathways involved in the pleasure circuit.

Effects Of Drugs Of Abuse On The Brain

Pleasure, which scientists call reward, is a very powerful biological force for our survival. If you do something pleasurable, the brain is wired in such a way that you tend to do it again. Life-sustaining activities, such as eating, activate a circuit of specialized nerve cells devoted to producing and regulating pleasure. One important set of these nerve cells, which uses a chemical

♣ It's A Fact!!

Results of autopsy studies show that patients with a history of chronic alcohol consumption have smaller, lighter, more shrunken brains than nonalcoholic adults of the same age and gender. This finding has been repeatedly confirmed in living alcoholics using structural imaging techniques, such as computed tomography (CT) and magnetic resonance imaging (MRI). Structural imaging reveals a consistent association between heavy drinking and physical brain damage, even in the absence of medical conditions previously considered to be clinical indicators of severe alcoholism (for example, chronic liver disease or alcohol-induced dementia).

Imaging reveals shrinkage to be more extensive in the folded outer layer (the cortex) of the frontal lobe, which is believed to be the seat of higher intellectual functions. In men, vulnerability to frontal lobe shrinkage increases with age. Current studies will determine if the same effect occurs in women. Repeated imaging of a group of alcoholics who continued drinking over a 5-year period showed progressive brain shrinkage that significantly exceeded normal age-related shrinkage. The rate of frontal cortex shrinkage in this study correlated approximately with the amount of alcohol consumed.

Shrinkage also occurs in deeper brain regions, including brain structures associated with memory, as well as in the cerebellum, which helps regulate coordination and balance. Limited research suggests that women may be more susceptible than men to alcohol-related brain shrinkage.

Excerpted from *Alcohol Alert*, No. 47, National Institute on Alcohol Abuse and Alcoholism, April 2000.

neurotransmitter called dopamine, sits at the very top of the brain-stem in the ventral tegmental area (VTA) (Figure 4.6). These dopamine-containing neurons relay messages about pleasure through their nerve fibers to nerve cells in a limbic system structure called the nucleus accumbens. Still other fibers reach to a related part of the frontal region of the cerebral cortex. So, the pleasure circuit, which is known as the mesolimbic dopamine system, spans the survival-oriented brainstem, the emotional limbic system, and the frontal cerebral cortex.

All drugs that are addicting can activate the brain's pleasure circuit. Drug addiction is a biological, pathological process that alters the way in which

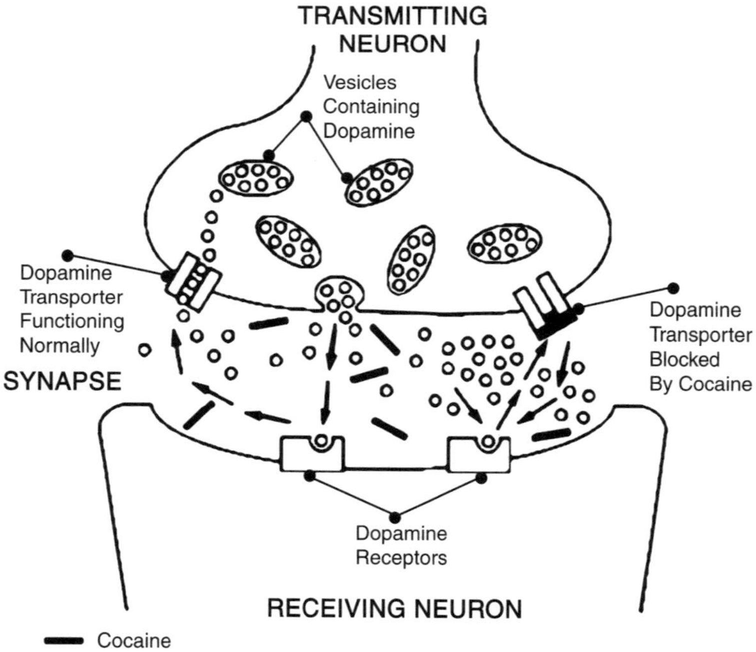

Figure 4.7. *When cocaine enters the brain, it blocks the dopamine transporter from pumping dopamine back into the transmitting neuron, flooding the synapse with dopamine. This intensifies and prolongs the stimulation of receiving neurons in the brain's pleasure circuits, causing a cocaine "high."*

the pleasure center, as well as other parts of the brain, functions. To understand this process, it is necessary to examine the effects of drugs on neurotransmission. Almost all drugs that change the way the brain works do so by affecting chemical neurotransmission. Some drugs, like heroin and LSD, mimic the effects of a natural neurotransmitter. Others, like PCP, block receptors and thereby prevent neuronal messages from getting through. Still others, like cocaine, interfere with the molecules that are responsible for transporting neurotransmitters back into the neurons that released them (Figure 4.7). Finally, some drugs, such as methamphetamine, act by causing neurotransmitters to be released in greater amounts than normal.

☞ Remember!!

Prolonged drug use changes the brain in fundamental and long-lasting ways. These long-lasting changes are a major component of the addiction itself. It is as though there is a figurative "switch" in the brain that "flips" at some point during an individual's drug use. The point at which this "flip" occurs varies from individual to individual, but the effect of this change is the transformation of a drug abuser to a drug addict.

Chapter 5

Preventing Drug Abuse

Since 1991, drug use has been increasing among America's youth. Unlike the late 1970s when drug use reached its peak, today we are in a unique position to intervene effectively by applying the results of more than 20 years of prevention research.

This research has helped identify the important factors that put young people at risk for or protect them from drug use. Intervention researchers have studied the effectiveness of various prevention approaches by using rigorous research designs and testing and implementing effective drug abuse prevention interventions in "real-world" settings. Now it is possible to describe the basic principles derived from drug abuse prevention research in simple direct terms so that they can be applied to successfully prevent drug use among young people.

Prevention Principles

- Prevention programs should be designed to enhance "protective factors" and move toward reversing or reducing known "risk factors."
- Prevention programs should target all forms of drug abuse, including the use of tobacco, alcohol, marijuana, and inhalants.

About This Chapter: Text in this chapter is excerpted from "Preventing Drug Use Among Children and Adolescents: A Research-Based Guide," National Institute on Drug Abuse, April 1997. Copies of this publication can be obtained free of charge from the National Clearinghouse for Alcohol and Drug Information (NCADI) at 800-729-6686.

- Prevention programs should include skills to resist drugs when offered, strengthen personal commitments against drug use, and increase social competency (for example, in communications, peer relationships, self-efficacy, and assertiveness), in conjunction with reinforcement of attitudes against drug use.
- Prevention programs for adolescents should include interactive methods, such as peer discussion groups, rather than instructional teaching techniques alone.
- Prevention programs should include a parents' or caregivers' component that reinforces what the children are learning—such as facts about drugs and their harmful effects—and that opens opportunities for family discussions about use of legal and illegal substances and family policies about their use.
- Prevention programs should be long-term, over the school career with repeat interventions to reinforce the original prevention goals. For example, school-based efforts directed at elementary and middle school students should include booster sessions to help with critical transitions from middle to high school.

✎ Weird Words

Intervention: An action that produces an effect or that is intended to change the course of a process.

Risk Factor: A characteristic statistically associated with, although not necessarily a cause of, an increased risk of sickness or death. (For example, smoking as a risk factor for heart disease.)

Self-Efficacy: An individual's estimate or personal judgment of his or her own ability to succeed in reaching a specific goal. (For example, quitting smoking or losing weight, or a more general goal, such as continuing to remain at a prescribed weight level.)

Source: From *Stedman's Medical Dictionary, 27th Edition*,

- Family-focused prevention efforts have a greater impact than strategies that focus on parents only or children only.
- Community programs that include media campaigns and policy changes, such as new regulations that restrict access to alcohol, tobacco, or other drugs, are more effective when they are accompanied by school and family interventions.
- Community programs need to strengthen norms against drug use in all drug abuse prevention settings, including the family, the school, and the community.
- Schools offer opportunities to reach all populations and also serve as important settings for specific subpopulations at risk for drug abuse, such as children with behavior problems or learning disabilities and those who are potential dropouts.
- Prevention programming should be adapted to address the specific nature of the drug abuse problem in the local community.
- The higher the level of risk of the target population, the more intensive the prevention effort must be and the earlier it must begin.
- Prevention programs should be age-specific, developmentally appropriate, and culturally sensitive.
- Effective prevention programs are cost-effective. For every dollar spent on drug use prevention, communities can save 4 to 5 dollars in costs for drug abuse treatment and counseling.

Risk Factors And Protective Factors

What are risk factors and protective factors?

Studies over the past two decades have tried to determine the origins and pathways of drug abuse—how the problem starts and how it progresses. Several factors have been identified that are different among those who use drugs and those who do not. Factors associated with greater potential for drug use are called "risk" factors, and those associated with reduced potential for such use are called "protective" factors.

✔ Quick Tip

Action Steps

- **Get media-wise.** Discuss and analyze popular movies, music videos, and television shows that promote and glamorize marijuana and other drugs. Contact the National Clearinghouse for Alcohol and Drug Information (NCADI) at 1-800-729-6686 (or on the Internet World Wide Web site at http://www.health.org) for information about media literacy resources for youth. Talk with parents and other trusted adults about these issues.
- **Get the facts about marijuana and other drugs.** Call your local health department, city or county substance abuse agency, or information clearinghouses such as NCADI or the Connecticut Clearinghouse at 1-800-232-4424 to get information about marijuana and other drugs. Ask librarians to help you get answers to your questions. Order materials for yourself, friends, parents and adults, and for distribution to clubs and groups.
- **Speak out on youth issues about drugs.** Make it a point to listen to and call in to radio stations with talk programs that discuss issues about drugs and related problems among youth. Throw your two cents in the barrel.
- **Influence the airwaves.** Call local radio stations and talk with the station manager if you object to the music being played. As a consumer, your opinion can make a difference.
- **Raise community awareness.** Bring information to the attention of parents, adults, and community leaders about problems faced by youth in the community, for example, the convenience store that allows underage youth to buy alcohol. Adults need to know what youth face on a day-to-day basis so they can rally to your support.
- **Promote drug-free youth.** Celebrate and acknowledge the drug-free lifestyle most youth already practice. Take your positive stories to newspapers, radio and TV stations, religious organizations, and other groups.

- **Develop teen spokespersons.** Organize a teen speakers bureau. Many adult groups and organizations are interested in involving youth in community prevention programs to help them develop programs that work.
- **Tap into the creative interests of youth.** Solicit the involvement of teens who are into the arts—dancers, actors, musicians, writers, and others—to help develop messages, slogans, posters, songs, print ads, T-shirts, buttons, speeches and articles that promote and address the benefits of non-use of marijuana and other drugs.
- **Create positive peer pressure.** Do not engage in any illegal marijuana or other drug use practices. Set an example for your friends and younger brothers and sisters. Remember, over 86 percent of youth ages 12- 17 have never tried marijuana.
- **Get in the game.** Sports and exercise help reduce the stress and strain of growing up. They keep you healthy and strong. When your mind and body are free from drugs, you have the performance edge.
- **The art of the matter.** Get involved in drama, music, writing, crafts, building things, or painting. You can express your thoughts and feelings through many different art forms and share them with the world. You can grow through your dreams and creativity.
- **Host a party.** Invite your friends to a drug-free social event and see how much fun you can have without marijuana and other drugs.
- **Share what you have learned.** Write an article for your school newspaper on the facts about marijuana. You can gather information from local libraries, NCADI, or the Connecticut Clearinghouse.

From: "Drugs and You: Action Steps for Youth," prepared by the Connecticut Clearinghouse, a program of Wheeler Clinic, Inc. © May 1997 Connecticut Clearinghouse, 334 Farmington Avenue, Plainville, CT 06062, 800-232-4424, 860-793-9791 (www.ctclearinghouse.org); reprinted with permission.

Research has revealed that there are many risk factors for drug abuse, each representing a challenge to the psychological and social development of an individual and each having a differential impact depending on the phase of development. For this reason, those factors that affect early development in the family are probably the most crucial, such as:

- chaotic home environments, particularly in which parents abuse substances or suffer from mental illnesses;
- ineffective parenting, especially with children with difficult temperaments and conduct disorders; and
- lack of mutual attachments and nurturing.

Other risk factors relate to children interacting with other socialization agents outside of the family, specifically the school, peers, and the community. Some of these factors are:

- inappropriate shy and aggressive behavior in the classroom;
- failure in school performance;
- poor social coping skills;
- affiliations with deviant peers or peers around deviant behaviors; and
- perceptions of approval of drug-using behaviors in the school, peer, and community environments.

Certain protective factors also have been identified. These factors are not always the opposite of risk factors. Their impact also varies along the developmental process. The most salient protective factors include:

- strong bonds with the family;
- experience of parental monitoring with clear rules of conduct within the family unit and involvement of parents in the lives of their children;
- success in school performance;
- strong bonds with prosocial institutions such as the family, school, and religious organizations; and
- adoption of conventional norms about drug use.

Other factors—such as the availability of drugs, trafficking patterns, and beliefs that drug use is generally tolerated—also influence the number of young people who start to use drugs.

How can prevention planners use risk and protective factors to develop programs?

- **Family Relationships.** Prevention programs can enhance protective factors among young children by teaching parents skills for better family communication, discipline, firm and consistent rulemaking, and other parenting skills. Research also has shown that parents need to take a more active role in their children's lives, including talking with them about drugs, monitoring their activities, getting to know their friends, and understanding their problems and personal concerns.
- **Peer Relationships.** Prevention programs focus on an individual's relationship to peers by developing social-competency skills, which involve improved communications, enhancement of positive peer relationships and social behaviors, and resistance skills to refuse drug offers.
- **The School Environment.** Prevention programs also focus on enhancing academic performance and strengthening students' bonding to school, by giving them a sense of identity and achievement and reducing the likelihood of their dropping out of school. Most curriculums include the support for positive peer relationships and a normative education component designed to correct the misperception that most students are using drugs. Research has found also that when children understand the negative effects of drugs (physical, psychological, and social) and when they perceive their friends' and families' social disapproval of drug use, they tend to avoid initiating drug use.
- **The Community Environment.** Prevention programs work at the community level with civic, religious, law enforcement, and governmental organizations to enhance antidrug norms and prosocial behavior through changes in policy or regulation, mass media efforts, and community-wide awareness programs. Community-based programs might include new laws and enforcement, advertising restrictions, and drug-free school zones—all designed to provide a cleaner, safer, drug-free environment.

Educating children about the negative effects of drugs, especially the most immediate adverse effects in their lives, is an important element in any prevention program. In addition, helping children become more successful in school behavior and performance helps them form strong prosocial bonds with their peers, the school, and the community.

What are the highest-risk periods for drug use among youth?

For most children, research has shown that the vulnerable periods are transitions, when they grow from one developmental stage to another. But exposure to risks can start even before a child is born; this is one reason that mothers are advised to abstain from drugs during pregnancy.

The first big transition for children is when they leave the security of the family and enter school. When they advance from elementary school to middle school or junior high, they often face social challenges, such as learning to get along with a wider group of peers. It is at this stage, early adolescence, that children are likely to encounter drug use for the first time.

Later on, when they enter high school, young people face social, psychological, and educational challenges as they prepare for the future, and these challenges can lead to use and abuse of alcohol, tobacco, and other drugs.

When young adults go on to college or get married or enter the workforce, they again face new risks from alcohol and other drug abuse in their new adult environments.

When does drug use start, and how does it proceed?

Studies indicate that children most often begin to use drugs at about age 12 or 13, and many researchers have observed young teens moving from the illicit use of legal substances (such as tobacco, alcohol, and inhalants) to the use of illegal drugs (marijuana is usually the first). The sequence from tobacco and alcohol use to marijuana use, and then, as children get older, to other drugs, has been found in almost all long-term studies of drug use. The order of drug use in this progression is largely consistent with social attitudes and norms and the availability of drugs. But it cannot be said that smoking and drinking at young ages are the cause of later drug use.

Nor does this sequencing imply that the progression is inevitable. It does say that for someone who ever smoked or drank, the risk of moving on to marijuana is 65 times higher than that for a person who never smoked or drank. The risk of moving on to cocaine is 104 times higher for someone who smoked marijuana at least once in his or her lifetime than for a person who never did (these figures are from an analysis of 1991–1993 data from the National Household Survey on Drug Abuse).

Scientists have hypothesized several reasons for this observed progression, including a possible biological cause. The research also suggests social or behavioral causes, such as early involvement with antisocial, drug-using people. Indeed, all these possibilities could play a part.

☞ Remember!!

"Drug abuse is a preventable behavior."

—Partnership for a Drug-Free America

Chapter 6

Learn To Resist Peer Pressure

Many adolescents find the need to fit in so strong that they will do virtually anything to be accepted. Some students, such as those who are not in sports or other school activities, may feel especially isolated and vulnerable to peer pressure. "The easiest group to belong to is the users," said Kris Van Hoof, a prevention specialist at Hazelden in Center City, Minn. "They accept pretty much anybody. As long as you drink or use, you're in."

The desire to "fit in," combined with young peoples easy access to illegal chemicals and parental indifference about alcohol use, means that kids need to learn specific skills in order to successfully resist peer pressure to drink or use.

"Parents, teachers and school counselors need to understand refusal skills and role-play with kids until it becomes a reality," Van Hoof said. "We need to start it as early as fourth grade, and it needs to be repeated every year. As adolescents grow and mature, they have different social situations in which peer pressure will come up."

About This Chapter: Text in this chapter is from "Young People Can Learn to Resist Peer Pressure to Use Drugs," Copyright © 2002 Hazelden. *Alive and Free* articles are reprinted with permission of Hazelden, a nonprofit agency based in Center City, MN, that offers a wide range of information and treatment services relating to addiction and recovery. For more resources on substance abuse, call Hazelden at (800) 257-7810 or check its web site at http://www.hazelden.org.

☞ **Remember!!**

Tips For Staying Drug Free

Healthy and helpful ways for you to stay drug and alcohol-free.

- *Make friends with kids who don't smoke, drink or use drugs*...Your friends have a lot of influence over you, both good and bad, so pick them carefully.
- *Make your own decisions*—that's an important part of becoming an adult. It's hard enough to make choices when you're straight—why make it harder by drinking or using drugs? It's important not to care what others think about you: what's important is what you think of yourself.
- *Don't try to please everyone*...you can never do it, so make taking care of yourself your No. 1 priority, rather than pleasing everybody else.
- *Talk to your parents* about things that bother you...CASA's surveys show that kids who spend time with their families, keep communications open, eat dinner and attend religious services together are less likely to smoke, drink or use drugs.
- *Get involved* in after-school activities such as sports, clubs or community service. Just hanging out with friends after school or being bored can lead to doing things that will hurt you, like smoking, drinking or using drugs.

Source: "CASA's Tips for Staying Drug Free," © 1996 The National Center on Addiction and Substance Abuse at Columbia University (CASA); reprinted with permission. Visit CASA online at http://www.casacolumbia.org.

The standard model for reversing peer pressure works for a variety of at-risk behaviors, including drug use and violence. Van Hoof offers a five-step model to resist peer pressure:

- **Ask questions.** Size up the situation before "going along." For example, a classmate might say, "Hey, lets go hang out at the mall" —and have shoplifting in mind. To be responsible, ask "What are we going to do? How long will we be there?" These questions will help you make informed decisions before getting into a problem situation.
- **Name the trouble.** After you identify the situation, you need to state the possible problem: "That sounds like trouble to me."
- **State the consequences.** Use the threat of punishment as an excuse not to drink. Say something such as, "My parents would ground me for months," or "I could get kicked off the soccer team."
- **Offer an alternative.** If a friend invites you to drink or use, suggest an alternative. "Lets go get pizza." If the friend pressures you more, walk away, but leave the door open. You could say, "Hey, that's fine. Go do your thing. You're welcome to join me later."
- **Getting out of trouble.** Should you find yourself in a problem situation, get out immediately and call a responsible adult for help.

Kathleen Dolan, a junior in the Peer-Helper Program at Hudson High School in Hudson, Wisconsin, says that peer pressure to smoke, drink and use marijuana is subtle, but strong, at her school. "It's not the in-your-face type pressure," she says. "Its usually like, Oh, come on with us to a party. It'll be great. Everyone's going to be there. When you get there, it's often an environment where alcohol and other drugs are available and being used. When you're exposed to that enough, it can build the expectation that it's okay to use or drink. It can really wear on you to the point where you might use."

Dolan has attended Hazelden's Peer Empowerment workshop, a two-day training that teaches young people communications, assertiveness, and refusal skills and empowers students to make healthy choices about their lives. She says the best thing is to stay away from parties where there's drinking and find chemical-free fun alternatives. "If you go to a party where there are substance abusers—people who may be addicted—in effect you're condoning their behavior by being there," she said.

Dolan is one of 35 peer helpers at her school who have pledged to remain drug-free. They serve as mentors for fellow students and share their knowledge about the dangers of drug use. They offer "care-frontation" —a compassionate intervention approach—to students at risk for chemical-use and other problems.

✔ Quick Tip

The National Clearinghouse for Alcohol and Drug Information offers a range of resources to help prevent adolescent substance abuse. One source is "Keeping Youth Drug-Free," a pamphlet that offers exercises on resisting peer pressure. To receive a free copy, call the Clearinghouse at (800) 729-6686. Hazelden offers educational materials and workshops, including a small-group curriculum called "From Peer Pressure to Peer Support" that teaches refusal skills. Call (800) 257-7810 for information.

Chapter 7

Chemical-Creativity Link May Be Folklore

The list of creative people who abused alcohol or other drugs is long. Among writers it includes Sinclair Lewis, Jack London, Thomas Wolfe, Truman Capote, F. Scott Fitzgerald, Eugene O'Neill, Hart Crane, John Cheever, John Berryman and William Faulkner. You can add numerous painters, musicians and other artists to that list.

Faulkner captured his fondness for alcohol when he remarked that "civilization begins with distillation." Fitzgerald said, "Drink heightens feeling. When I drink, it heightens my emotions and I put it in a story. My stories written when sober are stupid . . . all reasoned out, not felt."

Behind such comments is a theory about the nature of creativity. According to this theory, creativity is the ability to see ordinary things in an extraordinary way. Chemical use leads to altered states of consciousness and helps the artist look at everyday life with fresh eyes.

There's no disputing the genius of writers such as Hemingway, Fitzgerald, and others. However, in all probability, great artists create great works in spite of, not because of, their heavy use of alcohol. This conclusion is supported by empirical evidence, including a study led by Ernest Noble and associates from the Alcohol Research Center at the University of California, Los Angeles ("Creativity in Alcoholic and Nonalcoholic Families," published in the journal *Alcohol*, Vol 10, pp 317-322, 1993).

Noble's study found that, based on a battery of creativity tests, alcoholic fathers and sons had generally lower creativity scores than nonalcoholic fathers and sons. The alcoholic fathers and sons scored significantly lower on most of the personality questionnaires, which have been found to be reasonably valid measures of creativity.

The most consistent conclusion to be drawn from Noble's research and other studies examining the creativity-chemical link is summed up best in Noble's study: "Whereas creative people may sometimes be alcoholic, alcoholics are seldom creative."

✎ Weird Words

Consciousness: The state of being aware, or perceiving physical facts or mental concepts; a state of general wakefulness and responsiveness to environment.

Empirical: Founded on practical experience, rather than on reasoning alone; based on careful observational testing of a hypothesis.

Source: From *Stedman's Medical Dictionary, 27th Edition*,

In *The Thirsty Muse: Alcohol and the American Writer* (Ticknor and Fields, 1989), author Tom Dardis pokes holes at the creativity-chemical link. In his book, Dardis, a professor of English, reviews the work and lives of Hemingway, Faulkner, Fitzgerald and O'Neill. All were alcoholic. He suggests that addiction may have diminished the creativity of several writers from this group later in life.

Dardis argues that Hemingway's most notable writing ended during his 41st year with *For Whom the Bell Tolls*. And after the publication of *Go Down, Moses* when he was 44, Faulkner's work declined.

Often artists return to the work they did while intoxicated and end up disappointed.

Even Fitzgerald regretted that he wrote the second half of *Tender is the Night* while drinking.

In many cases, alcoholism and other drug use probably contributed to circumstances that ended the lives of artists. Hemingway committed suicide. So did London, Crane and Berryman.

Among the writers Dardis studied, O'Neill was the only one to choose the path of recovery. When he turned 38, the playwright decided that alcoholism would devour his writing talent and lead to suicide or insanity. He stopped drinking. During his years of sobriety he produced two classics of American drama: *The Iceman Cometh* and *Long Day's Journey Into Night*.

☞ **Remember!!**

In addiction we find a formula for creative burnout, rather than creative inspiration.

Part 2

Alcohol

Chapter 8

Drinking: Facts For Teens

If I were 21 no one would care if I drink.

Not true. Even adults get warnings about the risks of alcohol. The major difference is that buying or drinking alcohol is illegal for people under age 21. Also, the younger you start drinking, the earlier alcohol can affect how you feel now and how you'll feel when you're older.

It's not easy to "Just say no" when my friends are drinking.

Television and radio make it sound easy to "Just say no," but it may not be so simple for you. You're facing some real pressures: your friends may want you to drink with them, you may be stressed out at home, school or work, or you may think drinking is a way to make people like you. But remember, only you can make decisions about what you do or don't do. This is your chance to be your own person. If you feel you need help to say no, then get the support you need. Talk to your family doctor or another adult you can trust.

How much alcohol is really in a drink?

Beer usually has 3% to 5% alcohol. Wine has 9% to 16%. Hard liquor usually contains the highest levels (up to 50%). Most states consider an adult

About This Chapter: Text in this chapter is adapted with permission from *Information From Your Family Doctor*. Retrieved November 19, 2001 from http://www.familydoctor.org/handouts/273.html.

to be "under the influence" or intoxicated (meaning drunk) at 0.08% blood level of alcohol. But for people under 21, many states have lowered their definition of intoxication to .02% or lower. For a man who weighs 160 pounds, this might mean as few as one to two beers (12 ounce cans) in an hour. For a woman who weighs 120 pounds, this might mean less than one beer in an hour.

Why should I say no to a beer or a drink?

Because alcohol is a drug and you can become addicted to it. It changes the way your mind and body work. Even one beer can slow your reactions

✤ It's A Fact!!

- **Alcohol affects your brain.** Drinking alcohol leads to a loss of coordination, poor judgment, slowed reflexes, distorted vision, memory lapses, and even blackouts.
- **Alcohol affects your body.** Alcohol can damage every organ in your body. It is absorbed directly into your bloodstream and can increase your risk for a variety of life-threatening diseases, including cancer.
- **Alcohol affects your self-control.** Alcohol depresses your central nervous system, lowers your inhibitions, and impairs your judgment. Drinking can lead to risky behaviors, including having unprotected sex. This may expose you to HIV/AIDS and other sexually transmitted diseases or cause unwanted pregnancy.
- **Alcohol can kill you.** Drinking large amounts of alcohol can lead to coma or even death. Also, in 1998, 35.8 percent of traffic deaths of 15- to 20-year-olds were alcohol-related.
- **Alcohol can hurt you—even if you're not the one drinking.** If you're around people who are drinking, you have an increased risk of being seriously injured, involved in car crashes, or affected by violence. At the very least, you may have to deal with people who are sick, out of control, or unable to take care of themselves.

Source: Excerpted from "Tips for Teens: The Truth about Alcohol," National Clearinghouse for Alcohol and Drug Information (NCADI), online at www.health.org.

and confuse your thinking. This means anything that requires concentration and coordination—like driving—is more dangerous when you've had a drink.

Alcohol also changes the way you act. It can make you let go of your inhibitions—the feelings that normally keep you from doing things you know are risky or even dangerous. So a couple of beers might make it easier for you to talk to a cute guy or girl, or be the life of the party. But it can also lead you to make bad decisions—like having sex before you're ready, having unsafe sex, or driving when you've been drinking. You might try to tell yourself, "It won't happen to me." But we all know people who have said that and then ended up in the hospital, or worse.

What problems does alcohol cause?

Alcohol can ruin your health. The more you drink, the more damage is done. You can get alcohol poisoning if you drink too much too fast. As the level of alcohol in your blood rises, the chemicals in your body can cause vomiting or seizures, or you may pass out. This type of poisoning will make you sicker than you've probably ever been.

Cirrhosis of the liver is one of the most well-known effects of alcohol abuse. Cirrhosis stops the liver from being able to clean the toxins (poisons) out of your body, which can cause a type of poisoning. Alcohol can also cause stomach ulcers that can lead to internal bleeding. If you drink when you're pregnant, your baby could be born mentally retarded or with other birth defects.

✤ It's A Fact!!

What causes a hangover?

As you drink, your body tries to make up for the changes alcohol causes. It "turns up" all of its senses. When the alcohol begins to wear off, these heightened senses cause shakiness, headaches, and nausea. Everything may seem louder, bigger, and faster.

Other things alcohol can do:

- Make you gain weight
- Make you feel sick and dizzy

- Make your breath smell bad
- Make you throw up
- Make you clumsy and slur your speech
- Make your skin break out
- Make you feel out of control

> ✔ **Quick Tip**
>
> Don't believe the myth that coffee can make you sober. Coffee will only make you a wide-awake drunk. It won't help you think faster or speed up your reactions. And coffee may hold the hidden danger of making you think you're alert enough to drive when you really aren't.

When is drinking a problem?

Drinking is a problem if it causes trouble in your relationships, your school or social activities, or how you think or feel.

A drinking problem usually starts when you just drink now and then. People often start drinking when they feel stressed or because their friends drink. Drinking may make you think that you will forget about your problems or make you feel more liked by others. But after the party or the next day you're still the same person with the same problems. And you might have a new problem—needing a drink.

How do I know if I have a problem?

Ask yourself the following questions to find out if you have a problem with alcohol. If you answer yes to any one of them, you probably have a drinking problem.

1. Do you sometimes drink more than you mean to?
2. Have you tried and failed to cut back on your drinking?
3. Do you ever have hangovers?
4. Have your problems at school, work or with your relationships increased?
5. Do you keep drinking even though you know it's causing you problems?
6. Do you drink when you're stressed out?

7. Do you drink alone?

8. Can you drink more than you used to be able to?

9. Do you sometimes feel guilty about drinking?

10. Do you feel uncomfortable when you haven't had a drink?

11. Do you ever have blackouts after you've been drinking?

12. Do you regret things that you say or do when you've been drinking?

How can I stop drinking?

The first step is to admit you have a problem and to get help. Talk to your family doctor, a school counselor, your family, or your minister or priest. The phone book is a good resource to find contact information for Alcoholics Anonymous (AA) and other groups that help people quit.

✔ Quick Tip

How can you tell if a friend has a drinking problem?

Sometimes it's tough to tell. But there are signs you can look for. If your friend has one or more of the following warning signs, he or she may have a problem with alcohol:

- Getting drunk on a regular basis
- Lying about how much alcohol he or she is using
- Believing that alcohol is necessary to have fun
- Having frequent hangovers
- Feeling run-down, depressed, or even suicidal
- Having "blackouts"—forgetting what he or she did while drinking
- Having problems at school or getting in trouble with the law

Source: Excerpted from "Tips for Teens: The Truth about Alcohol," National Clearinghouse for Alcohol and Drug Information (NCADI), online at www.health.org.

What can you do to help someone who has a drinking problem?

Be a real friend. You might even save a life. Encourage your friend to stop or seek professional help. For information and referrals, call the National Clearinghouse for Alcohol and Drug Information at 800-729-6686.

For More Information

Al-Anon/Alateen

888-4AL-ANON (888-425-2666)

http://www.al-anon.org

Alcoholics Anonymous (AA)

212-870-3400 (or check your local phone book)

http://www.alcoholics-anonymous.org; or http://www.aa.org

Mothers Against Drunk Driving (MADD)

800-GET-MADD (800-438-6233)

http://www.madd.org

National Council on Alcoholism and Drug Dependence, Inc.

800-NCA-CALL (800-622-2255)

http://www.ncadd.org

Students Against Destructive Decisions (SADD)

877-SADD-INC (877-723-3462)

http://www.saddonline.com

Chapter 9

Some Good Reasons Young People Should Avoid Alcohol

> **✤ It's A Fact!!**
>
> Alcohol—the most widely used drug among youth—causes serious and potentially life-threatening problems for this population. Research indicates that drinking is associated with risk-taking and sensation-seeking behavior among adolescents. Alcohol has disinhibiting effects that may increase the likelihood of unsafe activities.
>
> Source: From "Consequences of Underage Alcohol Use," Substance Abuse and Mental Health Ser-

Adolescence can be a volatile time of life. Young people's physical and emotional states are in flux. They live in a society that places demands on them to "grow up fast."

Add alcohol to this mix and you have the potential for lifelong and life-threatening consequences.

Young people are especially vulnerable to the effects of drinking. They may think that because they're in good health now,

About This Chapter: Text in this chapter is from "Some Good Reasons Young People Should Avoid Alcohol," Copyright © 2002 Hazelden. *Alive and Free* articles are reprinted with permission of Hazelden, a nonprofit agency based in Center City, MN, that offers a wide range of information and treatment services relating to addiction and recovery. For more resources on substance abuse, call Hazelden at (800) 257-7810 or check its web site at http://www.hazelden.org.

drinking won't hurt. But it can have devastating consequences—today and later in life.

You can't ignore the facts. According to the *Ninth Special Report to the U.S. Congress on Alcohol and Health*, substance abuse may impair adolescents ability to make judgments about sex and contraception, placing them at increased risk for unplanned pregnancy, sexual assault, or becoming infected with a sexually transmitted disease, including HIV/AIDS.

According to a study released in December 1999 by the Center on Addiction and Substance Abuse (CASA) at Columbia University, teens 14 and younger who use alcohol are twice as likely to have sex than those who don't, and teens 15 and older who drink are seven times likelier to have sexual intercourse and twice as likely to have it with four or more partners than non-drinking teens. What's more, numerous studies have shown that adolescents are more likely to engage in unprotected sex when they drink alcohol than when they do not.

✤ It's A Fact!!

Alcohol-Related Fatalities

- In 1997, 21 percent of the young drivers 15 to 20 years old who were killed in crashes were intoxicated. For young drivers, alcohol involvement is higher among males than among females. In 1997, 25 percent of the young male drivers involved in fatal crashes had been drinking at the time of the crash, compared with 12 percent of the young female drivers involved in fatal crashes.
- According to national data, drowning is the leading cause of injury-related death among adolescents and young adults. Factors contributing to youth drowning include alcohol which can severely affect a swimmer's coordination and judgment. Forty to 50 percent of young males who drown were drinking when they died, and an equal percentage of all diving accidents are alcohol related.

Source: From "Consequences of Underage Alcohol Use," Substance Abuse and Mental Health Services Administration (SAMHSA).

Every year about three million teens are infected with a sexually transmitted disease. Among sexually active teens, those who average five or more drinks daily are nearly three times less likely to use condoms, thus placing them at greater risk for contracting sexually transmitted diseases. The Centers for Disease Control and Prevention estimates that fewer than one percent of AIDS cases occur in adolescents, whereas persons in their 20s account for 20 percent of all cases. Because of the incubation period between exposure to HIV and the onset of AIDS symptoms (as long as 10 years), the high rate of AIDS among people in their 20s may be a consequence of infection during the teen years.

There are other disturbing numbers. One national study of teenagers found that about half had been drinking and/or using drugs before the act of intercourse that resulted in unintended pregnancy. Each year about one million teenaged girls in this country become pregnant, and 80 percent of those pregnancies are unintended. Alcohol use during pregnancy may result in fetal alcohol syndrome or effect.

Alcohol use is implicated in more incidents of sexual violence than any single drug, according to the CASA study. Alcohol use—by the victim, the perpetrator or both—is implicated in 46 to 75 percent of date rape cases among teens and college students.

✤ It's A Fact!!

Academic Performance

- A lower dosage of alcohol will damage a young brain compared to a fully mature brain, and young brains are damaged more quickly. Alcohol exposure during adolescence is linked with a reduced ability to learn compared with those not exposed until adulthood.
- Alcohol is implicated in more than 40 percent of all college academic problems and 28 percent of all college dropouts. At both 2- and 4-year colleges, the heaviest drinkers make the lowest grades.
- High school students who use alcohol or other substances are five times more likely than other students to drop out of school or to believe that earning good grades is not important.

Source: From "Consequences of Underage Alcohol Use," Substance Abuse and Mental Health Services Administration (SAMHSA).

The use of alcohol and other drugs is associated with the leading causes of death and injury (such as motor-vehicle crashes, homicides and suicides) among teenagers and young adults. A 16-year-old is still more likely to die from an alcohol-related problem than any other cause.

In addition to the immediate dangers posed by young drinkers, underage alcohol use is a strong predictor of future alcohol abuse. A recent study found that people who begin drinking before age 15 are four times more likely to develop alcoholism than those who begin at 21.

✤ It's A Fact!!

Crime

- About half of college students who are victims of crime are drinking when they are victimized.
- In a high percentage of serious crimes, alcohol is found in the offender, the victim, or both, and alcohol-related problems are disproportionately found in both juvenile and adult offenders.
- Ninety-five percent of violent crime on college campuses is alcohol related, and 90 percent of college rapes involve alcohol use by the victim and/or assailant.

Source: From "Consequences of Underage Alcohol Use," Substance Abuse and Mental Health Services Administration (SAMHSA).

☞ Remember!!

It's clear that delaying alcohol use is beneficial to the health and development of young people. Increasing awareness of the potential consequences of alcohol use is one piece to helping young people make informed, healthy choices in their lives.

Chapter 10

Alcohol Abuse And Alcoholism

Is alcoholism a disease?

Yes, alcoholism is a disease. The craving that an alcoholic feels for alcohol can be as strong as the need for food or water. An alcoholic will continue to drink despite serious family, health, or legal problems.

Like many other diseases, alcoholism is chronic, meaning that it lasts a person's lifetime; it usually follows a predictable course; and it has symptoms. The risk for developing alcoholism is influenced both by a person's genes and by his or her lifestyle.

Is alcoholism inherited?

Research shows that the risk for developing alcoholism does indeed run in families. The genes a person inherits partially explain this pattern, but lifestyle is also a factor. Currently, researchers are working to discover the actual genes that put people at risk for alcoholism. Your friends, the amount of stress in your life, and how readily available alcohol is also are factors that may increase your risk for alcoholism.

But remember: Risk is not destiny. Just because alcoholism tends to run in families doesn't mean that a child of an alcoholic parent will automatically

About This Chapter: Text in this chapter is excerpted from "FAQs on Alcohol Abuse and Alcoholism," National Institute on Alcohol Abuse and Alcoholism (NIAAA), November 2001; available online at http://www.niaaa.nih.gov/faq/q-a.htm.

become an alcoholic too. Some people develop alcoholism even though no one in their family has a drinking problem. By the same token, not all children of alcoholic families get into trouble with alcohol. Knowing you are at risk is important, though, because then you can take steps to protect yourself from developing problems with alcohol.

✎ Weird Words

Alcoholism, also known as alcohol dependence, is a disease that includes the following four symptoms:

Craving: A strong need, or urge, to drink.

Loss Of Control: Not being able to stop drinking once drinking has begun.

Physical Dependence: Withdrawal symptoms, such as nausea, sweating, shakiness, and anxiety after stopping drinking.

Tolerance: The need to drink greater amounts of alcohol to get "high."

Source: National Institute on Alcohol Abuse and Alcoholism (NIAAA)

Can alcoholism be cured?

No, alcoholism cannot be cured at this time. Even if an alcoholic hasn't been drinking for a long time, he or she can still suffer a relapse. To guard against a relapse, an alcoholic must continue to avoid all alcoholic beverages.

Can alcoholism be treated?

Yes, alcoholism can be treated. Alcoholism treatment programs use both counseling and medications to help a person stop drinking. Most alcoholics need help to recover from their disease. With support and treatment, many people are able to stop drinking and rebuild their lives.

Which medications treat alcoholism?

A range of medications is used to treat alcoholism. Benzodiazepines (for example, Valium® and Librium®) are sometimes used during the first days after a person stops drinking to help him or her safely withdraw from alcohol.

These medications are not used beyond the first few days, however, because they may be highly addictive. Other medications help people remain sober. One medication used for this purpose is naltrexone (ReVia™). When combined with counseling naltrexone can reduce the craving for alcohol and help prevent a person from returning, or relapsing, to heavy drinking. Another medication, disulfiram (Antabuse®), discourages drinking by making the person feel sick if he or she drinks alcohol.

Through several medications help treat alcoholism, there is no "magic bullet." In other words, no single medication is available that works in every case and/or in every person. Developing new and more effective medications to treat alcoholism remains a high priority for researchers.

Does alcoholism treatment work?

Alcoholism treatment works for many people. But just like any chronic disease, there are varying levels of success when it comes to treatment. Some people stop drinking and remain sober. Others have long periods of sobriety with bouts of relapse. And still others cannot stop drinking for any length of time. With treatment, one thing is clear, however: the longer a person abstains from alcohol, the more likely he or she will be able to stay sober.

Do you have to be an alcoholic to experience problems?

No. Alcoholism is only one type of an alcohol problem. Alcohol abuse can be just as harmful. A person can abuse alcohol without actually being an alcoholic—that is, he or she may drink too much and too often but still not be dependent on alcohol. Some of the problems linked to alcohol abuse include not being able to meet work, school, or family responsibilities; drunk-driving arrests and car crashes; and drinking-related medical conditions. Under some circumstances, even social or moderate drinking is dangerous—for example, when driving, during pregnancy, or when taking certain medications.

Are specific groups of people more likely to have problems?

Alcohol abuse and alcoholism cut across gender, race, and nationality. Nearly 14 million people in the United States—one in every 13 adults—abuse alcohol or are alcoholic. In general, though, more men than women are alcohol dependent or have alcohol problems. And alcohol problems are

✤ It's A Fact!!

Alcohol Impairment Chart

This chart is intended as a guide, not a guarantee.

Alcohol affects individuals differently. Your blood alcohol level may be affected by your age, gender, physical condition, amount of food consumed, and any drugs or medication. In addition, different drinks may contain different amounts of alcohol, so it's important to know how much and the concentration of alcohol you consume.

For purposes of this guide, "one drink" is equal to 1.25 oz. of 80 proof liquor, 12 oz. of regular beer, or 5 oz. of table wine.

Table 10.1. Alcohol Impairment Chart for Men: Know Your Limits (This chart is intended as a guide, not a guarantee.)

MEN Approximate Blood Alcohol Percentage									
	Body Weight in Pounds								
Drinks	100	120	140	160	180	200	220	240	Impairment
0	0.00	0.00	0.00	0.00	0.00	0.00	0.00	0.00	Only Safe Driving Limit
1	0.04	0.03	0.03	0.02	0.02	0.02	0.02	0.02	Impairment Begins
2	0.08	0.06	0.05	0.05	0.04	0.04	0.03	0.03	Driving Skills Significantly Affected; Possible Criminal Penalties
3	0.11	0.09	0.08	0.07	0.06	0.06	0.05	0.05	
4	0.15	0.12	0.11	0.09	0.08	0.08	0.07	0.06	
5	0.19	0.16	0.13	0.12	0.11	0.09	0.09	0.08	
6	0.23	0.19	0.16	0.14	0.13	0.11	0.10	0.09	
7	0.26	0.22	0.19	0.16	0.15	0.13	0.12	0.11	Legally Intoxicated; Criminal Penalties
8	0.30	0.25	0.21	0.19	0.17	0.15	0.14	0.13	
9	0.34	0.28	0.24	0.21	0.19	0.17	0.15	0.14	
10	0.38	0.31	0.27	0.23	0.21	0.19	0.17	0.16	

Subtract .01% for each 40 minutes of drinking

One drink is 1.25 oz. of 80 proof liquor, 12 oz. of beer, or 5 oz. of table wine

A woman drinking an equal amount of alcohol in the same period of time as a man of an equivalent weight may have a higher blood alcohol level than that man. Therefore, women should refer to the female "Know Your Limits" chart.

Some states have set .08% Blood Alcohol Concentration (BAC) as the legal limit for Driving Under the Influence. For commercial drivers, a BAC of .04% can result in a DUI conviction nationwide.

- Impairment begins with your first drink.
- For safety's sake, never drive after drinking.

Table 10.2. Alcohol Impairment Chart for Women: Know Your Limits (This chart is intended as a guide, not a guarantee.)

WOMEN Approximate Blood Alcohol Percentage										
	Body Weight in Pounds									
Drinks	90	100	120	140	160	180	200	220	240	Impairment
0	0.00	0.00	0.00	0.00	0.00	0.00	0.00	0.00	0.00	Only Safe Driving Limit
1	0.05	0.05	0.04	0.03	0.03	0.03	0.02	0.02	0.02	Impairment Begins
2	0.10	0.09	0.08	0.07	0.06	0.05	0.05	0.04	0.04	Driving Skills Significantly Affected; Possible Criminal Penalties
3	0.15	0.14	0.11	0.10	0.09	0.08	0.07	0.06	0.06	
4	0.20	0.18	0.15	0.13	0.11	0.10	0.09	0.08	0.08	
5	0.25	0.23	0.19	0.16	0.14	0.13	0.11	0.10	0.09	
6	0.30	0.27	0.23	0.19	0.17	0.15	0.14	0.12	0.11	Legally Intoxicated; Criminal Penalties
7	0.35	0.32	0.27	0.23	0.20	0.18	0.16	0.14	0.13	
8	0.40	0.36	0.30	0.26	0.23	0.20	0.18	0.17	0.15	
9	0.45	0.41	0.34	0.29	0.26	0.23	0.20	0.19	0.17	
10	0.51	0.45	0.38	0.32	0.28	0.25	0.23	0.21	0.10	

Subtract .01% for each 40 minutes of drinking
One drink is 1.25 oz. of 80 proof liquor, 12 oz. of beer, or 5 oz. of table wine

Source: © Pennsylvania Liquor Control Board; reprinted with permission. Available online at http://www.health.org/nongovpubs/bac-chart/index.htm

highest among young adults ages 18–29 and lowest among adults ages 65 and older. We also know that people who start drinking at an early age—for example, at age 14 or younger—greatly increase the chance that they will develop alcohol problems at some point in their lives.

How can you tell if someone has a problem?

Answering the following four questions can help you find out if you or a loved one has a drinking problem:

- Have you ever felt you should cut down on your drinking?
- Have people annoyed you by criticizing your drinking?
- Have you ever felt bad or guilty about your drinking?
- Have you ever had a drink first thing in the morning to steady your nerves or to get rid of a hangover?

One "yes" answer suggests a possible alcohol problem. More than one "yes" answer means it is highly likely that a problem exists. If you think that you or someone you know might have an alcohol problem, it is important to see a doctor or other health care provider right away. They can help you determine if a drinking problem exists and plan the best course of action.

Can a problem drinker simply cut down?

It depends. If that person has been diagnosed as an alcoholic, the answer is "no." Alcoholics who try to cut down on drinking rarely succeed. Cutting out alcohol—that is, abstaining—is usually the best course for recovery. People who are not alcohol dependent but who have experienced alcohol-related problems may be able to limit the amount they drink. If they can't stay within those limits, they need to stop drinking altogether.

If an alcoholic is unwilling to get help, what can you do about it?

This can be a challenge. An alcoholic can't be forced to get help except under certain circumstances, such as a violent incident that results in court-ordered treatment or medical emergency. But you don't have to wait for someone to "hit rock bottom" to act. Many alcoholism treatment specialists suggest the following steps to help an alcoholic get treatment:

- **Stop all "cover ups."** Family members often make excuses to others or try to protect the alcoholic from the results of his or her drinking. It is important to stop covering for the alcoholic so that he or she experiences the full consequences of drinking.
- **Time your intervention.** The best time to talk to the drinker is shortly after an alcohol-related problem has occurred—like a serious family argument or an accident. Choose a time when he or she is sober, both of you are fairly calm, and you have a chance to talk in private.
- **Be specific.** Tell the family member that you are worried about his or her drinking. Use examples of the ways in which the drinking has caused problems, including the most recent incident.
- **State the results.** Explain to the drinker what you will do if he or she doesn't go for help—not to punish the drinker, but to protect yourself from his or her problems. What you say may range from refusing to go with the person to any social activity where alcohol will be served, to moving out of the house. Do not make any threats you are not prepared to carry out.
- **Get help.** Gather information in advance about treatment options in your community. If the person is willing to get help, call immediately for an appointment with a treatment counselor. Offer to go with the family member on the first visit to a treatment program and/or an Alcoholics Anonymous meeting.
- **Call on a friend.** If the family member still refuses to get help, ask a friend to talk with him or her using the steps just described. A friend who is a recovering alcoholic may be particularly persuasive, but any person who is caring and nonjudgmental may help. The intervention of more than one person, more than one time, is often necessary to coax an alcoholic to seek help.
- **Find strength in numbers.** With the help of a health care professional, some families join with other relatives and friends to confront an alcoholic as a group. This approach should only be tried under the guidance of a health care professional who is experienced in this kind of group intervention.

- **Get support.** It is important to remember that you are not alone. Support groups offered in most communities include Al-Anon, which holds regular meetings for spouses and other significant adults in an alcoholic's life, and Alateen, which is geared to children of alcoholics. These groups help family members understand that they are not responsible for an alcoholic's drinking and that they need to take steps to take care of themselves, regardless of whether the alcoholic family member chooses to get help.

✔ Quick Tip

1. Do you drink because you have problems? To relax?
2. Do you drink when you get mad at other people, your friends, or parents?
3. Do you prefer to drink alone, rather than with others?
4. Are your grades starting to slip? Are you goofing off on your job?
5. Did you ever try to stop drinking or drink less—and fail?
6. Have you begun to drink in the morning, before school or work?
7. Do you gulp your drinks?
8. Do you ever have loss of memory due to your drinking?
9. Do you lie about your drinking?
10. Do you ever get into trouble when you're drinking?
11. Do you get drunk when you drink, even when you don't mean to?
12. Do you think it's cool to be able to hold your liquor?

According to Alcoholics Anonymous (A.A.), a "yes" answer to any one of the above questions indicates that the person answering is probably in trouble with alcohol.

Source: The preceding twelve questions have been excerpted from material appearing in the pamphlet, "A Message to Teenagers," and have been reprinted with permission of Alcoholics Anonymous World Services, Inc. (A.A.W.S). Permission to reprint this material does not mean that A.A.W.S. has reviewed and/or endorses this publication. A.A. is a program for recovery from alcoholism only—use of A.A. material in any non-A.A. context does not imply otherwise.

How can a person get help for an alcohol problem?

There are many national and local resources that can help. The National Drug and Alcohol Treatment Referral Routing Service provides a toll-free telephone number, 1-800-662-HELP, offering various resource information. Through this service you can speak directly to a representative concerning substance abuse treatment, request printed material on alcohol or other drugs, or obtain local substance abuse treatment referral information in your state.

Chapter 11

Alcohol Poisoning: Drinking Too Much Can Kill You

When police found Bradley McCue, a student at the University of Michigan, they saw that he was unconscious, his nose was painted red, and the words "24 shots" were scribbled across his forehead.

An autopsy revealed that McCue had a blood alcohol level of .44 percent. Witnesses said that he drank 24 shots of liquor in less than two hours. He died of acute alcohol intoxication—also known as alcohol poisoning.

Friends had taken McCue out drinking to celebrate his 21st birthday.

Cases such as McCue's are rare. However, each year several alcohol poisoning deaths on college campuses gain national attention. And the National Council on Alcoholism and Drug Dependence (NCADD), Inc., reports that hundreds die each year from acute alcohol intoxication.

Research reveals that binge drinking—consuming five or more drinks in a row on a single occasion—is common among college students. In 1997, the Harvard School of Public Health published the results of its College Alcohol

About This Chapter: Text in this chapter is from "Alcohol Poisoning: Drinking Too Much Too Fast Can Kill You," Copyright © 2002 Hazelden. *Alive and Free* articles are reprinted with permission of Hazelden, a nonprofit agency based in Center City, MN, that offers a wide range of information and treatment services relating to addiction and recovery. For more resources on substance abuse, call Hazelden at (800) 257-7810 or check its web site at http://www.hazelden.org.

Study. The bottom line: one in five college students binge drinks frequently (at least three times every two weeks).

According to the NCADD, many students are surprised to learn that they can die from an overdose of alcohol. Often, the worst they expect from a night of binge drinking is a blackout and bad hangover.

Common attitudes toward binge drinking don't help: "It's a rite of passage." "If you pass out from drinking, you just sleep it off."

Changing these attitudes starts with knowing some facts. Blood alcohol levels skyrocket during binge drinking. When people who weigh 160 pounds take a single drink, their blood alcohol level rises .025 percent, on average. But for inexperienced drinkers, or those sensitive to alcohol, blood alcohol levels elevate faster and acute intoxication can result more quickly. Because of differences in body chemistry, women can overdose after drinking lesser amounts than men.

> **✎ Weird Words**
>
> Intoxication: A synonym for poisoning.
>
> Poison: Any substance, either taken internally or applied externally, that is injurious to health or dangerous to life.
>
> Source: From *Stedman's Medical Dictionary, 27th Edition*,

"If you binge drink six or eight drinks within an hour, this can take you to a blood alcohol level that is potentially fatal by sedating the breathing mechanism or causing cardiac irregularity," says Max Schneider, MD, chairman of NCADD's Board of Directors.

"Anywhere from four to five drinks a day is toxic to the body," Schneider adds. "Some students say, 'I won't drink every day; I'll just take six or seven drinks on Saturday night.' That's very toxic."

It's important to remember that the amount of alcohol in standard servings of wine (5 oz.), beer (12 oz.) and distilled spirits (1.5 oz., 80 proof) is the same. This fact refutes the myth that beer or wine present less danger to the binge drinker than "hard" liquor.

Alcohol poisoning quickly affects the bodily functions that sustain life. As a depressant, alcohol slows breathing, heart rate and blood pressure. If blood alcohol levels rise sharply in a short time, the areas of the brain that control these functions can be sedated—literally put to sleep. When that happens, people lose consciousness and can die. People who poison themselves with alcohol can also die from aspirating, or choking, on their own vomit.

We can respond to this problem on two levels. One is knowing appropriate emergency procedures. According to the NCADD, signs and symptoms of alcohol poisoning include:

- Unconsciousness or semi-consciousness
- Slow breathing—eight breaths or less per minute, or lapses of more than eight seconds between breaths

✤ It's A Fact!!

Did you know....

- Frequent binge drinkers were eight times more likely than non-binge drinkers to miss a class, fall behind in schoolwork, get hurt or injured, and damage property.
- More than 60 percent of college men and almost 50 percent of college women who are frequent binge drinkers report that they drink and drive.
- Binge drinking during college may be associated with mental health disorders such as compulsiveness, depression or anxiety, or early deviant behavior.
- In a national study, 91 percent of women and 78 percent of the men who were frequent binge drinkers considered themselves to be moderate or light drinkers.
- In schools with high binge drinking rates, 34 percent of non-binge drinkers reported being insulted or humiliated by binge drinkers; 13 percent reported being pushed, hit, or assaulted; 54 percent reported having to take care of a drunken student; 68 percent were interrupted while studying; and 26 percent of women experienced an unwanted sexual advance.

Source: Excerpted from "Binge Drinking in Adolescents and College Students," Substance Abuse and Mental Health Services Administration (SAMHSA).

- Cold, clammy, pale or bluish skin
- A strong odor of alcohol

If you encounter someone with these signs or symptoms, call 911. Then gently turn this person on his or her side. This helps to prevent choking after vomiting.

A second response is to prevent binge drinking. We can support campus policies that discourage drinking, such as providing alcohol-free residence halls and restricting pledging activities by fraternities and sororities. We can also reinforce abstinence from alcohol as the norm. The fact is that most college students drink moderately or not at all.

✔ Quick Tip

A pamphlet titled "Drinking Too Much Too Fast Can Kill You" is available from the National Council on Alcoholism and Drug Dependence (NCADD). Call (212) 269-7797 or visit their website at http://www.ncadd.org.

Chapter 12

Alcohol Treatment And Adolescents

Alcohol abuse and alcohol dependence are not only adult problems—they also affect a significant number of adolescents and young adults between the ages of 12 and 20, even though drinking under the age of 21 is illegal in every state. Alcohol use for some adolescents can lead to an abusive and addictive pattern that requires intervention. Diagnosis and treatment of alcohol abuse and dependence are more important because alcohol-related problems can have an enormous impact on the adolescent's future.[1]

Prevalence Of Adolescent Alcohol Abuse And Dependence Treatment

- In SAMHSA's Treatment Episode Data Set (TEDS), data indicate that about 80 percent of adult respondents receiving alcohol treatment reported that they first became intoxicated before the age of 18.[7]
- Within TEDS treatment admissions, the proportion of those under 18 has increased slightly from 7 percent in 1992 to 9 percent in 1997.[8]
- In 1996, nearly 182,000 adolescents or young adults under age 20 received treatment for substance abuse in the United States. Of those, 21 percent received treatment for alcohol abuse or dependence, and

About This Chapter: Information in this chapter is from "Alcohol Treatment and Adolescents," a fact sheet produced by the Substance Abuse and Mental Health Services Administration (SAMHSA), 1999.

approximately another 34 percent received treatment for alcohol and a secondary drug dependence.[9]

- Researchers and treatment professionals have found it useful to view adolescent substance use as occurring on a continuum that extends from experimentation through problem use to disorders of abuse and dependence. Adolescent substance use occurs with the severity of involvement with alcohol or other substances. Not all adolescents who use alcohol are, or will become, dependent.[10]

The Unique Needs Of Adolescents In Alcohol Treatment

Summary of Key Points from SAMHSA's Treatment Improvement Protocol on Treatment of Adolescents with Substance Abuse Disorders.[11]

- Adolescent alcohol use often stems from different causes than for adults. In treatment, adolescents must be approached differently from adults because of developmental issues, differences in values and belief systems, environmental considerations such as strong peer influences, and educational requirements.

✤ It's A Fact!!

- According to the Substance Abuse and Mental Health Services Administration (SAMHSA)'s most recent National Household Survey on Drug Abuse (NHSDA), there were 10.4 million drinkers ages 12 to 20 in 1998. Of these, 5.1 million were binge drinkers, meaning that they drank five or more drinks on at least one occasion in the month before the survey. Two million were heavy drinkers, binge drinking at least five times that month.[2]
- The average age when youth first try alcohol is 11 years for boys and 13 years for girls. According to research by the National Institute on Alcohol Abuse and Alcoholism, adolescents who begin drinking before age 15 are four times more likely to develop alcohol dependence than those who begin drinking at age 21.[3]

- Treatment approaches should also account for age, gender, ethnicity, cultural background, family structure, cognitive and social development, and readiness for change. Younger adolescents have different developmental needs than older adolescents, and treatment approaches should be developed appropriately for different age groups.
- Treatment should involve family members because family history may play a role in the origins of the problem and successful treatment cannot take place in isolation.
- Treatment providers should have specific training in the principles of adolescent development, and treatment programs should avoid mixing adult clients with adolescent clients.

Screening And Assessment

- Clinicians and researchers use various approaches to identify and assess alcohol problems in adolescents. One approach is the use of brief screening instruments—most commonly self-report questionnaires—to determine the possible presence of alcohol problems. Screening tools

- Generally, an adolescent's risk for alcohol dependence at some point in life decreases by 14 percent with each additional year that drinking onset is delayed.[4]
- Data from SAMHSA's National Household Survey on Drug Abuse indicates that while 915,000 youth ages 12 to 20 reported alcohol dependence in the past year, only 16 percent of them (148,000) received treatment.[5]
- Although national data on the prevalence of alcohol abuse and dependence among teenagers are not available, several large-scale school surveys suggest that 4 to 20 percent of teenagers have either a current or past diagnosis of alcohol abuse or alcohol dependence, based on *DSM* (*Diagnostic and Statistical Manual*) criteria.[6]

should be used with caution, as scores only indicate that an alcohol use disorder is likely or not. Some available screening tools for use with adolescents in screening for alcohol and other drug use disorders include the Adolescent Alcohol Involvement Scale, the Adolescent Drinking Index, the Personal Experience Screening Questionnaire, and the Rutgers Alcohol Problem Index. Research has generally supported the validity of these self-reports of alcohol within clinical settings.[12]

- If an initial screening indicates the need for further assessment, clinicians and researchers can employ diagnostic interviews to measure the nature and severity of alcohol problems and other drug use disorders. Some of these diagnostic interviews include the Adolescent Diagnostic Interview, the Customary Drinking and Drug Use Record, and the Diagnostic Interview for Children and Adolescents.[13]

✎ Weird Words

Aftercare: A continuing program of rehabilitation designed to reinforce the effects of the therapy; may include partial hospitalization, day hospital, or outpatient treatment.

Cognitive: Pertaining to the mental activities associated with thinking, learning, and memory.

Detoxification: 1. Recovery from the toxic effects of a drug; 2. Removal of the toxic properties from a poison.

Psycho-: A prefix relating to the mind and its processes (for example, psychoeducational refers to education and mental functioning; psychosocial refers to social interactions and mental functioning).

Rehabilitation: Restoration, following disease, illness, or injury, of the ability to function in a normal or near-normal manner.

Relapse: Return of the manifestations of a disease after an interval of improvement. Synonym: recurrence.

Screening: To examine, evaluate; to process a group to select or separate certain individuals from it.

Therapeutic Communities: Places where people live together for therapeutic purposes. Therapeutic means relating to the treatment, remediating, or curing of a disorder or disease.

Trigger: Term describing a system in which a relatively small input turns on a relatively large output, the magnitude of which is unrelated to the magnitude of the input.

Source: From *Stedman's Medical Dictionary, 27th Edition*,

Levels Of Treatment

- Treatment options can vary. Brief interventions, which involve screening, anticipatory guidance, and psychoeducational interventions, are primarily appropriate for adolescents in the low-to-middle range of the severity continuum. Brief interventions may also occur in primary care settings as part of a routine medical exam. Variations of brief interventions have been found effective for helping alcohol-abusing adults, but research is needed to evaluate its effectiveness with adolescents.[14]

- Treatment may also include various intensities of outpatient treatment, as well as 24-hour intensive inpatient care for adolescents requiring a high level of supervision. Inpatient care generally includes detoxification—a 3- to 5-day program with intensive medical monitoring and management of withdrawal symptoms. Residential treatment is a long-term model that includes psychosocial rehabilitation among its goals. The duration for residential treatment can range from 30 days to 1 year and is especially beneficial for adolescents with coexisting personality and substance abuse disorders.[15]

- Therapeutic communities are intensive and comprehensive treatment models. Although originally developed for adults, they have been modified successfully to treat adolescents with the most severe alcohol or substance use disorders for whom long-term care is indicated. The community itself is both therapist and teacher in the treatment process. The core goal is to promote a holistic lifestyle and identify behaviors that can lead to alcohol and substance abuse that need to be changed. The community provides a safe and nurturing environment within which adolescents can begin to experience healthy living. Duration within the community is typically 12 to 18 months.[16]

- Self-help groups such as Alcoholics Anonymous, Al-Anon, and Alateen are valuable adjuncts to outpatient services and residential programs for teenagers during the recovery process, both during and after primary treatment. Self-help groups offer positive role models, new friends who are learning to enjoy life free from substance use, people celebrating sober living, and a place to learn how to cope with stress and other relapse triggers. Many adolescents involved with these 12-step programs have a fellow member serve as a sponsor to provide guidance and help in times of crisis or when the urge to return to drinking becomes overwhelming.[17]

- Treatment programs can also include family therapy to bring about positive changes in the way family members relate to each other by examining the underlying causes of dysfunctional interactions. This type of therapy may help decrease family conflict and improve effectiveness of communication. Family members, both parents and youth, can learn how to listen to one another and solve problems through negotiation and compromise.[18]

- It is extremely important that adolescents are assessed for coexisting mental disorders, because progress in alcohol treatment may be stalled until coexisting conditions are addressed. Treatment providers use that information to develop a treatment plan that may include such services as individual, group, and family therapy.[19] Since problem drinking often occurs along with other behavior disorders, many providers offer skills training in impulse control, anger management, problem solving, assertiveness, time management, and stress management.[20]

> **✔ Quick Tip**
>
> If you would like additional information or need help finding treatment please call the National Clearinghouse for Alcohol and Drug Information at 1-800-729-6686 or visit http://www.health.org.

- During the final phase of treatment, providers work with adolescents to develop an aftercare plan to make sure they don't start drinking again. Continuing care programs are structured and time-limited outpatient care that helps the adolescent reduce his or her risk for relapse. Self-help groups may be valuable adjuncts to the treatment program during the recovery process. Group homes that offer transitional living arrangements with different levels of specificity of treatment planning and staff supervision may also provide an environment for successful recovery.[21]

About SAMHSA

SAMHSA, a public health agency in the Department of Health and Human Services, is the Federal Government's lead agency for improving the quality and availability of substance abuse prevention, addiction treatment, and mental health services in the United States. Further information about SAMHSA is available on the Internet at www.samhsa.gov.

Sources

1. Bukstein, Oscar G., "Treatment of Adolescent Alcohol Abuse and Dependence," *Alcohol Health and Research World*, 1994.

2. Substance Abuse and Mental Health Services Administration, *Summary Findings From the 1998 National Household Survey on Drug Abuse.* Bethesda, MD: Department of Health and Human Services, 1999.

3. Grant, Bridget F., National Institute of Alcohol Abuse and Alcoholism's Epidemiologic Bulletin No. 39 "The Impact of a Family History of Alcoholism on the Relationship Between Age at Onset of Alcohol Use and *DSM-IV* Alcohol Dependence, Results From the National Longitudinal Alcohol Epidemiologic Survey," *Alcohol Health and Research World*, Volume 22, No. 2, 1998.

4. Ibid.

5. Substance Abuse and Mental Health Services Administration, *Summary Findings From the 1998 National Household Survey on Drug Abuse.* Bethesda, MD: Department of Health and Human Services, 1999.

6. Martin, Christopher, S. and Ken C. Winters, "Diagnosis and Assessment of Alcohol Use Disorders Among Adolescents," *Alcohol Health and Research World*, Volume 22, No. # 2, 1998.

7. Substance Abuse and Mental Health Services Administration, Office of Applied Studies, Drug and Alcohol Services Information System Series:

S-5, National Admissions to Substance Abuse Treatment Services Treatment Episode Data Set (TEDS) 1992-1997, Rockville, MD: Department of Health and Human Services, DHHS Pub. No. (SMA) 99-3324, 1999.

8. Ibid.

9. Ibid.

10. Substance Abuse and Mental Health Services Administration, *Treatment of Adolescents With Substance Abuse Disorders*, Treatment Improvement Protocol (TIP) Series 32, Rockville, MD: Department of Health and Human Services, 1999.

11. Ibid.

12. Martin, Christopher, S. and Ken C. Winters, "Diagnosis and Assessment of Alcohol Use Disorders Among Adolescents," *Alcohol Health and Research World*, Volume 22, No. # 2, 1998.

13. Ibid.

14. Substance Abuse and Mental Health Services Administration, *Treatment of Adolescents With Substance Abuse Disorders*, Treatment Improvement Protocol (TIP) Series 32, Rockville, MD: U.S. Department of Health and Human Services, 1999.

15. Ibid.

16. Ibid.

17. Ibid.

18. Ibid.

19. Ibid.

20. Shoemaker, R.H., and Sherry, P., "Posttreatment factors influencing outcome of adolescent chemical dependency treatment," *Journal of Adolescent Chemical Dependency* 2(1): 1999.

21. Substance Abuse and Mental Health Services Administration, *Treatment of Adolescents With Substance Abuse Disorders*, Treatment Improvement Protocol (TIP) Series 32, Rockville, MD: Department of Health and Human Services, 1999.

Chapter 13

Alcoholism Tends To Run In Families

What's Important About Children Of Alcoholics?

Children of alcoholics (COAs):

- are at high risk for alcohol and other drug problems
- often live with pervasive tension and stress
- have higher levels of anxiety and depression
- do poorly in school
- experience problems with coping

The good news is that they can be helped to bounce back from the effects of their families' problems.

> ✔ **Quick Tip**
>
> When talking with anyone under 21 about alcohol and other drugs, urge them to "Be Smart! Don't Start!"

When family members (parents, grandparents, aunts/uncles), guardians, or other adults in charge of children are alcoholics, there is strong evidence that children in these families are more likely to develop the disease of alcoholism as well. The fact is, alcoholism tends to run in families.

About This Chapter: Text in this chapter is from "The Fact Is ... Alcoholism Tends to Run in Families," National Clearinghouse for Alcohol and Drug Information, DHHS Pub. No. (ADM) 92-1914, reprinted in 1993 and 1995. Available online at http://www.health.org/govpubs/ph318; accessed November 2001.

What Causes COAs To Have Increased Risk?

Children of alcoholics may or may not be raised by alcoholics. Either way, every COA is at risk for alcoholism or alcoholism-related problems.

Children Living With Alcoholics

Children who live with alcoholics are at increased risk because of genetic and/or environmental factors. They may be at more risk for alcoholism just as children of diabetics are at higher risk for diabetes. Children living with alcoholics often develop unhealthy living patterns. They may not learn how to trust themselves or others, how to handle uncomfortable feelings, or how to build positive relationships. COAs who lack these skills are also at higher risk for school failure, depression, increased anxiety, as well as trouble with alcohol and other drugs.

Adopted And Foster Children

Even COAs adopted by non-alcoholics (or do not live with their alcoholic parents for other reasons), may have a genetic predisposition to alcoholism, just as children born to parents with a history of heart disease are more at risk for heart disease.

Alcoholism can skip a generation. Some COAs never drink, but may pass on a genetic vulnerability and/or unhealthy living pattern to their own children.

COAs Do Not Have To Develop Problems

Genes can't be replaced. But unhealthy living patterns can be countered by the consistent caring of others. COAs can learn to trust, handle their feelings in healthy ways, and build positive, nurturing relationships. Anyone can help COAs understand their risks and learn better social and coping skills.

How Many COAs Are There? How Many Become Alcoholics?

There were an estimated 28.6 million COAs in the U.S. in 1991, nearly 11 million of them under age 18. Of the under-18 group, almost 3 million will develop alcoholism, other drug problems, and/or other serious coping problems. About half of COAs marry alcoholics and are likely to recreate the same kinds of highly stressful and unhealthy families in which they grew up, unless supportive interventions are provided to them in their formative years.

What About The Other COAs?

Based on stories from adult COAs in professional treatment and self-help programs, it appears all children are affected by family alcoholism. But, going back to the good news, many of them make positive adjustments to their families' alcoholism. Even COAs in high- risk environments with other chronic sources of stress—including poverty, racism, disrupted marriages, serious emotional problems, and histories of abuse and neglect—are often able to overcome these painful beginnings and create healthy, fulfilling lives for themselves.

How Can COAs Be Helped To Bounce Back?

This is where the good news is really exciting.

The child in an alcoholic home may be helped whether the alcoholic stops drinking or not. It is not necessary to do anything to change the adult's drinking behavior. And helping a COA does not require special training or skills.

☞ Remember!!

It is important not to label or stigmatize COAs or their families. If someone identifies himself or herself as a COA, be prepared to refer that person to school counselors or professional therapists for additional support.

Simple acts of kindness and compassion can make a big difference in the lives of COAs. Just by being there—to lend an ear, share normal interests and activities, talk about feelings, accept their mistakes, and support and encourage their friend-making efforts—YOU will be helping.

✤ **It's A Fact!!**

Fact #1

Alcoholism is a disease. Your parent is not a bad person; he or she has a disease that makes him or her lose control when drinking. Alcohol does that; when you drink too much, you do and say things that you normally wouldn't. Maybe the disease makes them do mean or stupid things that they would not do if they didn't drink.

Fact #2

You cannot control your parent's drinking. It is not your fault. Don't hide the bottle or try to be perfect; you can't do anything about your parent's drinking. You are not the reason why your parent drinks. You did not cause the disease.

Fact #3

You are not alone. There are lots of kids just like you. I'll bet there are some in your class at school—kids you would never think of might have a parent who drinks like yours. Maybe you know some of them because you've seen what goes on in their house. In fact, from all the surveys done in the United States, we know that there are about eleven million children with alcoholic parents living in our country. You really aren't alone.

Fact #4

You CAN talk about the problem. Find someone you trust who will talk to you. It could be a teacher, a friend's parent, a big brother or sister, or someone else who will listen to you. These are the 'safe people' in your life. Make a list called "People Who Can Help Me." Keep this list with you so that you can call someone if you feel like talking.

Also, there is a group for kids called Alateen. This group has meetings, like a club, and the kids there share tips on how to make their lives easier. Some schools have Alateen meetings on the school grounds during the day or after school. Maybe your teacher could help you find one. Or, you could look for the phone number of Alateen in the phone book or call directory assistance and ask for the number. (Sometimes you need to call Al-Anon or Alcoholics Anonymous to find Alateen meetings in your area.) Maybe someone you can trust will help you get to a meeting if transportation is a problem for you.

Source: From *Children of Alcoholics: Kit for Kids* by the National Association for Children of Alcoholics, 1st edition, 1996; 4th edition, 1999. Rockville, Maryland. Reprinted with permission.

What Else Helps COAs?

Tell them that they did not cause alcoholism and cannot cure or control it. But they can learn to cope with it. Make clear that children are not responsible for solving grown-up problems.

Understand that COAs often build up defenses against the pain, shame, guilt, or loneliness they may feel. They may show off, act tough, keep secrets, or hide. You may help by just accepting them for who they are. Encouraging them to share their thoughts and feelings will help them learn to trust others and accept and adjust to their lives.

Get them involved in something about which they feel good. It can be something small like taking care of a pet; or a hobby such as collecting rocks, or stamps, or comic books; or a sport. Go slow, don't push, but keep trying.

Do something with them on a regular basis, even if it's only twice a year, such as on the 4th of July or Martin Luther King's birthday. Providing some consistency and showing that adults can be counted on are important assurances for young people who may have experienced many broken promises and unpredictable parental behavior.

Gently help them get positive attention from others. Let them know they are wonderful, special, and cared about just because they are who they are. Again, go slowly, but tell them often.

Help them see life as really living even though there are times and situations that may be very painful. Help them see beyond their present circumstances. Help them feel connected to nature, art, and history; to heritage, culture, religion; to their community. Help them build a larger picture of their lives and their world than their families' current problems.

Help them understand that it is okay to ask for help. Assure them that getting help is a sign of strength. Offer some examples from your own life so they'll know how it's done and that it really is okay.

Follow through if a child asks for help, because it probably required a lot of courage for her/him to do so. Know the local number for Alateen and other sources of help you can offer as needed. Let them know they aren't alone; there are approximately 11 million COAs under the age of 18. Collect information about alcoholism to discuss with the child when it's comfortable for both of you to do so. Be aware and respectful of cultural differences, such as family structure, customs, values, and beliefs. Be aware that some COAs may have been mistreated and may be threatened by displays of affection, especially physical contact. Help them make discoveries, positive connections; instill enthusiasm for life and all its many possibilities.

Chapter 14

How To Talk To A Friend With A Drinking Problem

Alcoholics often deny that they have a drinking problem. Many will not seek help on their own. Left alone, these people often experience severe consequences of their drinking before getting help. Some literally drink themselves to death.

That's hard news if you're concerned about a friend or family member's drinking. But there's good news, too. By skillfully approaching this person, you can make a lifesaving difference.

"Most people who decide to enter treatment for alcoholism claim that it was the influence of a close friend or loved one that actually helped them make the decision," said Tim Sheehan, PhD, regional vice president of Minnesota Recovery Services for Hazelden in Center City, Minnesota.

According to a Gallup Poll, 94 percent of Americans believe it's their responsibility to intervene when a friend has a problem with alcohol or other drugs. But the poll also showed that only 38 percent feel "very confident and comfortable" in approaching that friend.

About This Chapter: Text in this chapter is from "How to Talk to a Friend with a Drinking Problem," Copyright © 2002 Hazelden. *Alive and Free* articles are reprinted with permission of Hazelden, a nonprofit agency based in Center City, MN, that offers a wide range of information and treatment services relating to addiction and recovery. For more resources on substance abuse, call Hazelden at (800) 257-7810 or check its web site at http://www.hazelden.org.

✤ It's A Fact!!

Are you a kid with a mom or dad that drinks too much? This is a letter that was written by a child of an alcoholic who is grown-up. No two families are exactly alike, but maybe you have some similar feelings.

Hello:

I'll bet you feel all alone when your mom or dad drinks too much, because maybe you think that no one else's mom or dad drinks like yours. Or maybe you think that no one knows how you feel. Do you know that there are plenty of kids your age who feel exactly like you, because their parents drink too much? I know how you feel, because one of my parents is an alcoholic too.

It's not easy. When I was your age, I felt so alone. Every time my parent started drinking, I had that funny feeling in my stomach that something wasn't right. I was scared to tell anyone. I wondered why I had a parent who drank so much.

I always wondered if I did anything to make my parent drink. None of my friends could spend the night at my house because I never knew when it would start. I didn't want my friends to know what went on in my house; besides, when my parent started to drink I never knew what would happen. I didn't want anyone to know what a mess it was when the drinking started. I felt ashamed, and believed my house was REALLY different from everybody else's.

When I grew up I moved away from my confusing house, and I began to meet other people who had alcoholic parents. I talked a lot to these people about how it was in my house, and I didn't feel embarrassed because they talked about what went on in their houses when their parents started drinking. I realized that other people had the same kinds of confusing things happen to them. Some people came from homes that were more messed up than mine, and other people came from homes that didn't have as many problems as mine did. But I realized one thing: that all the time when I was a kid, when I thought I was alone and the only one with parents who drank too much, I WASN'T.

You aren't the only one with parents who drink too much. There are a lot of us here.

Your friend,

An adult child of an alcoholic

Source: From *Children of Alcoholics: Kit for Kids* by the National Association for Children of Alcoholics, 1st edition, 1996; 4th edition, 1999. Rockville, Maryland. Reprinted with permission.

Using the following guidelines can help you gain the kind of influence needed to start a loved one on recovery:

- *Time your message carefully.* Talk to loved ones shortly after they've experienced a problem related to drinking. These problems could range from a family argument to divorce, loss of a job, or arrest for driving while intoxicated.

- *Avoid talking to people while they're intoxicated.* Wait until the following day when the person is clear-headed and when the problem related to his or her drinking is still fresh in mind. At that time you have a better chance of getting your message across.

- *Focus on consequences.* "It's usually best to talk to people about how their drinking is actually hurting them," said Sheehan. "Explain how their drinking behavior is self-defeating. Focus on the discomfort, the psychological distress, the emotional pain your loved one feels." You can say things like, "It really hurts me to see you go through all of this."

✔ Quick Tip

Hazelden Foundation offers a brochure titled "What can I say to get you to stop?" For a free copy, call 1-800-I-DO-CARE.

- *Avoid lecturing.* Some people assume that a direct, hard-edged confrontation is the only way they can convince a loved one to get help. But this strategy often backfires. Sermonizing or scolding people for their behavior may invite further resistance and denial. Instead, take a compassionate approach and show care and respect for the individual. Use nonjudgmental language and don't blame or criticize. Don't label the person as alcoholic or demand that they seek treatment. State your concerns and encourage your loved one to be assessed by an addiction professional.

- *Maintain rapport.* When approaching a loved one about a drinking problem, the most important thing you can do is to maintain rapport. If you make a comment that this person interprets as shaming or blaming, you weaken that rapport.

- *Expect the worst.* Your loved one might get angry, deny the drinking problem, and tell you to mind your own business. Don't take it personally; these are common reactions. Denial is one of the unfortunate symptoms of alcoholism. After loved ones cool down and experience more negative consequences from drinking, they might take your message to heart. You may have planted the seed for recovery.

☞ Remember!!

To find out more about getting help for alcoholism, check the Yellow Pages for a local AA group or call AA World Services at 212-870-3400. A 24-hour substance abuse treatment referral service hotline is offered by the Center for Substance Abuse Treatment at 1-800-662-HELP.

- *Offer assistance in getting help.* If your friend is ready for help, be prepared to refer that person to a source of help—an Alcoholics Anonymous group or treatment center. Escort them to the source of help and take part in the process as needed.

Part 3

Tobacco

Chapter 15

Cigarettes And Other Nicotine Products

Nicotine is one of the most heavily used addictive drugs in the United States. Cigarette smoking has been the most popular method of taking nicotine since the beginning of the 20th century. In 1998, 60 million Americans were current cigarette smokers (28 percent of all Americans aged 12 and older), and 4.1 million were between the ages of 12 and 17 (18 percent of youth in this age bracket).

In 1989, the U.S. Surgeon General issued a report that concluded that cigarettes and other forms of tobacco, such as cigars, pipe tobacco, and chewing tobacco, are addictive and that nicotine is the drug in tobacco that causes addiction. In addition, the report determined that smoking was a major cause of stroke and the third leading cause of death in the United States.

Nicotine is highly addictive. It is both a stimulant and a sedative to the central nervous system. The ingestion of nicotine results in an almost immediate "kick" because it causes a discharge of epinephrine (a hormone) from the adrenal cortex. This stimulates the central nervous system and other glands that secrete hormones into the blood stream, which causes a sudden release of glucose (blood sugar). Stimulation is then followed by depression and fatigue, leading the abuser to seek more nicotine. Nicotine is absorbed readily

About This Chapter: Text in this chapter is from "Cigarettes and Other Nicotine Products," National Institute on Drug Abuse (NIDA), InfoFax No. 13545, November 1999, updated September 2001.

from tobacco smoke in the lungs, and it does not matter whether the tobacco smoke is from cigarettes, cigars, or pipes.

Nicotine also is absorbed readily when tobacco is chewed. With regular use of tobacco, levels of nicotine accumulate in the body during the day and persist overnight. Thus, daily smokers or chewers are exposed to the effects of nicotine for 24 hours each day. Nicotine taken in by cigarette or cigar smoking takes only seconds to reach the brain but has a direct effect on the body for up to 30 minutes.

Research has shown that stress and anxiety affect nicotine tolerance and dependence. The stress hormone corticosterone reduces the effects of nicotine; therefore, more nicotine must be consumed to achieve the same effect. This increases tolerance to nicotine and leads to increased dependence. Studies in animals have also shown that stress can directly cause relapse to nicotine self-administration after a period of abstinence.

Other studies have shown that animals cannot discriminate between the effects of nicotine and the effects of cocaine. Studies have

✤ It's A Fact!!

When nicotine was isolated from tobacco leaves in 1828, scientists began studying its effects in the brain and body. This research eventually showed that, although tobacco contains thousands of chemicals, the main ingredient that acts in the brain and produces addiction is nicotine. More recent research has shown that the addiction produced by nicotine is extremely powerful and is at least as strong as addictions to other drugs such as heroin and cocaine.

When tobacco is smoked, nicotine enters the bloodstream through the lungs. When it is sniffed or chewed, nicotine passes through the mucous membranes of the mouth or nose to enter the bloodstream. Nicotine can also enter the bloodstream by passing through the skin.

Some of the effects of nicotine include changes in respiration and blood pressure, constriction of arteries, and increased alertness. Many of these effects are produced through its action on both the central and peripheral nervous system.

Source: Excerpted from *Mind Over Matter: Teacher's Guide*, National Institute on Drug Abuse, NIH Pub. No. 98-3592.

also shown that nicotine self-administration sensitizes animals to self-administer cocaine more readily. Addiction to nicotine results in withdrawal symptoms when a person tries to stop smoking. For example, a study found that when chronic smokers were deprived of cigarettes for 24 hours, they had increased anger, hostility, and aggression, and loss of social cooperation. Persons suffering from withdrawal also take longer to regain emotional balance following stress. During periods of abstinence and/or craving, smokers have shown reduced ability across a wide range of psychomotor and thinking processes, such as language comprehension.

Women who smoke generally have earlier menopause. If women smoke cigarettes and also take birth control pills, they are more prone to cardiovascular and cerebrovascular diseases than are other smokers; this is especially true for women older than 30.

Pregnant women who smoke cigarettes run an increased risk of having stillborn or premature infants or infants with low birthweight. Children of women who smoked while pregnant have an increased risk for developing conduct disorders. National studies of mothers and daughters have also found that when mothers smoked during pregnancy it increased the changes that their daughters would also be smokers.

Adolescent smokeless tobacco users are more likely than nonusers to become cigarette smokers. Behavioral research is beginning to explain how social influences, such as observing adults or other peers smoking, affect whether adolescents begin to smoke cigarettes. Research has shown that teens generally are not influenced by many kinds of anti-smoking messages.

In addition to nicotine, cigarette smoke is primarily composed of a dozen gases (mainly carbon monoxide) and tar. The tar in a cigarette, which varies from about 15 milligrams (mg) for a regular cigarette to 7 mg in a low-tar cigarette, exposes the user to a high risks of lung cancer, emphysema, and bronchial disorders. The carbon monoxide in the smoke increases the chance of cardiovascular diseases.

The Environmental Protection Agency has concluded that secondhand smoke causes lung cancer in adults and greatly increases the risk of respiratory illnesses in children and sudden infant death.

Promising Research

Research has shown that nicotine, like cocaine, heroin, and marijuana, increases the level of the neurotransmitter dopamine, which affects the brain pathways that control reward and pleasure. Scientists now have pinpointed a particular molecule as a critical component in nicotine addiction. Mice that lack this molecule fail to self-administer nicotine, implying that without the specific molecule, the mice do not experience the positive reinforcing properties of nicotine. This new finding identifies a potential site for targeting the development of anti-nicotine addiction medications.

Other new research found that individuals have greater resistance to nicotine addiction if they have a genetic variant that decreases the function of the enzyme CYP2A6. The decrease in CYP2A6 slows the breakdown of nicotine and protects individuals against nicotine addiction. Understanding the role of this enzyme in nicotine addiction gives a new target for developing more effective medications to help people stop smoking. Medications might be developed that can inhibit the function of CYP2A6, thus providing a new approach to preventing and treating nicotine addiction.

✎ Weird Words

Abstinence: Refraining from the use of certain articles of diet, alcoholic beverages, illegal drugs, or from sexual intercourse.

Adrenal Cortex: The outer part of the adrenal gland, consisting of three zones (called the zona glomerulosa, zona fasciculata, and zona reticularis); this part of the adrenal cortex yields steroid hormones such as corticosterone, deoxycorticosterone, and estrone.

Carbon Monoxide: a colorless, practically odorless, and poisonous gas formed by the incomplete combustion of carbon; it is toxic because it reduces oxygen transport and blocks the body's ability to use oxygen.

Cardiovascular: Relating to the heart and the blood vessels or the circulation.

Another study found dramatic changes in the brain's pleasure circuits during withdrawal from chronic nicotine use. These changes are comparable in magnitude and duration to similar changes observed during the withdrawal from other abused drugs such as cocaine, opiates, amphetamines, and alcohol. Scientists found significant decreases in the sensitivity of the brains of laboratory rats to pleasurable stimulation after nicotine administration was abruptly stopped. These changes lasted several days and may correspond to the anxiety and depression experienced by humans for several days after quitting smoking "cold turkey." The results of this research may help in the development of better treatments for the withdrawal symptoms that may interfere with individual's attempts to quit smoking.

Treatment

Research suggests that smoking cessation should be a gradual process because withdrawal symptoms are less severe in those who quit gradually than in those who quit all at once. Rates of relapse are highest in the first few weeks and months and diminish considerably after 3 months.

Central Nervous System: The brain and the spinal cord.

Cerebrovascular: Relating to the blood supply to the brain, particularly with reference to changes associated with disease.

Psychomotor: Relating to the psychologic processes associated with muscular movement and to the production of voluntary movements.

Respiration: A fundamental process of life, characteristic of both plants and animals, in which oxygen is used to oxidize organic fuel molecules, providing a source of energy as well as carbon dioxide and water (breathing).

Vascular: Relating to or containing blood vessels.

☞ Remember!!

Nicotine is a highly addictive drug. This can clearly be seen when one considers the vast number of people who continue to use tobacco products despite their well known harmful and even lethal effects. In fact, at least 90% of smokers would like to quit, but each year fewer than 10% who try are actually successful. But, while nicotine may produce addiction to tobacco products, it is the thousands of other chemicals in tobacco that are responsible for its many adverse health effects.

Smoking either cigarettes or cigars can cause respiratory problems, lung cancer, emphysema, heart problems, and peripheral vascular disease. In fact, smoking is the largest preventable cause of premature death and disability. Cigarette smoking kills at least 400,000 people in the United States each year and makes countless others ill, including those who are exposed to secondhand smoke. The use of smokeless tobacco is also associated with serious health problems.

Chewing tobacco can cause cancers of the oral cavity, pharynx, larynx, and esophagus. It also causes damage to gums that may lead to the loss of teeth. Although popular among sports figures, smokeless tobacco can also reduce physical performance.

Source: Excerpted from *Mind Over Matter: Teacher's Guide*, National Institute on Drug Abuse, NIH Pub. No. 98-3592. To obtain a copy of this publication, call the National Clearinghouse for Alcohol and Drug Abuse Information at 800-729-6686.

Studies have shown that treatment using medications combined with psychological treatment, including psychological support and skills training to overcome high-risk situations, results in some of the highest long-term abstinence rates.

Behavioral economic studies find that alternative rewards and reinforcers can reduce cigarette use. One study found that the greatest reductions in cigarette use were achieved when smoking cost was increased in combination with the presence of alternative recreational activities.

Nicotine chewing gum is one medication approved by the Food and Drug Administration (FDA) for the treatment of nicotine dependence. Nicotine in this form acts as a nicotine replacement to help smokers quit the smoking habit.

The success rates for smoking cessation treatment with nicotine chewing gum vary considerably across studies, but evidence suggests that it is a safe means of facilitating smoking cessation if chewed according to instructions and restricted to patients who are under medical supervision.

Another approach to smoking cessation is the nicotine transdermal patch, a skin patch that delivers a relatively constant amount of nicotine to the person wearing it. A research team at NIDA's Division of Intramural Research studied the safety, mechanism of action, and abuse liability of the patch that was consequently approved by FDA. Both nicotine gum and the nicotine patch, as well as other nicotine replacements such as sprays and inhalers, are used to help people fully quit smoking by reducing withdrawal symptoms and preventing relapse while undergoing behavioral treatment.

Another tool in treating nicotine addiction is a medication that goes by the trademark Zyban. This is not a nicotine replacement, as are the gum and patch. Rather, this works on other areas of the brain, and its effectiveness is in helping to make controllable nicotine craving or thoughts about cigarette use in people trying to quit.

In the future, a nicotine vaccine may be an effective method for preventing and treating tobacco addiction. The vaccine would prevent nicotine from reaching the brain so as to reduce its effects and help keep people from becoming addicted.

Scientists recently developed an experimental nicotine vaccine consisting of a nicotine derivative attached to a large protein. The scientists injected a single dose of nicotine into vaccinated rats and found that the amount of nicotine reaching the brain was reduced by 64%. Further, the researchers found that administering doses of nicotine antibodies similar to those that are ordinarily produced by the vaccine greatly reduced the rise in blood pressure produced by a nicotine injection. The antibodies also completely prevented the increased movements ordinarily seen when rats are injected with nicotine.

The next steps will be to conduct additional safety studies, followed by clinical trials with the vaccine in human volunteers.

Extent Of Use

Monitoring The Future Study (MTF)

Prevalence rates for smoking among young people remain high, in spite of the demonstrated health risk associated with smoking. Since 1975, cigarettes have consistently been the substance the greatest number of high school students use daily.

Between 1998 and 1999, however, past month smoking decreased significantly among 8th graders, from 19.1 percent to 17.5 percent, and rates of use were stable or slightly decreased for 10th graders (25.7 percent) and seniors (34.6 percent). Lifetime and daily use also leveled off in 1999 among all grades, as did use of smokeless tobacco. (Lifetime refers to use at least once during a respondent's lifetime. Past month refers to an individual's drug use at least once during the month preceding their response to the survey.)

The MTF survey is conducted by the University of Michigan's Institute for Social Research and is funded by National Institute on Drug Abuse, National Institutes of Health; it has tracked 12th graders' illicit drug use and related attitudes since 1975. In 1991, 8th and 10th graders were added to the study. For the 1999 study, 45,000 students were surveyed from a representative sample of 433 public and private schools nationwide. The latest survey data are available at NIDA's website, http://www.drugabuse.gov, and at the University of Michigan website, http://www.monitoringthefuture.org.

✔ Quick Tip

Count The Cost

The typical smoker spends about $700 a year on cigarettes. Think of what you could do with all that dough:

- Play 2,800 video-arcade games.
- Have the world's greatest slumber party: Take your 40 best friends to the movies, then order 19 pizzas (with everything, of course) to munch on while reading your 162 new comic books.
- Talk on the phone to your friend in another state for 126 hours and 22 minutes.
- Make a donation to your favorite charity. That way you could really help others.
- Buy 1,400 seedlings to plant three acres of oak, hickory, walnut, or ash trees.
- It's boring, we know, but if you put $700 every year in a bank account earning 5 percent interest, you'd have $25,003.47 after 20 years. With a sum like that you could really have some fun.

Source: U.S. Surgeon General's Office, text online at http://www.health.org/features/kidsarea/pubs/sgr4kids/upsmoke.htm; accessed November 2001.

National Household Survey On Drug Abuse (NHSDA)

Each year, the NHSDA reports on the nature and extent of drug use among the American household population aged 12 and older. In 1998, an estimated 60 million Americans, or 28 percent of all Americans aged 12 and older, were current smokers. Approximately 18 percent (4.1 million) of youths 12 to 17 years old were current smokers in 1998.

The 1998 survey shows that current smokers are more likely to drink heavily and use illicit drugs than non-smokers.

NHSDA is an annual survey conducted by the Substance Abuse and Mental Health Services administration. Copies of the latest survey are available from the National Clearinghouse for Alcohol and Drug Information at 1-800-729-6686

Table 15.1. Cigarette Use by Students, 1999 (Monitoring the Future Study)

	8th-Graders	10th-Graders	12th-Graders
Ever Used	44.1%	57.6%	64.6%
Used in Past Month	17.5	25.7	34.6
Pack + per Day	3.3	7.6	13.2

Chapter 16

Teens And Tobacco

Facts: Not Fiction

- Nearly 4 million adolescents in the United States smoke cigarettes.[1] Each day, about 6,000 young people try a cigarette, and more than 3,000 of these young people become regular smokers—that's more than one million new smokers a year.[2]
- Of all young people in the United States who are currently younger than age 18, more than 5 million will die prematurely from a smoking-related disease.[3]
- Teen smoking rates have increased each year since 1992. In 1996, 22.2% of high school seniors smoked daily—up from 17.2% in 1992. Between 1991 and 1996, the percentage of students who had smoked a cigarette during the past month increased from 14.3% to 21.0% among eighth graders and from 20.8 to 30.4% among tenth graders.[4]
- The percentage of male African-American high school students who reported smoking a cigarette in the past month has nearly doubled in recent years, from 14.1% in 1991 to 27.8% in 1995. However, among female African-American high school students, this rate has remained relatively stable (11.3% in 1991 and 12.2% in 1995).[5]

About This Chapter: The text in this chapter is from "Boyz II Men—Teens and Tobacco Facts Not Fiction," Centers for Disease Control and Prevention (CDC), 1997, reviewed April 2001.

- In 1996, an estimated 6 million U.S. teenagers aged 14 to 19—4.3 million males and 1.7 million females—had smoked at least one cigar within the past year. Teenagers who used other tobacco products (for example, cigarettes or smokeless tobacco) were more likely to report smoking cigars.[6]

- Smokeless tobacco use among young people is a continuing problem. Data from recent school-based surveys indicate that about one in every five male students in 9th through 12th grades uses smokeless tobacco.[7] Smokeless tobacco can cause gum disease and cancer of the mouth, pharynx, esophagus, and pancreas.[8,9] It may also increase the risk of heart disease and stroke.[10]

- Starting smoking at an early age greatly increases the risk of lung cancer. A person's risk for most other smoking-related cancers also rises with the length of time that a person smokes.[11]

- Among adults, cigarette smoking causes heart disease and stroke. Studies have shown that early signs of these diseases can be found in adolescents who smoke.[12] Teenage smokers suffer from shortness of breath almost three times as often and produce phlegm more than twice as often as teens who don't smoke.[13]

- Several studies have found nicotine to be addictive in ways similar to those of heroin, cocaine, and alcohol.[14] The transition from experimentation to dependence occurs just as frequently among young smokers as it does among users of cocaine and heroin.[15]

- Young people tend to underestimate the addictiveness of nicotine. Of people who were daily smokers in high school but who planned to stop smoking, almost 75 percent were still smoking 5 or 6 years later.[16]

- Cigarette products are among the most heavily advertised and promoted products in the United States. In 1994, tobacco companies spent an estimated $5 billion—or more than $13 million a day—to advertise and promote cigarettes.[17]

- Teen smoking is often an early warning sign of future problems. Teens who smoke are three times as likely as nonsmokers to use alcohol,

✤ It's A Fact!!

What's In A Cigarette?

Cigarette smoke contains over 4,000 toxic substances, many of which are known to cause cancer in humans. In addition to the very addictive nicotine, cigarettes contain:

- Arsenic: used in rat poison.
- Acetic Acid: hair dye and developer.
- Acetone: main ingredient in paint and fingernail (polish) remover.
- Ammonia: a typical household cleaner.
- Benzene: rubber cement.
- Cadmium: found in batteries and artists' oil paint.
- Carbon Monoxide: poison.
- Formaldehyde: used to embalm dead bodies.
- Hydrazine: used in jet and rocket fuels.
- Hydrogen Cyanide: poison in gas chambers.
- Naphthalenes: used in explosives, moth balls, and paint pigments.
- Nickel: used in the process of electroplating.
- Phenol: used in disinfectants and plastics.
- Polonium: radiation dosage, equal to 300 chest X-rays in one year.
- Styrene: found in insulation material.
- Toluene: embalmers glue.
- Vinyl Chloride: ingredient found in garbage bags.

These toxic ingredients don't just harm the smoker. Nonsmokers exposed to second-hand smoke have in their body fluids significant amounts of nicotine, carbon monoxide, and other evidence of secondhand smoke exposure.

Source: From "What's in a Cigarette?" © 1997 Youth Media Network (Prunedale, CA); reprinted with permission.

eight times as likely to use marijuana, and 22 times as likely to use cocaine. Smoking is also associated with numerous other risky behaviors, including fighting and having unprotected sex.[18]

✤ It's A Fact!!

- Most people start using tobacco before they finish high school. This means that if you stay smoke-free in school, you will probably never smoke.
- Most teens who smoke are addicted to nicotine. They want to quit smoking, but they can't. When they try to quit, they experience nasty withdrawal symptoms—just like adults.
- Tobacco is often the first drug used by kids who use alcohol and illegal drugs like marijuana.
- Kids who start smoking are more likely to get lower grades in school. They tend to hang out with other kids who smoke. They may have a low self-image and they don't know how to say no to tobacco.
- Cigarette advertisements are designed to make people think that smoking is cool and that everybody does it. These misleading ads appear to increase kids' risk of smoking.
- Finally, here's some good news: People working in their communities—kids who warn each other about the dangers of smoking, for example, and programs that make it harder for stores to sell cigarettes to kids—are helping to keep kids away from tobacco.

Source: U.S. Surgeon General's Office, text online at http://www.health.org/features/kidsarea/pubs/sgr4kids/6facts.htm; accessed November 2001.

References

1. Substance Abuse and Mental Health Services Administration. *Preliminary Results from the 1996 National Household Survey on Drug Abuse*. Office of Applied Studies, August 1997.

2. Pierce JP, Fiore MC, Novotny TE, et al. Trends in Cigarette Smoking in the United States, Projections to the Year 2000. *Journal of the American Medical Association*, 1989, Vol. 261, pp. 61–65.

3. Centers for Disease Control and Prevention. Projected Smoking-Related Deaths Among Youth—United States. *Morbidity and Mortality Weekly Report*, 1996, Vol. 45, pp. 971–974.

4. The University of Michigan. "Cigarette Smoking Among American Teens Rises Again in 1996" (press release), December 19, 1996.

5. Centers for Disease Control and Prevention. Tobacco Use and Usual Source of Cigarettes Among High School Students—United States, 1995. *Morbidity and Mortality Weekly Report*, 1996, Vol. 45, pp. 413–418.

6. Centers for Disease Control and Prevention. Cigar Smoking Among Teenagers—United States, Massachusetts, and New York, 1996. *Morbidity and Mortality Weekly Report*, 1997, Vol. 46, pp. 433–440.

7. Centers for Disease Control and Prevention. Tobacco Use and Usual Source of Cigarettes Among High School Students—United States, 1995. *Morbidity and Mortality Weekly Report*, 1996, Vol. 45, pp. 413–418.

8. Centers for Disease Control and Prevention. *Preventing Tobacco Use Among Young People: A Report of the Surgeon General*. Atlanta: U.S. Department of Health and Human Services, Centers for Disease Control and Prevention, 1994, p. 39.

9. National Cancer Institute. *Smokeless Tobacco or Health: An International Perspective* (Monograph 2). U.S. Department of Health and Human Services, Public Health Service. NIH Pub. Number 95-3461, 1992, pp. 109, 114, and 115.

10. Bolinder G, Alfredsson L, Englund A, de Faire U. Smokeless Tobacco Use and Increased Cardiovascular Mortality among Swedish Construction Workers. *American Journal of Public Health* 1994, Vol. 84, pp. 399–404.

11. Centers for Disease Control and Prevention. *Preventing Tobacco Use Among Young People: A Report of the Surgeon General*. Atlanta: U.S. Department of Health and Human Services, Centers for Disease Control and Prevention, 1994, p. 29.

12. Centers for Disease Control and Prevention. *Preventing Tobacco Use Among Young People: A Report of the Surgeon General.* Atlanta: U.S. Department of Health and Human Services, Centers for Disease Control and Prevention, 1994, p. 25.

13. Arday DR, Giovino GA, Schulman J, Nelson DE, Mowery P, Samet JM. Cigarette Smoking and Self-Reported Health Problems Among U. S. High School Seniors. *American Journal of Health Promotion*, 1995, Vol. 10, pp. 111–116.

14. Centers for Disease Control and Prevention. *Preventing Tobacco Use Among Young People: A Report of the Surgeon General.* Atlanta: U.S. Department of Health and Human Services, Centers for Disease Control and Prevention, 1994, p.31.

15. Anthony JC, Warner LA, Kessler RC. Comparative Epidemiology of Dependence on Tobacco, Alcohol, Controlled Substances and Inhalants: Basic Findings from the National Comorbidity Survey. *Experimental and Clinical Psychopharmacology*, 1994, Vol. 2, pp. 244–268.

16. Centers for Disease Control and Prevention. Reasons for Tobacco Use and Symptoms of Nicotine Withdrawal Among Adolescent and Young Adult Tobacco Users-United States, 1993. *Morbidity and Mortality Weekly Report*, 1994, Vol. 43, pp. 746–750.

17. Federal Trade Commission Report to Congress, Pursuant to the Federal Cigarette Labeling and Advertising Act. Issued 1996.

18. Centers for Disease Control and Prevention. *Preventing Tobacco Use Among Young People: A Report of the Surgeon General.* Atlanta: U.S. Department of Health and Human Services, Centers for Disease Control and Prevention, 1994, pp. 34–38

Chapter 17

Teen Smokers Risk Getting Hooked Early On

The conventional wisdom has been that teens usually become addicted to nicotine slowly, only after months or even years of daily smoking. But researchers at the University of Massachusetts Medical School in Worcester found that teens can experience the first symptoms of nicotine dependence within just a few weeks of occasional use.

Dr. Joseph R. DiFranza and colleagues studied nicotine use among 681 Massachusetts seventh-graders ages 12 to 13, interviewing these students three times during a year. Among the students in this study, 95 said they smoked at least one cigarette in each of the last two months. Twenty percent of these monthly smokers developed symptoms of nicotine dependence within four weeks of starting to smoke. Some showed the symptoms within two weeks, including strong urges to smoke and feeling anxious when unable to smoke.

This study, published in the September 2000 issue of *Tobacco Control*, sends an urgent message to teenagers: Experimenting with nicotine is even more dangerous than we thought. Some young people can become addicted almost immediately.

✤ It's A Fact!!

Nicotine Addiction In Adolescence

- Nicotine dependency through cigarette smoking is the most common form of drug addiction and causes more death and disease than all other addictions combined.[1]
- Forty percent of teenagers who smoke daily have tried to quit and failed.[2]
- Although nicotine is not normally associated with intoxication, its ability to addict users is much higher than so-called "harder" drugs. The risk of becoming dependent on alcohol with regular use is one in nine. For crack or cocaine used intravenously, the chance is one in four. However, the risk of becoming addicted to nicotine is between one in four and one in three.[3]
- More than 80% of young people who smoke one pack or more of cigarettes per day report that they "need" or are dependent on cigarettes.[4]
- Nicotine is as addictive as heroin, cocaine, and alcohol. Moreover, because the typical tobacco user receives daily and repeated doses of nicotine, addiction is more common among all tobacco users than among other drug users.[4]
- Among addictive behaviors, cigarette smoking is the one most likely to take hold during adolescence.[5]
- The younger people start smoking cigarettes, the more likely they are to become strongly addicted to nicotine.[5]
- Each year, only 3% of all smokers who try to quit smoking have long-term success.[4]
- 42% of young people who smoke as few as three cigarettes go on to become regular smokers.[6]
- 50% of all smokers who have lost a lung because of cancer or have undergone major heart surgery cannot quit for more than a few weeks.[4]
- Young people who try to quit smoking suffer the same nicotine withdrawal symptoms as adults who try to quit.[7]
- Among young people who are daily smokers, more than half smoke their first cigarette within 30 minutes of waking in the morning.[8]

- About two-thirds of adolescent smokers say they want to quit smoking, and 70% say they would not have started if they could choose again.[9]
- Three-fourths of young people who use tobacco daily report that they use it because "it's really hard to quit." Findings were the same for cigarette smokers and for smokeless tobacco users.[10]
- Over 90% of young people who use tobacco daily (cigarettes or smokeless tobacco) experienced at least one symptom of nicotine withdrawal when they tried to quit.[10]

References

1. Surgeon General's Report (SGR), *Preventing Tobacco Use Among Young People*, p.30.
2. SGR, *Preventing Tobacco Use Among Young People*, p.78.
3. *Comparative epidemiology of dependence on tobacco, alcohol, controlled substances and inhalants: basic findings from the National Comorbidity Survey*, Anthony, J.C., Warner, L.A., Kessler, R.C., 1994, 2:244-68.
4. SGR, *Preventing Tobacco Use Among Young People*, p.31.
5. SGR, *Preventing Tobacco Use Among Young People*, p.9.
6. Office on Smoking and Health (OSH), unpublished data from *Teenage Attitudes and Practices Surveys-II* (TAPS-II), 1994.
7. SGR, *Preventing Tobacco Use Among Young People*, p.33.
8. "Epidemiology of Tobacco Use and Symptoms of Nicotine Addiction in the United States: A compilation of data from large national surveys," Presentation for the Food and Drug Administration, Drug Abuse Advisory Committee, Giovino, G.A., Zhu, B.P., Tomar, S., August 2, 1994.
9. George, H., Gallup International Institute, *Teen-age attitudes and behavior concerning tobacco: Report of the findings*, Princeton, New Jersey, 1992.
10. CDC, Reasons for tobacco use and symptoms of nicotine withdrawal among adolescent and young adult tobacco users, United States, 1993, *MMWR*, 1994, 43:745-750.

Add this to what we already know about teens and smoking:

- About 15 percent of young people 12 to 17 years old are current smokers.
- Teens who try to quit smoking can experience the same withdrawal symptoms as adults who try to quit.
- Teens who start smoking are more likely to get lower grades.
- Compared with nonsmokers, kids who smoke are three times more likely to use alcohol, eight times more likely to smoke marijuana, and 22 times more likely to use cocaine.

However, there's good news: If teens can stay nicotine-free during high school, they will probably never smoke. This shifts the discussion to prevention.

Prevention really needs to take a comprehensive, community-wide approach to decrease smoking incidence, said Judy Knapp, executive director of the Minnesota Smoke-Free Coalition in St. Paul, Minnesota. You have to look at the many different segments of society that influence young people—their peers, parents, and the media. Kids need to get the proper message in school, at home, and in the community. Establishing that smoking is socially unacceptable has the greatest impact, and you do that by concentrating on widespread policy changes and media advocacy designed to promote non-use of tobacco as a

✔ Quick Tip

Here's a concrete way to refuse tobacco.

1. *Ask questions* to find out if a social situation will include tobacco use.
2. *Name the problem*: If we hang out with those kids, we could end up smoking.
3. *State consequences*: If I smoke, my clothes will smell and my parents will find out.
4. *Suggest an alternative*: I'm going home to watch a video. Want to come with me?
5. *Act on the alternative*. Walk away from any situation that could lead to tobacco use.

When you've got a plan for how they're going to say no, you're are less likely to get caught unaware.

social norm. This includes limiting access to tobacco products, broadening the areas where smoking is banned, and raising taxes.

One of the most effective ways to deter use is by imposing an excise tax on cigarettes. People think of it as a sin tax, said Knapp, but studies have shown that for each 10 percent increase in retail price, there is about a five percent decrease in demand for cigarettes. And because young people generally have less disposable income, the decreased consumption may double for them.

Parents can have a powerful influence on prevention. Kay Provine, a community education specialist for Hazelden, emphasizes three actions.

"One thing we know that works is parents telling kids that they expect no tobacco use," Provine says. "Set a no-use standard early on—as early as third grade."

Second, talk to young people about short-term consequences of tobacco use. Emphasize that young people are unattractive to friends if they smoke—they smell bad, their breath stinks, their teeth get yellow. Talking about long-term consequences, such as heart disease and lung cancer, has less impact, because young people are unable to think that far into the future.

Chapter 18

Smoking May Lead To Anxiety Disorders And Depression

Using a wealth of data obtained through a 25-year longitudinal study, NIDA-funded researcher Dr. Judith Brook of the Mount Sinai School of Medicine in New York, Dr. Patricia Cohen of Columbia University in New York, and their colleagues have documented adverse effects of smoking in several critical areas of functioning during young adulthood. Most recently, the team has reported a connection between tobacco use by adolescents and young adults and the likelihood that they will develop agoraphobia (fear of leaving home or of the outdoors), generalized anxiety disorder, or panic disorder. Analyzing data from their Children in the Community study, funded by the National Institute of Drug Abuse (NIDA) and the National Institute of Mental Health (NIMH), the researchers were able to separate the effects of smoking from the effects of age, gender, childhood temperament, alcohol and other drug abuse, and depression among the adolescents, as well as parents' smoking, education, and behavioral and/or mental health problems.

Adolescents who smoked heavily were 6.8 times more likely to develop agoraphobia, 5.5 times more likely to develop generalized anxiety disorder, and 15.6 times more likely to develop a panic disorder as young adults than

About This Chapter: Text in this chapter is from " Smoking May Lead to Anxiety Disorders in Adolescents and Young Adults," in *NIDA Notes*, Volume 16, Number 1 (March, 2001), National Institute on Drug Abuse (NIDA). *NIDA Notes* is available online at http://www.nida.nih.gov/NIDA_Notes.

were their counterparts who smoked fewer than 20 cigarettes a day or not at all. The investigators speculate that impaired respiration and the potentially damaging effects of nicotine on blood vessels to the brain may help explain why the adolescents who smoked heavily were at increased risk of developing anxiety disorders.

The long-held notion that depression causes some adolescents to smoke may be true. But Dr. Brook's study suggests the opposite may also be true—that smoking increases the risk of depression in this population. Dr. Brook and her team recommend that future research examine further the possible relationships between various anxiety disorders and smoking.

Source

Johnson, J.G.; Cohen, P.; Pine, D.S.; Klein, D.F.; Kasen, S.; and Brook, J.S. The association between cigarette smoking and anxiety disorders during adolescence and early adulthood. *Journal of the American Medical Association* 284(18):2348-2351, 2000.

✎ Weird Words

Agoraphobia: A mental disorder characterized by an irrational fear of leaving the familiar setting of home, or venturing into the open, so pervasive that a large number of external life situations are entered into reluctantly or are avoided; often associated with panic attacks.

Depression: A temporary mental state or chronic mental disorder characterized by feelings of sadness, loneliness, despair, low self-esteem, and self-reproach; accompanying signs withdrawal from social contact and states such as loss of appetite and insomnia.

Generalized Anxiety Disorder: Chronic, repeated episodes of anxiety reactions; a psychological disorder in which anxiety or morbid fear and dread accompanied by involuntary changes in certain body functions (for example, heart rate and sweating) are prominent features.

Longitudinal Study: Studied over a period of time (as opposed to the study of something in a population at a single point in time)

Source: From *Stedman's Medical Dictionary, 27th Edition*,

✤ It's A Fact!!

The researchers interviewed 688 youths and their mothers in 1983, between 1985 and 1986, and again between 1991 and 1993. A total of 69 of the youths smoked heavily—at least 20 cigarettes every day—and experienced an anxiety disorder during adolescence, early adulthood, or both. Of these 69 youths, 29 (42 percent) began smoking before they were diagnosed with an anxiety disorder. The remaining 40 youths were split between those who were diagnosed with anxiety disorders before they reported heavy smoking (13, or 19 percent) and those who reported smoking and were diagnosed with anxiety disorders at the same interview session (27, or 39 percent).

Chapter 19

Boyz II Men Answer Questions About Smoking

Boyz II Men Answer Your Smoke-Free Questions

What advice would you give teens who want to smoke?

It's really easier NOT to start, than to stop. Once you begin smoking, your body gets addicted to the nicotine, making it extra hard to quit. Smoking is a real drag, please be a strong individual and don't give in to all the false advertisement or peer pressure.

Does any of your family smoke?

Yes, unfortunately, we all have family members or friends who smoke. One of the reasons Boyz II Men are so involved in getting the smoke-free message out is that we hope to influence our loved ones to quit.

If you could say five words to everyone on the planet about smoking, what would they be?

Smoking cigarettes is addictive and will kill you. (That's eight, sorry.)

About This Chapter: This chapter includes text from "Boyz II Men Answer Your Smoke-Free Questions," and "Interview with the Boyz," Centers for Disease Control and Prevention (CDC), last reviewed April 2001. The full text is available online at http://www.cdc.gov/tobacco/askboyz2men.htm and /b2mq&a.htm.

What do you think of secondhand smoking?

We think secondhand smoke is dangerous and causes a lot of sickness. Wanya got a throat infection in Japan from secondhand smoke, and we had to cancel portions of our tour. Most people don't realize that secondhand smoke causes cancer.

Do you think peer pressure is why most teens begin smoking?

We think that peer pressure is definitely an influence. However, did you know that the three most heavily advertised brands of cigarettes, Marlboro, Camel, and Newport, are the ones kids smoke the most? Makes you kind of wonder, doesn't it?

Do you know any singers who smoke?

Yes, we know several. But guess what, we know more singers who DON'T smoke than do! Smoking can ruin your voice, not to mention your health.

What are some strategies you use to get people to stop smoking?

We never force our opinions on anyone, but we do make it known that our staff/band cannot smoke around us. We also participate in health campaigns, like the Centers for Disease Control's Teen Media contest, and we make posters and television commercials with smoke-free messages.

Are your concerts smoke-free?

We try to perform in smoke-free venues, but not all of them are. Have you seen our commercial we air before our shows? It's a nice way of reminding the audience that smoking can affect our voices, and we hope it gives them a big hint.

My parents smoke. My mom has tried the patch and stopped for awhile, but started up again. My dad stopped just last week. Why can't she stop?

We think it's great that BOTH of your parents are trying to quit and recognize that smoking is harmful. Remember that the nicotine in cigarettes is VERY addicting, and some people have a more difficult time than others. Be patient and offer your mom lots of support (don't nag her). Now that your dad has quit, he can be a motivating partner as well.

How would it look if you guys just smoked just once in a while?

Pretty stupid. First, tobacco is addictive...the nicotine is a drug. So, smoking just once in a while can be deadly and habit-forming. We sing, and tobacco affects our voices...plus, we don't want to have gross teeth and smell bad for all the special ladies in our lives.

What is your opinion on other celebrities smoking. Do you think they are setting terrible examples?

BIIM hopes that all smokers, regardless of whether or not they are celebrities, realize the harmful effects of smoking and quit. However, not everyone chooses to be smoke-free, and we don't condemn our friends, we try to help them. As for celebrities setting terrible examples, BIIM believe the best examples for kids are their parents; however, we are aware that young people look up to singers/actors/models/athletes and try to be like them. There are many celebrities who do provide positive role modeling, but like any group, there are always those who, because of their poor choices, give everyone a bad name.

My science teacher says smoking is only a psychological addiction. I say it's physical, too. Who is correct?

We had to check our sources at the CDC but you, and not your science teacher, are correct. (We'd like to be flies on the wall when you share this information.) Addiction to cigarettes is a biological addiction, not just a psychological one. Basically, because nicotine has been scientifically proven to be addictive, and because nicotine exists in all tobacco products, then tobacco use or consumption can be physically addictive. We think you ought to get an extra credit point for this.

Have you been pressured to smoke/drink?

Sure, we were pressured to smoke and drink; however, the key is that we all have choices, and every choice we make has a consequence. We always wanted to sing, and we all have spiritual backgrounds. Our health, as well as knowing the difference between right and wrong guided us through those very tough teen years.

Have you ever chewed chewing tobacco?

No, none of us has ever used or tried chewing tobacco. It's really gross.

I don't smoke, but I want my friends to stop. How do I go about telling them their breath smells like an ash tray?

You may want to offer them gum or breathsavers. When your friends ask why, politely tell them that when you get near them, all you can smell is stale cigarette smoke from their breath, and that it doesn't smell very nice. Most importantly, is your encouragement to get them to stop smoking altogether. You need to be supportive, but don't nag. Usually nagging makes people angry, and they tune you out.

✔ Quick Tip

You can get more information about tobacco, including facts about quitting smoking, from the Centers from Disease Control and Prevention (CDC). Check out:

TIPS (Tobacco Information and Prevention Source) at www.cdc.gov/tobacco

Tips4Youth at www.cdc.gov/tobacco/tips4youth.htm

What made you decide to back this 'Smoke-Free' idea?

We decided to become role models for our fans by promoting a smoke-free lifestyle because BIIM believe that this is a healthy lifestyle choice. There are a lot of people dying from tobacco-related illnesses, and there are a lot of underage kids smoking cigarettes. We hope we can prevent our fans from starting. We also sing in front of large crowds. Sometimes, the smoke from other people's cigarettes irritates our throats. We've even had to cancel some shows because we've gotten so sick from secondhand smoke. We wanted to make our feelings known to the public.

Do you think you will have a big impact on teens who smoke?

We're not sure BIIM can influence kids who have started to quit (although we hope so) but there are a lot of young people who really enjoy our music and look up to us. Even if we can prevent just one fan from ever starting to smoke, then we will feel proud because we believe we will have helped to save a life.

What other things as teens do you think we can do to help prevent other teens from smoking?

Teens have more influence than they think...perhaps the first thing you can do is set a good example and be smoke-free. You don't have to be critical of your friends who do smoke, but talking to them privately (never in front of a group of people) about the dangers of smoking and why, as a friend, you would hope they stop because you care about their health is a first step. Additional activities can include volunteering for your local heart, lung, or cancer society or writing to your local representatives to encourage them to support smoke-free ordinances and laws that protect kids from secondhand smoke. Stay smoke-free and good luck.

Why do kids smoke when they know it is bad for them?

Kids smoke for many reasons, not just one. Peer pressure, stress, lack of positive role models, low self-esteem are among some of the reasons. Most kids today DO KNOW that smoking is bad, but they DON'T know how addictive the nicotine is. Kids believe they can quit down the road, but by the time they are mature enough to realize the habit is nasty, expensive, and harmful, they are unfortunately already hooked. That's why Boyz II Men wants to get the word out so kids never start.

Interview With The Boyz

What does Boyz II Men think about teen smoking?

We think smoking is an unhealthy choice. We believe that teens who smoke risk missing out on a full, healthy, and productive life.

Have any members of Boyz II Men ever smoked? Have you ever considered smoking?

No, because singing is so important for us. We couldn't do what we do if we smoked. Our sound depends on taking care of our voices. The worst thing for voices is taking in cigarette smoke.

Do you believe your campaign, "Smoke-Free—It's the New Evolution," will help teen smokers give up smoking?

We hope the campaign will inspire teen smokers to take the necessary steps toward quitting—even better, we hope to give teens another reason not to start smoking in the first place. Tobacco use is very addictive because of the nicotine, and once you start smoking, quitting can be a challenge.

How has smoking personally touched the group?

Some of us have lost relatives to cancer caused by smoking. Several of our family members and friends smoke, and we hope that someday they will quit. We prefer to limit smoking around us. We are very sensitive to smoke. A smoke-filled concert stage prevents us from performing at the level that our fans expect from us.

Do you think other entertainers and music artists will get involved in the smoke-free issue?

Some athletes, entertainers, models, and other public figures have already spoken out. We are hoping that our participation will inspire others in the entertainment industry to take a stand against teen tobacco use.

What would Boyz II Men say to teens who believe smoking is cool?

The way we see it, becoming ill or risking an early death from cigarette smoking is the farthest thing from cool. Being cool is living life to your full potential.

☞ Remember!!

If you want to do your best—whether it's singing, sports, acting, or even being a super-model—smoke-free is definitely the way to go.

Chapter 20

If You Chew, Quit

Smokeless tobacco use in the United States continues to increase each year. It may be smokeless, but it isn't harmless. Why should you care? Keep reading.

Smokeless Tobacco

Tooth Abrasion: Grit and sand in smokeless tobacco products scratches teeth and wears away the hard surface or enamel. Premature loss of tooth enamel can cause added sensitivity and may require corrective treatment.

Gum Recession: Constant irritation to the spot in the mouth where a small wad of chewing tobacco is placed can result in permanent damage to periodontal tissue. It also can damage the supporting bone structure. The injured gums pull away from the teeth, exposing root surfaces and leaving teeth sensitive to heat and cold. Erosion of critical bone support leads to loosened teeth that can be permanently lost.

Increased Tooth Decay: Sugar is added to smokeless tobacco during the curing and processing to improve its taste. The sugar reacts with bacteria found naturally in the mouth, causing an acid reaction, which leads to decay.

About This Chapter: Text in this chapter is from "If You Chew, Quit," © 2000 California Dental Association. Reprinted with permission. For more information visit the website of the California Dental Association at www.cda.org.

✤ It's A Fact!!

Teens And Smokeless Tobacco

1. Adolescents who use smokeless tobacco are more likely than those who don't to smoke cigarettes, drink alcohol, and use marijuana.
2. The top five selling brands of snuff are: Copenhagen, Skoal fine cut, Kodiak, Hawken, Skoal bandits. The top three sellers, Copenhagen, Skoal fine cut and Kodiak, contain significantly higher levels of nicotine than the other brands of snuff.
3. Snuff-dippers may be exposed to more N-nitrosamines (shown in a number of laboratory studies to be powerful cancer causing chemicals) than a one-pack-a-day cigarette smoker.
4. The three best selling brands of snuff, Copenhagen, Skoal fine cut, and Kodiak, have statistically significant higher levels of nicotine than do Hawken and Skoal Bandits, the number four and five brands. The higher nicotine snuff also has a higher pH enabling enhanced absorption of nicotine.
5. Use of smokeless tobacco among men 18-24 years old increased from 2.2% in 1970 to 8.4% in 1991, an increase of nearly 300%.
6. Consumption of moist snuff has increased every year in the United States since 1979.
7. Among high school seniors who have ever tried smokeless tobacco, 73% did so by the ninth grade (age 14).
8. The smokeless tobacco prevalence was much higher among male (15.8%) than among female (1.5%) students in the United States.
9. White male students (20.6%) were significantly more likely to use smokeless tobacco than any other subgroup of high school students.
10. In 1997, African-American male high school students (3.2%) were less likely to use smokeless tobacco products than white male (20.6%) and Hispanic male (5.1%) high school students.

Source: Excerpted from "Smokeless Tobacco," full text including resources and statistics available online at http://www.ymn.org/newstats/smokeless.shtml.

Tooth Discoloration and Bad Breath: Common traits of long-term smokeless tobacco users are stained teeth and bad breath. Moreover, the habit of continually spitting can be both unsightly and offensive.

Nicotine Dependence: Nicotine blood levels achieved by smokeless tobacco use are similar to those from cigarette smoking. Nicotine addiction can lead to an artificially increased heart rate and blood pressure. In addition, it can constrict the blood vessels that are necessary to carry oxygen-rich blood throughout the body. Athletic performance and endurance levels are decreased by this reaction.

Unhealthy Eating Habits: Chewing tobacco lessens a person's sense of taste and ability to smell. As a result, users tend to eat more salty and sweet foods, both of which are harmful if consumed in excess.

Oral Cancer: With the practice of "chewing" and "dipping," tobacco and its irritating juices are left in contact with gums, cheeks and/or lips for prolonged periods of time. This can result in a condition called leukoplakia. Leukoplakia appears either as a smooth, white patch or as leathery-looking wrinkled skin. It results in cancer in 3 percent to 5 percent of all cases.

☞ **Remember!!**

Danger Signs

If you use smokeless tobacco, or have in the past, you should be on the lookout for some of these early signs of oral cancer:

- A sore that does not heal
- A lump or white patch
- A prolonged sore throat
- Difficulty in chewing
- Restricted movement of the tongue or jaws
- A feeling of something in the throat

Pain is rarely an early symptom. For this reason, all tobacco users need regular dental check-ups.

Other Cancers: All forms of smokeless tobacco contain high concentrations of cancer-causing agents. These substances subject users to increased cancer risk not only of the oral cavity, but also the pharynx, larynx and esophagus.

Chapter 21

Cigars And Pipes

Cigar smoking is on the foul-smelling rise. Over 4.5 billion cigars were consumed in the United States in 1996 and pipes aren't smoldering far behind in this dangerous trend. A century ago, "Robber Barons" of the Gilded Age adopted the cigar as a symbol of conspicuous consumption and masculine power. In recent times, manufacturers of cigars and related paraphernalia have sought to recreate this image of privilege, exclusivity, and wealth. Encouraged by advertising efforts of the cigar and pipe tobacco industry, men and women are urged to attend "smokers" or "cigar seminars" to learn arcane information about cigars, but not to learn the most important fact of all: cigars kill. Cigars and pipe tobacco are dangerous to one's health as is tobacco in any other form.

Pipe tobacco and cigars are made from the dried leaves and stems of the tobacco plant, *Nicotiana tabacum*. Originally native to North America, the plant is now cultivated and grown around the world. One of the chemicals contained in tobacco is nicotine, a powerful and toxic nerve stimulant. Two or three drops of nicotine, if taken all at once, could kill an average person.

Pipe tobacco is shredded tobacco leaf in loose form, it may be aged, it may also be sprayed with chemicals or flavorings. Cigar construction differs

About This Chapter: Text in this chapter is reprinted with permission from "FactLine on Cigar and Pipe Smoking," by the Indiana Prevention Resource Center at Indiana University.

from that of cigarettes in that the wrappers are made from whole tobacco leaf, rather than paper, and are filled with shredded tobacco, or, as is said of cheaper "stogies," "sweepings off the floor." Some cigars have filter tips or plastic holders built in, some are long and narrow. A large cigar may have as much tobacco in volume as an entire pack of cigarettes.

A False Impression Of Glamour, A False Impression Of Safety

The tobacco industry, Hollywood, and advertising concerns are capitalizing on what they perceive as the "sophistication, glamour, power, and sexiness"

✤ It's A Fact!!

What's In A Cigar?

Cigars are made from tobacco fillers in a tobacco wrapping. Though most premium cigars contain only pure tobacco and no additives, the smoke from cigars contains 23 poisons and 43 carcinogens. A comparison between filter cigarettes and cigars shows a marked difference in quantities:[1]

	Filter Cigarette	Regular Cigar
Weight (approximately)	.68 g	8 g
Nicotine	.5–1.4 mg	1.7–5.2 mg
Tar	.5–18 mg	16–110 mg
Carbon Monoxide	.5–18 mg	90–120 mg

The Health Hazards Of Cigar Use

- Cigars burn cooler resulting in an increased carbon monoxide content of up to 25 times that of cigarette smoke[2]
- Smokers of 5 or more cigars per day are 2–3 times more likely to contract lung cancer than nonsmokers[3]

of smoking cigars. Manufacturers of small cigars called "blunts" also wink at the practice of users removing part of the tobacco from their products and filling the cigars with marijuana, even to the extent of making clothing and paraphernalia with the brand names of the cigars.

Celebrities smirk publicly about smoking illegally imported Cuban cigars. Slick magazines, such as *Cigar Aficionado* combine advertising copy with articles on gambling, sports, alcohol, and interviews of celebrity cigar smokers. Cigars are smelly, and the breath, hair, and clothing of smokers as well as their surroundings reek of the odor. They are profitable however, and restaurants have added "cigar bars," as those who congregate to add to the

- The same cigar smokers double their risk of stroke and heart-attack over nonsmokers[4]
- Because the smoke from cigars is alkaline (rather than slightly acidic as in cigarette smoke) the nicotine and other chemicals in it can be absorbed directly through the tissues of the mouth[1]
- Cigar smokers have a 4 to 10 times higher risk of dying from laryngeal, oral, and esophageal cancers than nonsmokers[3]
- Cigar smokers are 1.3 to 3.6 times more likely to die from emphysema than nonsmokers[5]

References

1. American Health Foundation

2. James Repace, Environmental Protection Agency, *Los Angeles Times*, October 17, 1996

3. U.S. Dept. of Health and Human Services, *The Health Consequences of Smoking: Cancer, A Report of the Surgeon General*, Rockville, MD, 1982

4. U.S. Office on Smoking and Health, August 14, 1996

5. U.S. Dept. of Health and Human Services, *The Health Consequences of Smoking: Chronic Obstructive Lung Disease, A Report of the Surgeon General*, Atlanta GA, 1994

clouds of smoke will pay $5 on up for a cigar and drink expensive brands of hard liquor while not requiring the overhead and personnel for food services.

When compared to non-smokers the cigar smoker has about a four times greater risk of dying of lung cancer. Non-smokers are also unlikely to develop cancers of the mouth, lips, palate and larynx. Cigar tobacco has a higher pH than cigarette tobacco because of aging and certain treatments. The more alkaline nature of the tobacco makes it easier for nicotine to be directly absorbed by the body, in the same manner that cigarette tobacco has been adulterated with ammonia-forming compounds to make cigarette smoke like "freebase" nicotine.

✎ Weird Words

pH: Symbol for a measurement of the hydrogen ion concentration (measured in moles per liter); a solution with pH 7.00 is neutral at 22°C, one with a pH value of more than 7.00 is alkaline, and one with a pH lower than 7.00 is acid.

Vasoconstriction: Narrowing of the blood vessels.

Source: From *Stedman's Medical Dictionary, 27th Edition*, Copyright © 2000 Lippincott Williams & Wilkins. All rights reserved.

Pipe and pipe tobacco manufactures are attempting to cash in on the current popularity of cigars by creating their own glossy magazines and online forums. Pipe sellers have an advantage over cigar manufactures in that old used pipes can be resold, marketed as "estate pipes." The downside of pipes, as an article singing their praises in *Fortune* magazine says, "is death."

A Danger To Youth

A recent report published by the Centers for Disease Control and Prevention (CDC) indicated that 6 million youth ages 14-19 had smoked a cigar in the past year, 1.7 million of these youth were females. Students in grades 9-12 who used other tobacco products were most likely to report smoking cigars. Youth who answered surveys conducted in New York state also reported no difficulty in buying cigars. Cigars may well become the next "gateway drug." Youth, like adults, may believe that because no Surgeon General's warning appears on cigars, that they are safe.

Health Issues

Cigars come in many different sizes, so comparisons are difficult, but cigars can contain 7 times more tar and 4 times more nicotine than cigarettes. Particle emissions from one cigar may be more than those of three cigarettes, and the amount of carbon monoxide produced by one cigar can be 30 times higher than cigarettes.

Cardiovascular Health

Nicotine can cause irregular or skipped heart beats, an increase in blood pressure, a decreased tolerance for exercise or exertion, a tendency for clotting, and vasoconstriction. One study showed that pipe smokers had almost the same coronary heart disease risk as cigarette smokers. Another study demonstrated that pipe smokers had a higher mortality rate from coronary heart disease, and 40% more deaths from all causes.

Chronic Cough And Phlegm, Lung Function, And Emphysema

Cigar and pipe smokers have increased rates of chronic cough and phlegm. Cigar smokers have up to twice the rate of cough and phlegm as nonsmokers. Use of tobacco can cause or worsen the effects of chronic obstructive pulmonary disease (COPD), asthma, and emphysema, and decrease lung function.

✤ It's A Fact!!

Federal Food and Drug Administration (FDA) regulations now require vendors that sell tobacco products to ask for proof of age from any purchaser who appears to be 26 years of age or younger.

Oral And Dental Health

Tobacco secretions stain teeth and cause sores in the mouth and gums. These lesions can be precancerous, including leukoplakia (also called "smoker's white patch") and erythroplakia (a red, velvety lesion). Cigar and pipe smoking may also cause "hairy tongue."

Cancer

In 1996 alone over 8,000 people died from oral cancer, the primary causes of which are tobacco and alcohol use. The National Cancer Institute says that were it not for tobacco use, oral cancer would be almost nonexistent as a cause of death. Oral cancer, the sixth most common cancer in the world can develop in any part of the mouth, most commonly on the lips, tongue, roof, or floor of the mouth, pharynx or esophagus. Pipe smokers are particularly prone to cancer of the lip.

Cigars and pipes use black (air-cured) tobacco, which carries a higher risk of causing esophageal cancer than the tobacco used for cigarettes. Even for pipe and cigar smokers who say they "don't inhale," the risk of lung cancer is still four times greater than that of nonsmokers.

One study showed a significant increase in colon and rectal cancer, not only in cigarette, but in pipe and cigar smokers. The study suggests that tobacco is responsible for 16% of colon cancer and 22% of rectal cancer deaths.

☞ Remember!!

Cigars and pipes are not a safe alternative to cigarettes. Like other forms of tobacco, use of cigars and pipes brings risks of lung, breast, pancreatic, prostate, colorectal, liver, and oral cancer, lung disease, stroke, and heart attack. Tobacco smoking is the principal cause of death from chronic obstructive pulmonary disease (COPD) and lung cancer. Smoke from cigars and pipes also causes respiratory infections, headaches, and burning eyes.

Chapter 22

Secondhand Smoke

Secondhand smoke is the name for the sickening, poisonous smoke given off by a burning cigarette, cigar, or pipe. Smokers may claim to have a right to smoke, but nonsmokers have a more important right to breathe safe air. So the next time one of your friends lights up in front of you, fire off these facts about secondhand smoke.

- Secondhand smoke can produce six times the pollution of a busy highway when in a crowded restaurant.
- Secondhand smoke causes 30 times as many lung cancer deaths as all regulated pollutants combined.
- Secondhand smoke makes clothes and hair stink.
- Secondhand smoke causes wheezing, coughing, colds, earaches, and asthma attacks.
- Secondhand smoke fills the air with many of the same poisons found in the air around toxic waste dumps.
- Secondhand smoke wrecks the smell and taste of food.
- Secondhand smoke causes reddening, itching, and watering of the eyes.

About This Chapter: Text in this chapter is excerpted from "Facts You Should Know," Centers for Disease Control and Prevention (CDC), November 2000. Full text is available online at http://www.cdc.gov/tobacco/tips_4_youth/facts.htm.

- Secondhand smoke kills about 3,000 nonsmokers each year from lung cancer.
- Secondhand smoke causes up to 300,000 lung infections (such as pneumonia and bronchitis) in infants and young children each year.

Table 22.1. Estimated Annual Deaths And Illnesses Among Nonsmokers Exposed To Secondhand Smoke.

Illnesses/Diseases	Number of People or Cases in the U.S.
Developmental Defects	
Low birth weight (cases)	9,700–18,600
Sudden infant death syndrome (SIDS) deaths	1,900–27,000
Respiratory Effects in Children	
Middle ear infection (physician office visits)	700,000–1.6 million
Asthma exacerbation (children)	400,000–1 million
Bronchitis or pneumonia in infants and toddlers (18 months and younger)	150,000–300,000 cases
	7,500–15,000 hospitalizations
	135–212 deaths
Cancer	
Lung	3,000 deaths
Cardiovascular Effects	
Heart attack and stroke	35,000–62,000 deaths

Source: Office of Environmental Health Hazard Assessment; from "Effects of Secondhand Smoke," © 1997 Youth Media Network (Prunedale, CA); reprinted with permission.

✤ It's A Fact!!

Other Health Effects Of Secondhand Smoke

- Children are particularly susceptible to the harmful effects of secondhand smoke; children who are exposed have higher rates of colds, asthma and other respiratory ailments. (*The Health Consequences of Involuntary Smoking: A Report of the U.S. Surgeon General*, 1986.)
- EPA estimates that every year, between 150,000 and 300,000 children under 1-1/2 years of age get bronchitis or pneumonia from breathing secondhand tobacco smoke, resulting in thousands of hospitalizations. ("Setting the Record Straight: Secondhand Smoke is A Preventable Health Risk." Environmental Protection Agency Report (EPA), June 1994.)
- Children exposed to tobacco smoke in their homes have more colds, flu, bronchitis and pneumonia and miss 7 million more school days a year than other kids. (*USA Today*, Health, 5/13/96.)

Source: From "Effects of Secondhand Smoke," © 1997 Youth Media Network (Prunedale, CA); reprinted with permission.

Part 4

Other Abused Drugs And Chemicals

Chapter 23

Anabolic Steroids

Anabolic-androgenic steroids are man-made substances related to male sex hormones. "Anabolic" refers to muscle-building, and "androgenic" refers to increased masculine characteristics. "Steroids" refers to the class of drugs. These drugs are available legally only by prescription, to treat conditions that occur when the body produces abnormally low amounts of testosterone, such as delayed puberty and some types of impotence. They are also used to treat body wasting in patients with AIDS and other diseases that result in loss of lean muscle mass. Abuse of anabolic steroids, however, can lead to serious health problems, some irreversible.

Today, athletes and others abuse anabolic steroids to enhance performance and also to improve physical appearance. Anabolic steroids are taken orally or injected, typically in cycles of weeks or months (referred to as "cycling"), rather than continuously. Cycling involves taking multiple doses of steroids over a specific period of time, stopping for a period, and starting again. In addition, users often combine several different types of steroids to maximize their effectiveness while minimizing negative effects (a practice referred to as "stacking").

About This Chapter: This chapter contains excerpts from "Steroids (Anabolic-Androgenic)," National Institute on Drug Abuse (NIDA), Infofax No. 13557, November 1999; "Anabolic Steroids," *Community Drug Alert Bulletin*, NIDA, September 2001; and "Tips for Teens: The Truth About Steroids," National Clearinghouse for Alcohol and Drug Information, December 2000.

Health Hazards

The major side effects from abusing anabolic steroids can include liver tumors and cancer, jaundice (yellowish pigmentation of skin, tissues, and body fluids), fluid retention, high blood pressure, increases in LDL (bad cholesterol), and decreases in HDL (good cholesterol). Other side effects include kidney tumors, severe acne, and trembling. In addition, there are some gender-specific side effects:

- For men—shrinking of the testicles, reduced sperm count, infertility, baldness, development of breasts, increased risk for prostate cancer.
- For women—growth of facial hair, male-pattern baldness, changes in or cessation of the menstrual cycle, enlargement of the clitoris, deepened voice.

✤ It's A Fact!!

Did You Know...

- Steroids affect your heart. Steroid abuse has been associated with cardiovascular disease, including heart attack and stroke. These heart problems can even happen to athletes under the age of 30.
- Steroids affect your appearance. In both sexes, steroids can cause male-pattern baldness, cysts, acne, and oily hair and skin.
- Steroids affect your mood. Steroids can make you angry and hostile for no reason. There are recorded cases of murder attributed to intense anger from steroid use.
- Steroids increase your risk of infection. Sharing needles or using dirty needles to inject steroids puts you at risk for diseases such as HIV/AIDS and hepatitis.
- Most teens aren't using steroids. Among teenage males, where most steroid use is concentrated, past year use was reported by 2.2 percent of 8th graders, 3.6 percent of 10th graders, and 2.5 percent of 12th graders. (*Monitoring the Future Survey*. U.S. Department of Health and Human Services (HHS). Press Release, *2000 Monitoring the Future Survey Released: Moderating Trend Among Teen Drug Use Continues*. December 14, 2000.)

- For adolescents—growth halted prematurely through premature skeletal maturation and accelerated puberty changes. This means that adolescents risk remaining short the remainder of their lives if they take anabolic steroids before the typical adolescent growth spurt.

In addition, people who inject anabolic steroids run the added risk of contracting or transmitting HIV/AIDS or hepatitis, which causes serious damage to the liver.

Scientific research also shows that aggression and other psychiatric side effects may result from abuse of anabolic steroids. Many users report feeling good about themselves while on anabolic steroids, but researchers report that extreme mood swings also can occur, including manic-like symptoms leading to violence. Depression often is seen when the drugs are stopped and may contribute to dependence on anabolic steroids. Researchers also report that users may suffer from paranoid jealousy, extreme irritability, delusions, and impaired judgment stemming from feelings of invincibility.

> **✎ Weird Words**
>
> Slang terms for steroids include: Arnolds, Gym Candy, Pumpers, Stackers, Weight Trainers, and Juice. Other slang terms associated with steroid use include:
>
> Roid Rages: Uncontrolled outbursts of anger, frustration, or combativeness that may result from using anabolic steroids.
>
> Shotgunning: Taking steroids on an inconsistent basis.
>
> Stacking: Using a combination of two or more anabolic steroids.

Questions And Answers About Steroids

Are steroids addictive?

Yes, they can be. Withdrawal symptoms include mood swings, suicidal thoughts and/or attempts, fatigue, restlessness, loss of appetite, and sleeplessness.

How long do steroids stay in your system?

The length of time that steroids stay in the body varies from a couple of weeks to more than 18 months.

What is pyramiding?

Pyramiding is the practice of taking anabolic steroids in cyclic dosage regimens. At the beginning of a cycle, the person starts with low doses of the stacked substances and then gradually increases the doses for 6 to 12 weeks. In the second half of the cycle, the doses are slowly decreased to zero. This is sometimes followed by a second cycle during which the person continues to train, but without drugs. Abusers believe that pyramiding allows the body time to adjust to the high doses, and the drug-free cycle allows time for the body's hormonal system to recuperate. As with stacking, the perceived benefits of pyramiding have not been substantiated scientifically.

✔ Quick Tip

How can you tell if a friend is abusing steroids?

Sometimes it's hard to tell. But there are signs you can look for. If your friend has one or more of the following warning signs, he or she may be abusing steroids:

For Guys

- Baldness
- Development of breasts
- Impotence

For Girls:

- Growth of facial hair
- Deepened voice
- Breast reduction

For Both:

- Jaundice (yellowing of the skin)
- Swelling of feet or ankles
- Aching joints
- Bad breath
- Mood swings
- Nervousness
- Trembling

What can you do to help someone who is abusing steroids? Be a real friend. You might even save a life. Encourage your friend to stop or seek professional help. For information and referrals, call the National Clearinghouse for Alcohol and Drug Information at 800-729-6686.

What can I do to excel in sports if I don't use steroids?

Focus on getting proper diet, rest, and good overall mental and physical health. These things are all factors in how your body is shaped and conditioned. Excelling in sports is achievable and done by millions of athletes without relying on steroids.

For More Information About Anabolic Steroids

To learn more about steroids or obtain referrals to programs in your community

- Contact the National Clearinghouse for Alcohol and Drug Information (NCADI) at 1-800-729-6686 (or online at http://www.health.org) for free National Institute on Drug Abuse (NIDA) publications.
- Access NIDA's specialized Web site, http://www.steroidabuse.org. Additional information on other illicit drugs can be accessed through NIDA's home page on the World Wide Web: http://www.drugabuse.gov.

✤ It's A Fact!!

Anabolic steroids are different from steroidal supplements. In the United States, supplements such as dehydroepiandrosterone (DHEA) and androstenedione (street name Andro) can be purchased legally without a prescription through many commercial sources including health food stores. They are often taken because the user believes they have anabolic effects.

☞ Remember!!

If you know someone who abuses steroids, urge him or her to get help. If you're abusing them—stop! The longer you ignore the facts, the more chances you take with your life.

Chapter 24

Caffeine And High Energy Drinks

What do high-caffeine energy drinks consist of and why are those ingredients present?

The caffeine-containing energy drinks usually contain a wide range of ingredients with different brands having similar, but not identical, formulations. One ingredient they all have in common is a form of sugar such as sucrose (table sugar) or glucose. Many also include a range of vitamins (especially B group vitamins). Some have amino acids (for example, taurine) while herbal supplements such as Gingko biloba, Echinacea, Ginseng, and St. John's Wort are present in many. They also usually include guarana (a caffeine-containing extract from a South American plant). In the next five paragraphs the most likely reasons for the inclusion of these ingredients are discussed, together with an appraisal of their probable value (or otherwise) to health and fitness.

Sugar is present as a source of energy and also because it has an appealing taste. Sugar is rapidly digested and absorbed into the body, so the kilojoules of energy it provides are quickly made a available for physical work. The inclusion of sugar in the drink is therefore sound from the physiological point of view.

About This Chapter: Text in this chapter is from "FAQ on Caffeine and High Energy Drinks," by Nutrition Australia, © 2001, The Australian Nutrition Foundation, Inc. Reproduced with permission of The Australian Nutrition Foundation, Inc. Additional information is available online at www.nutritionaustralia.org.

B group vitamins are used by the body to release energy from food, but a well-balanced diet provides adequate intake of these vitamins, so they are probably not an important component of these drinks.

The rationale for providing amino acids (components of protein) such as taurine is unclear. It is believed that taurine plays a role in muscle contraction, especially in the heart, but the typical Western diet is relatively high in protein, so few people are likely to be deficient in taurine.

Herbal supplements are often touted as providing health benefits, but there isn't much scientific evidence supporting most such claims. Also, the Therapeutic Goods Administration [Australian] has warned that high intakes of these supplements can be harmful, and that some can interfere with the effectiveness of—or interact in harmful ways with—medicines.

✤ It's A Fact!!

Caffeine can change the way a medicine works or lead to unintended side effects. Here are a few examples:

- Consuming caffeine while taking some kinds of antibiotics can lead to excitability and nervousness.
- Caffeine may lessen the effects of anti-anxiety drugs by causing excitability, nervousness, and hyperactivity.
- Caffeine may compound the effects of some bronchodilators (which are used to treat lung conditions like asthma and emphysema).

Also, food and beverages with caffeine may irritate the stomach. They should be avoided if a person is taking medicines for ailments such as heartburn, indigestion, and gas.

Source: U.S. Food and Drug Administration

Guarana is usually present in these drinks as the main source of caffeine. Caffeine is there as a stimulant, that is, to give a stimulus to both physical and cognitive (mental) performance. But a stimulant can be a doubled-edged sword. As explained in detail below, excessive stimulation due to caffeine can have a detrimental effect not only on physical performance, but also on aspects of metabolism that influence health (such as blood pressure and heart rate).

How much caffeine do energy drinks contain and how does this compare with other caffeine-containing beverages?

The typical energy drink provides about 80 mg of caffeine per can (although this varies between brands). This is about the same as the amount of caffeine provided by an average strength cup of coffee and about twice that in a cup of tea. It is also about twice the level of caffeine found in a can of carbonated, cola-flavored soft drink.

What are the possible effects on health from the amount of caffeine in these drinks?

The caffeine level in most of these drinks is only equivalent to that in coffee, but because many typical consumers are young—and quite high levels of consumption are common—there is at least the potential for health risks associated with energy drinks.

Many parents would not allow their young children to drink coffee or strong tea—because they know that these drinks contain caffeine. The same may not apply to energy drinks. For example an Australian survey found that 27% of boys aged 8–12 had consumed high-caffeine energy drinks in the two-week period prior to the survey.

This may be at least partly because the quantity of caffeine isn't always stated on the label of energy drinks, and many people aren't aware of how much caffeine constitutes "high-caffeine" anyway. Parents, guardians, and other people in positions of responsibility (for example, sports coaches) should be aware that young children could have disturbed sleeping patterns, suffer bed-wetting, and show symptoms of anxiety from ingesting the caffeine in just one can of energy drink. It is clear that pre-teens should not consume high caffeine drinks and it is highly desirable to discourage their use by people in their early teens.

Some people are especially sensitive to caffeine, showing symptoms of caffeine sensitivity (tremors, sleep disturbances, gastrointestinal upsets) following consumption of relatively small doses of caffeine. Those who suffer these adverse reactions to caffeine-containing drinks such as coffee should not consume energy drinks. People with heart disease should avoid large intakes of caffeine. The sudden 'jolt' to metabolism caused by caffeine (which is a stimulant) can be enough to trigger a heart attack in people with pre-existing heart conditions. Pregnant women are also well advised to avoid high-caffeine beverages. During the first trimester (three months) of pregnancy, consuming as little as 100 mg of caffeine per day was associated with an increased risk of spontaneous abortion [miscarriage] in studies conducted in Sweden.

✤ It's A Fact!!

Caffeine And Diet Products Can Be Dangerous

In 1995 after receiving reports of adverse reactions, the U.S. Food and Drug Administration issued a warning against using diet products that contained Ma huang (ephedrine) and caffeine. Reported reactions included heart attack, strokes, seizures, and even some deaths.

Source: U.S. Food and Drug Administration

Finally, these drinks are sometimes consumed in conjunction with alcoholic beverages. Even on their own, high-caffeine drinks will cause diuresis (increased urine production). The combined effect of alcohol and caffeine will be to dehydrate people to an even greater extent than occurs with either caffeine or alcohol alone.

Do these drinks really provide a "boost" to physical and/or cognitive performance?

There is no doubt that caffeine is an effective ergogenic aid (enhances physical performance) and an aid to cognitive performance as it stimulates cardiac output and the central nervous system. Due to this, the International Olympic Committee (IOC) has banned its use above a certain level (as detected in the athlete's urine).

But as with so many substances, if a little is good, more is NOT better. In the Australian survey, some teenagers were reported to be consuming up to five cans of energy drink (up to about 400 mg of caffeine, depending on the brand) before sporting events. This is more than is needed to safely gain a boost to performance and carries with it a risk of increased blood pressure, anxiety, shaking, elevated heart rate, and increased urine production (increasing the risk of dehydration).

Do these high-caffeine energy drinks have the same function in sports as "sports drinks"?

High-caffeine energy drinks do not have the same role to play in sports as sports drinks (that is, carbohydrate/electrolyte solutions). Caffeine is a stimulant, so it provides a short sharp boost to performance. On the other hand, sports drinks do not contain stimulants—only carbohydrate and salts (to replace those lost in sweat).

Also, the quantity of sugar present in energy drinks is often much higher (for example 10–12%) than in sports drinks (which are usually 6–8% sugar).

☞ Remember!!

In summary, a can of high-caffeine energy drink generally provides about as much caffeine as a cup of coffee. When taken in small quantities (up to two or three cans per day) these drinks are as unlikely to be harmful to most adolescents and adults as drinking two or three cups of coffee.

There is convincing evidence that young children, caffeine-sensitive people, pregnant women, and people with heart disease should avoid the high caffeine intakes that would result from consuming these drinks (or from consuming coffee).

Although caffeine does provide a boost to physical and mental performance, consuming many cans of these energy drinks shortly before physical activity is more likely to be detrimental than beneficial to athletes or other active people.

High sugar concentration can slow absorption of water into the body, making these drinks unsuitable as rehydration drinks during prolonged and vigorous physical exercise. Sports drinks are the most appropriate hydration fluid during vigorous activity (especially if it is conducted in the heat).

Can energy drinks be used as a satisfactory meal replacement?

Although high-caffeine energy drinks do provide some energy (in the form of sugar) and vitamins (some brands), this does not mean that they constitute a suitable meal replacement. They contain very little protein or minerals and no dietary fiber. They are drinks, not meal replacers.

Reference

Wahlquist, M.L., "Food and Nutrition—Australia, Asia, and the Pacific," Allen and Unwin Pty Ltd., NWS, 1997.

Chapter 25

Cocaine

Cocaine is a powerfully addictive drug of abuse. Once having tried cocaine, an individual cannot predict or control the extent to which he or she will continue to use the drug.

The most common ways drug users take cocaine are sniffing or snorting, injecting, and smoking (including free-base and crack cocaine). Snorting is the process of inhaling cocaine powder through the nose where it is absorbed into the bloodstream through the nasal tissues. Injecting is the act of using a needle to release the drug directly into the bloodstream. Smoking involves inhaling cocaine vapor or smoke into the lungs where absorption into the bloodstream is as rapid as by injection.

"Crack" is the street name given to cocaine that has been processed from cocaine hydrochloride to a free base for smoking. Rather than requiring the more volatile method of processing cocaine using ether, crack cocaine is processed with ammonia or sodium bicarbonate (baking soda) and water and heated to remove the hydrochloride, thus producing a form of cocaine that can be smoked. The term "crack" refers to the crackling sound heard when the mixture is smoked (heated), presumably from the sodium bicarbonate.

About This Chapter: This chapter includes excerpts from "Crack and Cocaine," National Institute on Drug Abuse (NIDA), Infofax No. 13546, October 2001; "Straight Facts about Drugs and Alcohol," Center for Substance Abuse Prevention, Substance Abuse and Mental Health Services Administration (SAMHSA); and "Tips for Teens: The Truth About Cocaine," National Clearinghouse for Alcohol and Drug Information (NCADI), 1998.

There is great risk whether cocaine is ingested by inhalation (snorting), injection, or smoking. It appears that compulsive cocaine use may develop even more rapidly if the substance is smoked rather than snorted. Smoking allows extremely high doses of cocaine to reach the brain very quickly and brings an intense and immediate high. The injecting drug user is at risk for transmitting or acquiring HIV infection/AIDS if needles or other injection equipment are shared.

The Straight Facts About Cocaine And Crack

> **✎ Weird Words**
> Slang terms used for cocaine include: coke, dust, toot, snow, blow, sneeze, powder, lines, and rock (used for crack).

Cocaine is a white powder that comes from the leaves of the South American coca plant. Cocaine belongs to a class of drugs known as stimulants, which tend to give a temporary illusion of limitless power and energy that leave the user feeling depressed, edgy, and craving more. Cocaine and crack are highly addictive. This addiction can erode physical and mental health and become so strong that these drugs dominate all aspects of an addicts life.

Physical risks associated with using any amount of cocaine and crack include:

- Increases in blood pressure, heart rate, breathing rate, and body temperature
- Heart attacks, strokes, and respiratory failure
- Hepatitis or AIDS through shared needles
- Brain seizures
- Reduction of the body's ability to resist and combat infection

Psychological risks associated with using cocaine include:

- Violent, erratic, or paranoid behavior
- Hallucinations and "coke bugs"—a sensation of imaginary insects crawling over the skin

- Confusion, anxiety and depression, loss of interest in food or sex
- "Cocaine psychosis"—losing touch with reality, loss of interest in friends, family, sports, hobbies, and other activities

Questions And Answers About Cocaine

Is cocaine really still a problem?

Yes. While the number of cocaine users has decreased from what was witnessed in the mid-1980's, there have been nearly 2 million cocaine users every year since 1992.

Isn't crack less addictive than cocaine because it doesn't stay in your body very long?

No. Both cocaine and crack are powerfully addictive. The length of time it stays in your body doesn't change that.

Don't some people use cocaine to feel good?

Any positive feelings are fleeting and are usually followed by some very bad feelings, like paranoia and intense cravings. Cocaine may give users a temporary illusion of power and energy, but it often leaves them unable to function emotionally, physically, and sexually.

✤ It's A Fact!!

- Some cocaine users spend hundreds or thousands of dollars on cocaine and crack each week and will do anything to support their habit. Many turn to drug selling, prostitution, or other crimes.
- Cocaine and crack use has been a contributing factor in a number of drownings, car crashes, falls, burns, and suicides.
- Cocaine and crack addicts often become unable to function sexually.
- Even first time users may experience seizures or heart attacks, which can be fatal.

Extent Of Use

Monitoring The Future Study

Monitoring the Future (MTF) is an annual survey on drug use and related attitudes of America's adolescents that began in 1975. The survey is conducted by the University of Michigan's Institute for Social Research and is funded by NIDA. Copies of the latest survey are available from the National Clearinghouse for Alcohol and Drug Information at 1-800-729-6686. The MTF assesses the extent of drug use among adolescents and young adults across the country.

The proportion of high school seniors who have used cocaine at least once in their lifetimes has increased from a low of 5.9 percent in 1994 to 9.8 percent in 1999. However, this is lower than its peak of 17.3 percent in 1985. Current (past month) use of cocaine by seniors decreased from a high of 6.7 percent in 1985 to 2.6 percent in 1999. Also in 1999, 7.7 percent of 10th-graders had tried cocaine at least once, up from a low of 3.3 percent in 1992. The percentage of 8th-graders who had ever tried cocaine has increased from a low of 2.3 percent in 1991 to 4.7 percent in 1999.

Of college students 1 to 4 years beyond high school, in 1995, 3.6 percent had used cocaine within the past year, and 0.7 percent had used cocaine in the past month.

✤ It's A Fact!!

- *Cocaine affects your brain.* The word "cocaine" refers to the drug in both a powder (cocaine) and crystal (crack) form. It is made from the coca plant and causes a short-lived high that is immediately followed by opposite, intense feelings of depression, edginess, and a craving for more of the drug. Cocaine may be snorted as a powder, converted to a liquid form for injection with a needle, or processed into a crystal form to be smoked.
- *Cocaine affects your body.* People who use cocaine often don't eat or sleep regularly. They can experience increased heart rate, muscle spasms, and convulsions. If they snort cocaine, they can also permanently damage their nasal tissue.
- *Cocaine affects your emotions.* Using cocaine can make you feel paranoid, angry, hostile, and anxious, even when you're not high.
- *Cocaine is addictive.* Cocaine interferes with the way your brain processes chemicals that create feelings of pleasure, so you need more and more of the drug just to feel normal. People who become addicted to cocaine start to lose interest in other areas of their life, like school, friends, and sports.
- *Cocaine can kill you.* Cocaine use can cause heart attacks, seizures, strokes, and respiratory failure. People who share needles can also contract hepatitis, HIV/AIDS, or other diseases.

Community Epidemiology Work Group

Community Epidemiology Work Group CEWG is a NIDA-sponsored network of researchers from 20 major U.S. metropolitan areas and selected foreign countries who meet semiannually to discuss the current epidemiology of drug abuse.

Although demographic data continue to show most cocaine users as older, inner-city crack addicts, isolated field reports indicate new groups of users: teenagers smoking crack with marijuana in some cities; Hispanic crack users in Texas; and in the Atlanta area, middle-class suburban users of cocaine hydrochloride and female crack users in their thirties with no prior drug history.

✔ Quick Tip

How can you tell if a friend is using cocaine? Sometimes it's tough to tell. But there are signs you can look for. If your friend has one or more of the following warning signs, he or she may be using cocaine or other illicit drugs:

- Red, bloodshot eyes
- A runny nose or frequently sniffing
- A change in eating or sleeping patterns
- A change in groups of friends
- A change in school grades or behavior
- Acting withdrawn, depressed, tired, or careless about personal appearance
- Losing interest in school, family, or activities he or she used to enjoy
- Frequently needing money

What can you do to help someone who is using cocaine? Be a real friend. Save a life. Encourage your friend to stop or seek professional help. For information and referrals, call the National Clearinghouse for Alcohol and Drug Information at 800-729-6686.

✤ It's A Fact!!

Added Danger: Cocaethylene

When people mix cocaine and alcohol consumption, they are compounding the danger each drug poses and unknowingly forming a complex chemical experiment within their bodies. Researchers have found that the human liver combines cocaine and alcohol and manufactures a third substance, cocaethylene, that intensifies cocaine's euphoric effects, while possibly increasing the risk of sudden death.

National Household Survey On Drug Abuse

National Household Survey on Drug Abuse (NHSDA) is an annual survey conducted by the Substance Abuse and Mental Health Services Administration. Copies of the latest survey are available from the National Clearinghouse for Alcohol and Drug Information at 1-800-729-6686.

In 1998, about 1.7 million Americans were current (at least once per month) cocaine users. This is about 0.8 percent of the population age 12 and older; about 437,000 of these used crack. The rate of current cocaine use in 1998 was highest among Americans ages 18 to 25 (2.0 percent). The rate of use for this age group was significantly higher in 1998 than in 1997, when it was 1.2 percent.

Treatment

The widespread abuse of cocaine has stimulated extensive efforts to develop treatment programs for this type of drug abuse.

The National Institute on Drug Abuse (NIDA)'s top research priority is to find a medication to block or greatly reduce the effects of cocaine, to be used as one part of a comprehensive treatment program. NIDA-funded researchers are also looking at medications that help alleviate the severe craving that people in treatment for cocaine addiction often experience. Several medications are currently being investigated to test their safety and efficacy in treating cocaine addiction.

In addition to treatment medications, behavioral interventions, particularly cognitive behavioral therapy, can be effective in decreasing drug use by patients in treatment for cocaine abuse. Providing the optimal combination of treatment services for each individual is critical to successful treatment outcome.

☞ **Remember!!**

If you know someone who has a problem with cocaine, urge him or her to get help. If you use it—stop. The longer you ignore the real facts, the more chances you take with your health and well-being.

To learn more about cocaine or obtain referrals to programs in your community, contact:

National Clearinghouse for Alcohol and Drug Information
Toll Free: 800-729-6686
TDD 800-487-4889
Linea gratis en Español 877-767-8432
Web site: www.health.org

Chapter 26

Ecstasy, GHB, Rohypnol, And Other Club Drugs

Across the country, teens and young adults enjoy all-night dance parties known as "raves" and increasingly encounter more than just music. Dangerous substances known collectively as club drugs—including Ecstasy, GHB, and Rohypnol—are gaining popularity. These drugs aren't "fun drugs."

Although users may think these substances are harmless, research has shown that club drugs can produce a range of unwanted effects, including hallucinations, paranoia, amnesia, and, in some cases, death. When used with alcohol, these drugs can be even more harmful. Some club drugs work on the same brain mechanisms as alcohol and, therefore, can dangerously boost the effects of both substances. Also, there are great differences among individuals in how they react to these substances and no one can predict how he or she will react. Some people have been known to have extreme, even fatal, reactions the first time they use club drugs. And studies suggest club drugs

About This Chapter: This chapter includes excerpts from "Club Drugs Aren't 'Fun Drugs,'" by Alan I. Leshner, Ph.D., Director, National Institute on Drug Abuse (NIDA), National Institutes of Health, January 2001; "Club Drugs," *Community Drug Alert*, NIDA, January 2001; "Tips for Teens: The Truth About Club Drugs," National Clearinghouse for Alcohol and Drug Information, 1999; "Club Drugs: Ecstasy," *PREVENTION Alert*, Vol. 3, No. 25, July 28, 2000, "Club Drugs: Ketamine," *PREVENTION Alert*, Vol. 3, No. 28, September 1, 2000; and "Club Drugs: Rohypnol," *PREVENTION Alert*, Vol. 3, No. 26, August 4, 2000. *PREVENTION Alert*, which is available online at http://www.health.org/govpubs/prevalert/ is supported by the Center for Substance Abuse Prevention of the Substance Abuse and Mental Health Services Administration.

found in party settings are often adulterated or impure and thus even more dangerous.

Because some club drugs are colorless, tasteless, and odorless, they are easy for people to slip into drinks. Some of these drugs have been associated with sexual assaults, and for that reason they are referred to as "date rape drugs."

An Introduction To Club Drugs

"X," "Adam," and "MDMA" are slang names for Ecstasy, which is a stimulant and a hallucinogen. Young people may use Ecstasy to improve their moods or get energy to keep dancing; however, chronic abuse of Ecstasy appears to damage the brain's ability to think and regulate emotion, memory, sleep, and pain.

"G," "Liquid Ecstasy," "Georgia Home Boy" or Gamma-hydroxybutyrate (GHB) may be made in homes by using recipes with common ingredients. At lower doses, GHB can relax the user, but, as the dose increases, the sedative effects may result in sleep and eventual coma or death.

"Roofie" or "Roche" (Rohypnol) is tasteless and odorless. It mixes easily in carbonated beverages. Rohypnol may cause individuals under the influence of the drug to forget what happened. Other effects include low blood pressure, drowsiness, dizziness, confusion, and stomach upset.

✎ Weird Words

Slang Terms For Some Common Club Drugs

Ecstasy: E, X, XTC, Adam, MDMA

GHB: G, Liquid Ecstasy, Liquid X, Grievous Bodily Harm, Georgia Home Boy

Ketamine: K, Special K, Ket, Vitamin K, Kit Kat

Methamphetamine: Speed, Ice, Chalk, Meth

Rohypnol: Roofies, Roche, R-2

"Special K" or "K" (Ketamine) is an anesthetic. Use of a small amount of ketamine results in loss of attention span, learning ability, and memory. At higher doses, ketamine can cause delirium, amnesia, high blood pressure, depression, and severe breathing problems.

"Speed," "Ice," "Chalk," "Meth" (Methamphetamine) is often made in home laboratories. Methamphetamine use can cause serious health concerns, including memory loss, aggression, violence, psychotic behavior, and heart problems.

Questions And Answers About Club Drugs

✤ It's A Fact!!

Because some club drugs are colorless, tasteless, and odorless, they can be added unobtrusively to beverages by individuals who want to intoxicate or sedate others. In recent years, there has been an increase in reports of club drugs used to commit sexual assaults.

If you were in a club and somebody slipped a club drug into your drink, wouldn't you realize it immediately?

Probably not. Most club drugs are odorless and tasteless. Some are made into a powder form that makes it easier to slip into a drink and dissolve without a person's knowledge. That is why some of these drugs have been called "date rape" drugs—because there have been increasing reports of club drugs being used in sexual assaults.

Are there any long-term effects of taking ecstasy?

Yes. Studies on both humans and animals have proven that regular use of ecstasy produces long-lasting, perhaps permanent damage to the brain's ability to think and store memories.

If you took a club drug at a rave, wouldn't you just dance off all of its effects?

Not necessarily. The stimulant effects of drugs like ecstasy that allow the user to dance for long periods of time, combined with the hot, crowded conditions usually found at raves, can lead to extreme dehydration and even heart or kidney failure. In addition, some of ecstasy's effects, like confusion, depression, anxiety, paranoia, and sleep problems, have been reported to occur even weeks after the drug is taken.

Ecstasy

Ecstasy is the street name for methylene-dioxymethamphetamine (MDMA), a chemical substance that combines methamphetamines with hallucinogenic properties. It is also known as X-TC, Adam, Clarity, and Lover's Speed.

Like all club drugs, Ecstasy is a combination of other illicit drugs. Because many different recipes are used to make Ecstasy, the risk of death and permanent brain damage are heightened when some substances are combined. It is available in tablet, capsule, or powder form; some manufacturers of the drug package it in capsules or generic tablets to imitate prescription drugs. The average cost is between $7 and $30 per pill.

Among the variations of the drug is a new substance, Herbal Ecstasy, that is composed of ephedrine (ma huang) or pseudoephedrine and caffeine from the kola nut. Sold in tablet form, this drug may cause permanent brain damage and death.

What Side Effects Are Produced By Ecstasy?

Ecstasy's effects can last up to 24 hours. The drug produces immediate side effects, and some—such as confusion, depression, sleep problems, anxiety, and paranoia—can occur weeks after it is taken.

Because Ecstasy alters serotonin levels in the brain, researchers have found that chronic use can lead to long-term or permanent damage to those parts of the brain critical to thought, memory, and pleasure.

Psychological Effects

Psychological effects are confusion, depression, sleep problems, severe anxiety and paranoia, euphoria, enhanced mental and emotional clarity, hallucinations, sensations of lightness and floating, depression, paranoid thinking, and violent, irrational behavior.

Physical Effects

Physical effects are muscle tension, involuntary teeth clenching, nausea, blurred vision, faintness, chills/sweating, dehydration, hypertension, loss of control over voluntary body movements, tremors, reduced appetite, kidney failure, heart attack, stroke, seizure, and malignant hyperthermia (increase in body temperature).

✤ It's A Fact!!

- *Club drugs affect your brain.* The term "club drugs" refers to a wide variety of drugs often used at all-night dance parties ("raves"), nightclubs, and concerts. Club drugs can damage the neurons in your brain, impairing your senses, memory, judgment, and coordination.
- *Club drugs affect your body.* Different club drugs have different effects on your body. Some common effects include loss of muscle and motor control, blurred vision, and seizures. Club drugs like ecstasy are stimulants that increase your heart rate and blood pressure and can lead to heart or kidney failure. Other club drugs, like GHB, are depressants that can cause drowsiness, unconsciousness, or breathing problems.
- *Club drugs affect your self-control.* Club drugs like GHB and Rohypnol are used in "date rape" and other assaults because they are sedatives that can make you unconscious and immobilize you. Rohypnol can cause a kind of amnesia—users may not remember what they said or did while under the effects of the drug, making it easier for others to take advantage of them.
- *Club drugs are not always what they seem.* Because club drugs are illegal and often produced in makeshift laboratories, it is impossible to know exactly what chemicals were used to produce them and where they came from. How strong or dangerous any illegal drug is varies each time.
- *Club drugs can kill you.* Higher doses of club drugs can cause severe breathing problems, coma, or even death.

Gamma-Hydroxybutyrate (GHB)

GHB can be produced in clear liquid, white powder, tablet, and capsule forms, and it is often used in combination with alcohol, making it even more dangerous. GHB has been increasingly involved in poisonings, overdoses, "date rapes," and fatalities. The drug is used predominantly by adolescents and young adults, often when they attend nightclubs and raves.

- GHB is usually abused either for its intoxicating/sedative/euphoriant properties or for its growth hormone-releasing effects, which can build muscles.
- Some individuals are synthesizing GHB in home laboratories. Ingredients in GHB, gamma-butyrolactone (GBL) and 1,4-butanediol, can also be converted by the body into GHB.
- GHB is a central nervous system depressant that can relax or sedate the body. At higher doses it can slow breathing and heart rate to dangerous levels.
- GHB's intoxicating effects begin 10 to 20 minutes after the drug is taken. The effects typically last up to 4 hours, depending on the dosage. At lower doses, GHB can relieve anxiety and produce relaxation; however, as the dose increases, the sedative effects may result in sleep and eventual coma or death.
- Overdose of GHB can occur rather quickly, and the signs are similar to those of other sedatives: drowsiness, nausea, vomiting, headache, loss of consciousness, loss of reflexes, impaired breathing, and ultimately death.
- GHB is cleared from the body relatively quickly, so it is sometimes difficult to detect in emergency rooms and other treatment facilities.

Ketamine

Ketamine (ketamine hydrochloride) is a central nervous system depressant that produces a rapid-acting dissociative effect. It was developed in the 1970s as a medical anesthetic for both humans and animals. Ketamine is often mistaken for cocaine or crystal methamphetamine because of a similarity in appearance.

✔ **Quick Tip**

How can you tell if a friend is using club drugs? Sometimes it's tough to tell. But there are signs you can look for. If your friend has one or more of the following warning signs, he or she may be using club drugs:

- Problems remembering things they recently said or did
- Loss of coordination, dizziness, fainting
- Depression
- Confusion
- Sleep problems
- Chills or sweating
- Slurred speech

What can you do to help someone who is using club drugs? Be a real friend. Save a life. Encourage your friend to stop or seek professional help. For information and referrals, call the National Clearinghouse for Alcohol and Drug Information at 800-729-6686.

Also known as K, Special K, Vitamin K, Kit Kat, Keller, Super Acid, and Super C, Ketamine is available in tablet, powder, and liquid form. So powerful is the drug that, when injected, there is a risk of losing motor control before the injection is completed. In powder form, the drug can be snorted or sprinkled on tobacco or marijuana and smoked. The effects of Ketamine last from 1 to 6 hours, and it is usually 24–48 hours before the user feels completely "normal" again.

What Are The Side Effects Of Ketamine?

Psychedelic effects are produced quickly by low doses (25–100 mg) of Ketamine. Higher doses (1 gram or more) can cause convulsions and death. As with most anesthetics, eating or drinking before taking Ketamine can produce vomiting. Other reported side effects are:

Physical Effects

Ketamine can cause slurred speech, increased heart rate, increased blood pressure, lack of coordination, muscle rigidity, bronchodilation, respiratory distress, paralysis, increased cardiac output (leading to risk of heart attack or stroke), coma, and death.

Psychological Effects

Psychological effects of ketamine include hallucinations, dreamlike states, feelings of invulnerability, psychological near-death experiences, paranoia, and aggressive behavior.

Rohypnol

Rohypnol, the trade name for flunitrazepam, is a member of the benzodiazepine family, which includes Valium, Halcyon, Xanax, and Versed. These drugs are known for their sedative effects. On the street, Rohypnol is called roofies, rophies, roche, and the forget-me pill.

Manufactured in tablet form, Rohypnol can be easily crushed and dissolved in liquid. It is tasteless and odorless, and can thus be slipped into people's drinks without their knowledge. A single dose of Rohypnol, as small as 1 mg., can produce effects for 8-12 hours after ingestion.

☞ **Remember!!**

"Raves" or all-night dance parties continue to attract teens and young adults who may think Ecstasy, GHB, Rohypnol, and other club drugs are harmless. This is not true. While researchers continue to study club drugs with a sense of urgency, treatment and prevention strategies are being developed. And the bottom line is simple: even experimenting with club drugs is an unpredictable and dangerous thing to do.

If you know someone who uses club drugs, urge him or her to get help. If you're using them—stop. The longer you ignore the real facts, the more chances you take with your life.

For more information, visit the National Institute on Drug Abuse's special web site at http://www.clubdrugs.org or call:

National Clearinghouse for Alcohol and Drug Information
1-800-729-6686
TDD 800-487-4889
linea gratis en Español 877-767-8432
Web site: www.health.org

What Are The Side Effects Of Rohypnol?

Among the immediate effects of taking Rohypnol are feelings of intoxication, muscle relaxation, and drowsiness. Users under the influence may exhibit slurred speech, impaired judgment, and difficulty in walking. The drug causes "anterograde amnesia," whereby individuals are unable to remember events they experienced while under its effects.

Other adverse effects of Rohypnol include respiratory distress, blackouts that can last up to 24 hours, decreased blood pressure, hallucinations, dizziness, confusion, gastrointestinal disturbances, urinary retention, headaches, and muscle pain. Some users may display aggressive behavior.

Rohypnol can produce physical and psychological dependence. As a result, chronic users can experience withdrawal effects and seizures. When used in combination with alcohol and other depressants, Rohypnol can be fatal.

Methamphetamine

Methamphetamine is a toxic, addictive stimulant that affects many areas of the central nervous system. The drug is often made in clandestine laboratories. It is being used by diverse groups, including young adults who attend raves, in many regions of the country.

Available in many forms, methamphetamine can be smoked, snorted, injected, or orally ingested.

Facts About Methamphetamine

- Methamphetamine is a white, odorless, bitter-tasting crystalline powder that easily dissolves in beverages.
- Methamphetamine is not sold in the same way as many other illicit drugs; it is typically sold through networks, not on the street.
- Methamphetamine use is associated with serious health consequences, including memory loss, aggression, violence, psychotic behavior, and potential cardiac and neurological damage.
- Methamphetamine abusers typically display signs of agitation, excited

speech, decreased appetite, and increased physical activity levels.

- Methamphetamine is neurotoxic. Methamphetamine abusers may have significant reductions in dopamine transporters.
- Methamphetamine use can contribute to higher rates of transmission of infectious diseases, especially hepatitis and HIV/AIDS.

Chapter 27

Hallucinogens

LSD

LSD (lysergic acid diethylamide) is one of the major drugs making up the hallucinogen class. LSD was discovered in 1938 and is one of the most potent mood-changing chemicals. It is manufactured from lysergic acid, which is found in ergot, a fungus that grows on rye and other grains.

LSD, commonly referred to as "acid," is sold on the street in tablets, capsules, and, occasionally, liquid form. It is odorless, colorless, and has a slightly bitter taste and is usually taken by mouth. Often LSD is added to absorbent paper, such as blotter paper, and divided into small decorated squares, with each square representing one dose.

The Drug Enforcement Administration (DEA) reports that the strength of LSD samples obtained currently from illicit sources ranges from 20 to 80 micrograms of LSD per dose. This is considerably less than the levels reported during the 1960s and early 1970s, when the dosage ranged from 100 to 200 micrograms, or higher, per unit.

About This Chapter: Text in this chapter includes excerpts from "LSD," National Institute on Drug Abuse (NIDA), Infofax No. 13550, October 2001; "PCP (Phencyclidine)," NIDA, Infofax No. 13554, October 2001; "The Hallucinogen PMA: Dancing With Death," *Drug Intelligence Brief*, Drug Enforcement Administration (DEA), October 2000; "4-Bromo-2,5-dimethoxyphenethylamine," *Drugs and Chemicals of Concern*, Diversion Control Program, DEA, August 2001; and "Tips for Teens: The Truth About Hallucinogens," National Clearinghouse for Alcohol and Drug Information, 1999.

Health Hazards

The effects of LSD are unpredictable. They depend on the amount taken; the user's personality, mood, and expectations; and the surroundings in which the drug is used. Usually, the user feels the first effects of the drug 30 to 90 minutes after taking it. The physical effects include dilated pupils, higher body temperature, increased heart rate and blood pressure, sweating, loss of appetite, sleeplessness, dry mouth, and tremors.

Sensations and feelings change much more dramatically than the physical signs. The user may feel several different emotions at once or swing rapidly from one emotion to another. If taken in a large enough dose, the drug produces delusions and visual hallucinations. The user's sense of time and self changes. Sensations may seem to "cross over," giving the user the feeling of hearing colors and seeing sounds. These changes can be frightening and can cause panic.

Users refer to their experience with LSD as a "trip" and to acute adverse reactions as a "bad trip." These experiences are long—typically they begin to clear after about 12 hours.

Some LSD users experience severe, terrifying thoughts and feelings, fear of losing control, fear of insanity and death, and despair while using LSD. Some fatal accidents have occurred during states of LSD intoxication.

Many LSD users experience flashbacks, recurrence of certain aspects of a person's experience, without the user having taken the drug again. A flashback occurs suddenly, often without warning, and may occur within a few days or more than a year after LSD use. Flashbacks usually occur in people who use hallucinogens chronically or have an underlying personality problem; however, otherwise healthy people

Weird Words

Slang Terms For Hallucinogens

Ecstasy: E, X, XTC

Lysergic Acid Diethylamide: LSD, Acid, Blotter

Phencyclidine: PCP, Angel Dust, Boat, Ozone, Wack

Psilocybin: Magic Mushrooms, Shrooms

who use LSD occasionally may also have flashbacks. Bad trips and flashbacks are only part of the risks of LSD use. LSD users may manifest relatively long-lasting psychoses, such as schizophrenia or severe depression. It is difficult to determine the extent and mechanism of the LSD involvement in these illnesses.

Most users of LSD voluntarily decrease or stop its use over time. LSD is not considered an addictive drug since it does not produce compulsive drug-seeking behavior as do cocaine, amphetamine, heroin, alcohol, and nicotine. However, like many of the addictive drugs, LSD produces tolerance, so some users who take the drug repeatedly must take progressively higher doses to achieve the state of intoxication that they had previously achieved. This is an extremely dangerous practice, given the unpredictability of the drug. The National Institute on Drug Abuse (NIDA) is funding studies that focus on the neurochemical and behavioral properties of LSD. This research will provide a greater understanding of the mechanisms of action of the drug.

Extent Of Use

Monitoring The Future Study

Monitoring the Future (MTF) is an annual survey on drug use and related attitudes of America's adolescents that began in 1975. The survey is conducted by the University of Michigan's Institute for Social Research and is funded by NIDA. Copies of the latest survey are available from the National Clearinghouse for Alcohol and Drug Information at 1-800-729-6686.

Since 1975, MTF researchers have annually surveyed almost 17,000 high school seniors nationwide to determine trends in drug use and to measure attitudes and beliefs about drug abuse. Over the past 2 years, the percentage of seniors who have used LSD has remained relatively stable. Between 1975 and 1997, the lowest lifetime use of LSD was reported by the class of 1986, when 7.2 percent of seniors reported using LSD at least once in their lives. In 1997, 13.6 percent of seniors had experimented with LSD at least once in their lifetimes. The percentage of seniors reporting use of LSD in the past year nearly doubled from a low of 4.4 percent in 1985 to 8.4 percent in 1997.

In 1997, 34.7 percent of seniors perceived great risk in using LSD once or twice, and 76.6 percent said they saw great risk in using LSD regularly.

More than 80 percent of seniors disapproved of people trying LSD once or twice, and almost 93 percent disapproved of people taking LSD regularly.

Almost 51 percent of seniors said it would have been fairly easy or very easy for them to get LSD if they had wanted it.

✣ It's A Fact!!

Hallucinogens affect your brain. Hallucinogens alter how the brain perceives time, reality, and the environment around you. They also affect the way you move, react to situations, think, hear, and see. This may make you think that you're hearing voices, seeing images, and feeling things that don't exist.

Hallucinogens affect your heart. The use of hallucinogens leads to an increase in heart rate and blood pressure. Hallucinogens can put you in a coma. They can also cause heart and lung failure. Hallucinogens affect your well-being. The use of hallucinogens may change the way you feel emotionally. They may cause you to feel confused, suspicious, and disoriented. Use of PCP may interfere with hormones related to normal growth as well as with the learning process.

Hallucinogens affect your self-control. The impact of hallucinogens varies from time to time, so there is no way to know how much self-control you might maintain. They can cause you to mix up your speech, lose control of your muscles, make meaningless movements, and do aggressive or violent things.

National Household Survey On Drug Abuse

The National Household Survey on Drug Abuse (NHSDA) is an annual survey conducted by the Substance Abuse and Mental Health Services Administration. Copies of the latest survey are available from the National Clearinghouse for Alcohol and Drug Information at 1-800-729-6686.

NHSDA reports the nature and extent of drug use among the American household population aged 12 and older. In the 1996 NHSDA estimates, the percentage of the population aged 12 and older who had ever used LSD (the lifetime prevalence rate) had increased to 7.7 percent from 6.0 percent in 1988. Among youths 12 to 17 years old, the 1996 LSD lifetime prevalence rate was 4.3 percent, and for those aged 18 to 25, the rate was 13.9 percent. The rate for past-year use of LSD among the population ages 12 and older was 1 percent in 1996. Past-year prevalence was highest among the age groups 12 to 17 (2.8 percent) and 18 to 25 (4.6 percent). The rate of current LSD use in 1996 for those aged 18 to 25 was 0.9 percent, and it was 0.8 percent for 12- to 17-year-old youths.

PCP (Phencyclidine)

PCP (phencyclidine) was developed in the 1950s as an intravenous anesthetic. Use of PCP in humans was discontinued in 1965, because it was found that patients often became agitated, delusional, and irrational while recovering from its anesthetic effects. PCP is illegally manufactured in laboratories and is sold on the street by such names as "angel dust," "ozone," "wack," and "rocket fuel." "Killer joints" and "crystal supergrass" are names that refer to PCP combined with marijuana. The variety of street names for PCP reflects its bizarre and volatile effects.

PCP is a white crystalline powder that is readily soluble in water or alcohol. It has a distinctive bitter chemical taste. PCP can be mixed easily with dyes and turns up on the illicit drug market in a variety of tablets, capsules, and colored powders. It is normally used in one of three ways: snorted, smoked, or eaten. For smoking, PCP is often applied to a leafy material such as mint, parsley, oregano, or marijuana.

Health Hazards

PCP is addicting; that is, its use often leads to psychological dependence, craving, and compulsive PCP-seeking behavior. It was first introduced as a street drug in the 1960s and quickly gained a reputation as a drug that could cause bad reactions and was not worth the risk. Many people, after using the drug once, will not knowingly use it again. Yet others use it consistently and regularly. Some persist in using PCP because of its addicting properties. Others cite feelings of strength, power, invulnerability and a numbing effect on the mind as reasons for their continued PCP use.

Many PCP users are brought to emergency rooms because of PCP's unpleasant psychological effects or because of overdoses. In a hospital or detention setting, they often become violent or suicidal, and are very dangerous to themselves and to others. They should be kept in a calm setting and should not be left alone.

At low to moderate doses, physiological effects of PCP include a slight increase in breathing rate and a more pronounced rise in blood pressure and pulse rate. Respiration becomes shallow, and flushing and profuse sweating occur. Generalized numbness of the extremities and muscular incoordination also may occur. Psychological effects include distinct changes in body awareness, similar to those associated with alcohol intoxication. Use of PCP among adolescents may interfere with hormones related to normal growth and development as well as with the learning process.

✤ It's A Fact!!

It's easy to quickly develop a tolerance to hallucinogens so that it takes more and more of the drug each time to get the same effect. This is dangerous because taking more and more of the same drug may lead to an overdose with severe effects.

At high doses of PCP, there is a drop in blood pressure, pulse rate, and respiration. This may be accompanied by nausea, vomiting, blurred vision, flicking up and down of the eyes, drooling, loss of balance, and dizziness. High doses of PCP can also cause seizures, coma, and death (though death more often results from accidental injury or suicide during PCP intoxication). Psychological effects at high doses include illusions and hallucinations. PCP can cause effects that mimic the full range of symptoms of schizophrenia, such as delusions, paranoia, disordered thinking, a sensation of distance from one's environment, and catatonia. Speech is often sparse and garbled.

People who use PCP for long periods report memory loss, difficulties with speech and thinking, depression, and weight loss. These symptoms can persist up to a year after cessation of PCP use. Mood disorders also have been reported. PCP has sedative effects, and interactions with other central nervous system depressants, such as alcohol and benzodiazepines, can lead to coma or accidental overdose.

Extent Of Use

Monitoring The Future Study

NIDA's 1997 MTF shows that use of PCP by high school seniors has declined steadily since 1979, when 7.0 percent of seniors had used PCP in the year preceding the survey. In 1997, however, 2.3 percent of seniors used PCP at least once in the past year, up from a low of 1.2 percent in 1990. Past month use among seniors decreased from 1.3 percent in 1996 to 0.7 percent in 1997.

National Household Survey On Drug Abuse

According to the 1996 NHSDA, 3.2 percent of the population aged 12 and older have used PCP at least once. Lifetime use of PCP was higher among those aged 26 through 34 (4.2 percent) than for those 18 through 25 (2.3 percent) and those 12 through 17 (1.2 percent).

Paramethoxyamphetamine (PMA)

Paramethoxyamphetamine (PMA), also known as 4-methoxy-amphetamine, is a potent and potentially lethal synthetic hallucinogen, which was placed into Schedule I of the Controlled Substances Act in 1973. The drug has been sold in tablet, capsule, and powder form, and its appearance and cost are comparable to MDMA. Until recently, illicit abuse of PMA was briefly encountered during the early 1970s in the United States and Canada. However, since February 2000, PMA has reemerged in Florida, Illinois, Michigan, Virginia, and Canada. Moreover, since May 2000, PMA ingestion has been associated with three deaths in Chicago, Illinois, and seven deaths in central Florida. Common street names for PMA are "Death" and "Mitsubishi Double-Stack."

Effects

The effects associated with PMA vary depending on the dose and whether other drugs are present. PMA typically is administered orally in pill or capsule form. PMA powder, although uncommon, may be inhaled or injected to accelerate the response. Ingesting a dose of less than 50 milligrams—usually one pill or capsule—without other drugs or alcohol, induces symptoms reminiscent of MDMA. Such effects include increased pulse rate and blood pressure, increased and labored respiration, elevated body temperature, erratic eye movements, muscle spasms, nausea, and heightened visual stimulation. Doses over 50 milligrams are considered potentially lethal, especially when taken with other drugs, such as amphetamine derivatives, cannabis, cocaine, prescription medications like fluoxetine (Prozac), and alcohol. Higher doses can produce cardiac arrhythmia and arrest, breathing problems, pulmonary congestion, renal failure, hyperthermia, vomiting, convulsions, coma, and death.

✤ It's A Fact!!
Hallucinogens can cause flashbacks. Effects of the drugs, including hallucinations, can occur weeks, months, even years after use.

Cause For Concern

Currently, illicit PMA distributors in the United States have targeted dealers primarily at rave clubs. Dealers may be unaware that they are buying or selling PMA rather than other club drugs like MDMA.

The increasing popularity associated with designer drugs increases the risk that users may inadvertently ingest substances such as PMA, which is similar in appearance to MDMA but is more toxic. The continued presence of PMA in Australia and the recent appearance in Canada, Europe, and the United States are causes for concern that PMA will be associated with additional overdoses and deaths.

4-Bromo-2,5-Dimethoxyphenethylamine

4-Bromo-2,5 dimethoxyphenethylamine (4-bromo-2,5- DMPEA) is an illicit, synthetic Schedule I hallucinogen. The structure of the compound is similar to a number of other clandestinely manufactured controlled substances. The compound is commonly referred to as "bromo", 2C-B, Nexus, 2's or Two's. Clandestine manufacturing imposes additional risks to the user due to impurities, instability, and uncertain dosage forms. In late 2000 and 2001, there has been a resurgence of 2C-B among the club and "circuit" party scene.

There is no accepted medical use in treatment for 4-bromo-2,5-DMPEA. The psychedelics have enjoyed periodic popularity in the United States. 4-bromo-2,5-DMPEA probably originated in Australia but soon showed up in seizures in Texas and California in the early 1970s. 4-bromo-2,5-DMPEA was manufactured in South Africa under the name Nexus, and imported domestically in late 1993. Distributed initially as a non-controlled substance of natural origin, it was promoted as a "New Age" aphrodisiac, sleep aid, and stimulant. It was purported to contain brominated cathinine, a fictional derivative of the khat plant.

Chemistry/Pharmacology

4-bromo-2,5-dimethoxyphenethylamine or 2-(4-bromo, 2,5-dimethoxyphenyl)-1-aminoethane (4-bromo-2,5-DMPEA) is a psychoactive substance which produces in human subjects, euphoria and perceptual enhancement (i.e., increased receptiveness of visual, auditory, olfactory, and tactile sensations). The effects can last up to 6-8 hours. The low dose effects of 4-bromo-2,5-DMPEA are separate and distinct from those typically referred to as hallucinogenic. Rather than showing signs of excitation, the subject becomes passive and relaxed and is aware of an integration of sensory perception with emotional states. There is considerable euphoria with an increased body awareness. Higher doses (20–40 mg) are likely to produce typical LSD-like hallucinations. Doses greater than 50 mg have produced extremely fearful hallucinations and morbid delusions.

4-bromo-2,5-DMPEA has been sold in "blotter" or "stamp" delivery systems. The drug has been misrepresented by distributors and sold as other clandestinely manufactured hallucinogenics, including DOB, LSD, and MDMA.

The availability of 4-bromo-2,5-DMPEA while not as widespread as LSD, is used by the same population as those using Ecstasy: high school and college students and other young adults. It is considered a "club drug" similar to GHB (gamma hydroxybutyrate), ketamine, and MDMA, which are distributed in "rave clubs" or upscale urban nightclubs.

Questions And Answers About Hallucinogens

Do hallucinogens have long-term effects?

Yes. In addition to flashbacks, long-term effects may include decreased motivation, prolonged depression, anxiety, increased delusions and panic, and psychosis.

Can I predict if I will have a "bad trip"?

There is no way to predict a "bad trip." There is no consistency in hallucinogenic drugs, so each "trip" may differ depending on the drug's strength and purity. The psychological effects of the hallucinogen are also dependent on the user's frame of mind.

How can I help someone through a bad trip?

Don't try to handle this situation on your own; call 911 and a trusted adult immediately. While waiting, address the person by name, remind them who and where they are, talk to them calmly, make sure they're safe, and don't leave them alone.

To Learn More

For additional information about hallucinogens or referrals for help, contact:

National Clearinghouse for Alcohol and Drug Information
800-729-6686
TDD 800-487-4889
linea gratis en Español 877-767-8432
Web site: www.health.org

✔ Quick Tip

How can you tell if a friend is using hallucinogens? Sometimes it's tough to tell. But there are signs you can look for. If your friend has one or more of the following warning signs, he or she may be using hallucinogens:

- Depression
- Weakness and lack of muscular coordination
- Anxiety or paranoia
- Trembling
- Nausea
- Dizziness
- Facial flushing
- Dilated pupils

What can you do to help someone who is using hallucinogens? Be a real friend. Encourage your friend to stop or seek professional help. For information and referrals, call the National Clearinghouse for Alcohol and Drug Information at 800-729-6686.

Chapter 28

Herbal And Other "Natural" Products

Products marketed as "dietary supplements" include a wide range of products, from traditional nutrients, such as vitamins or minerals, to other substances that often have no scientifically recognized role in nutrition. Some terms used to identify these other substances include "high-potency free amino acids," "botanicals," "enzymes," "animal extracts," and "bioflavonoids."

Dietary supplements are often sold without undergoing the same kind of safety review that is used for medicines. Because of concern about these products, the U.S. Food and Drug Administration (FDA) started identifying dietary supplements for which serious adverse reactions had been documented. This chapter includes information about some herbal and other "natural" products sold as dietary supplements that have been associated with serious safety problems. All hazardous ingredients in dietary supplements are not included, however, so the fact that something is not listed does not mean it is safe.

Herbals

Herbal and other botanical (made from plants) ingredients in dietary supplements include processed or unprocessed plant parts (bark, leaves, flowers,

About This Chapter: Information in this chapter includes text adapted from " Illnesses and Injuries Associated With the Use of Selected Dietary Supplements," Center for Food Safety and Applied Nutrition, U. S. Food and Drug Administration (FDA), 1993; and "FDA Statement on Street Drugs Containing Botanical Ephedrine," U.S. Department of Health and Human Services, April 1996. The text was reviewed and updated by David Cooke, M.D., in May 2002.

fruits, and stems), as well as extracts and essential oils. They are available in a variety of forms, including teas, powders, tablets, capsules, and elixirs, and may be marketed as single substances or in combination with other materials, such as vitamins, minerals, amino acids, and non-nutrient ingredients.

Chaparral (*Larrea tridentata*)

Chaparral, commonly called the creosote bush, is a desert shrub with a long history of use as a traditional medicine by Native Americans. Chaparral is marketed as a tea, as well as in tablet, capsule, and concentrated extract form. It has been promoted as a natural antioxidant "blood purifier," cancer cure, and acne treatment.

✎ Weird Words

Alkaloids: Originally, any one of hundreds of plant and fungal products distinguished by alkaline (basic) reactions, but now used in a more restricted way to refer to a specific type of these products. (Their common names usually end in -ine; for example, morphine). Alkaloids are made by plants and are found in the leaf, bark, seed, or other parts. They are a loosely defined group, but may be classified according to the chemical structure of their main nucleus. For medicinal purposes, due to improved water solubility, the salts of alkaloids (for example, morphine sulfate or codeine phosphate) are usually used.

Antioxidant: An agent, including certain natural body products and nutrients, that can neutralize the oxidant effect (combining with oxygen) of free radicals and other substances. Free radicals are substances in the body that have been implicated in various types of tissue damage, particularly those involved in atherosclerosis, the aging process, and the development of cancer. Free radicals are normally removed from tissues by antioxidant enzymes. Although a high intake of antioxidant nutrients from food sources appears to offer some health advantages, there is presently no clear evidence that any antioxidant nutrient, when taken in excess of normal dietary amounts, has value in the prevention or treatment of cardiovascular disease, cancer, or any other abnormal process (except in cases of obvious nutritional or vitamin deficiency). In fact, although naturally occurring antioxidant nutrients are vital dietary components, they can cause adverse effects when large amounts are taken for a long time.

Several cases of acute non-viral hepatitis (rapidly developing liver damage) have been associated with the consumption of chaparral as a dietary supplement. In most of the cases, the injury to the liver healed over time, after discontinuation of the product. In at least two patients, however, there is evidence that chaparral consumption caused irreversible liver damage. One patient suffered terminal liver failure requiring liver transplant.

Most of these cases are associated with the consumption of single ingredient chaparral capsules or tablets; however, a few of the more recent cases appear to be associated with consumption of multi-ingredient products (capsules, tablets or teas) that contain chaparral as one ingredient. Chemical analyses have identified no contaminants in the products associated with the

Chelation: A chemical process involving a metal ion. Chelation can be used to remove an ion from participation in biological reactions.

Cirrhosis: Endstage liver disease characterized by damage to a certain type of cell in the liver; associated with failure in the function of liver cells and interference with blood flow in the liver, frequently resulting in jaundice and other signs of liver failure.

Elixir: A clear, sweetened type of liquid intended for oral use (to be taken by mouth).

Poultice: A soft mush prepared by wetting various powders or other absorbent substances with oily or watery fluids, sometimes medicated, and usually applied hot to the surface.

Scleroderma: Thickening and hardening of the skin caused by new collagen (a form of protein) formation

Sedative: 1. Calming; quieting; 2. A drug that quiets nervous excitement.

Tincture: A type of liquid solution prepared from vegetable materials or from chemical substances. The proportions of drug represented in the different tinctures are not uniform, but vary according to the established standards for each.

Source: From *Stedman's Medical Dictionary, 27th Edition*,

cases of hepatitis. Products from at least four different distributors and from at least two different sources have been implicated thus far.

After FDA's health warning, many distributors of chaparral products voluntarily removed the products from the market in December of 1992. Some chaparral products remain on the market, however, and other distributors who removed their products from the market are seeking to clarify the status of these products.

Comfrey (common comfrey: *Symphytum officinale*; prickly comfrey: *S. asperum*; Russian comfrey: *S. X uplandicum*)

Preparations of comfrey, a fast-growing leafy plant, are widely sold in the United States as teas, tablets, capsules, tinctures, medicinal poultices, and lotions. Since 1985, at least seven cases of hepatic veno-occlusive disease—obstruction of blood flow from the liver with potential scarring (cirrhosis)—including one death, have been associated with the use of comfrey products.

Comfrey contains a toxic alkaloid that has been associated with hepatic veno-occlusive disease in other parts of the world. This disease is usually acute (sudden) and may result in fatal liver failure. In less severe cases, liver disease may progress to a chronic form. Even after apparent recovery, chronic liver disease, has been noted. Individuals who eat or drink small amounts of the toxic alkaloid for a prolonged period may also be at risk for development of hepatic cirrhosis (liver scarring).

Factors such as the age of the user, gender, body weight, liver function, and how much of the alkaloid is consumed probably influence how much injury the substance causes. Infants in general appear to be particularly susceptible to adverse effects. (There are reports of infants developing hepatic veno-occlusive disease following exposure of less than one week.)

Four countries (the United Kingdom, Australia, Canada, and Germany) have restricted the availability of products containing comfrey, and other countries permit use of comfrey only with a physician's prescription.

Yohimbe (*Pausinystalia yohimbe*)

Yohimbe is a tree bark containing a variety of chemicals that have an effect on the body. It is marketed in a number of products for body building and "enhanced male performance." Serious adverse effects, including kidney failure, seizures and death, have been reported.

The major identified alkaloid in yohimbe is yohimbine, a chemical that causes a widening of the blood vessels, thereby lowering blood pressure. Yohimbine is also a prescription drug in the United States. Side effects are well recognized and may include central nervous system stimulation that causes anxiety attacks. At high doses, yohimbine is a monoamine oxidase (MAO) inhibitor. MAO inhibitors can cause serious adverse effects when taken at the same time as foods that contain tyramine (for example, liver, cheeses, red wine).

Yohimbe should also be avoided by people with hypotension (low blood pressure), diabetes, and heart, liver or kidney disease. Symptoms of overdosage include weakness and nervous stimulation followed by paralysis, fatigue, stomach disorders, and ultimately death.

Lobelia (*Lobelia inflata*)

Lobelia, also known as Indian tobacco, contains pyridine-derived alkaloids, primarily lobeline. These alkaloids have actions on the body that are similar to nicotine, although they are less potent. There have been several reported cases of adverse reactions associated with consumption of dietary supplements containing lobelia.

Depending on the dose, lobeline can cause either autonomic nervous system stimulation or depression. At low doses, it produces bronchial dilation and increased respiratory rate. Higher doses result in respiratory depression, as well as sweating, rapid heart rate, hypotension, and even coma and death. As little as 50 milligrams of dried herb or a single milliliter of lobelia tincture has caused these reactions.

Because of its similarity to nicotine, lobelia may be especially dangerous to some people, including children, pregnant women, and people with cardiac disease.

Germander (*Teucrium* genus)

Germander is the common name for a group of plants that are contained in medicinal teas, elixirs, and capsules or tablets, either singly or in combination with other herbs, and marketed for weight loss and the treatment of obesity.

Since 1986, at least 27 cases of acute nonviral hepatitis (liver disease), including one death, have been associated with the use of commercially available germander products in France. These cases show a relationship between ingestion of germander and onset of hepatitis, as well as the resolution of symptoms when the use of germander was stopped. In 12 cases, re-administration of germander was followed by prompt recurrence of hepatitis. Recovery occurred gradually in most cases, approximately two of six months after withdrawal of germander. Although the substance in germander that is responsible for causing hepatitis has not been identified, germander contains several chemicals, including polyphenols, tannins, diterpenoids, and flavonoids. The French Ministry of Health has forbidden the use of germander in drugs. Its use has been restricted in other countries.

Willow Bark (*Salix* species)

Willow bark has long been used as a medicine. Its pain-killing (analgesic) and fever-reducing (antipyretic) properties are well known. Willow bark is widely promoted as an "aspirin-free" analgesic, including in dietary supplement products for children. Because it shares the same chemical properties and the same adverse effects as aspirin, this claim is highly misleading. The "aspirin-free" claim is particularly dangerous on products marketed, without warning labels, for use by children and other aspirin-sensitive individuals.

The component in willow bark that works as a medicine in the body is called "salicin"; it is a compound that is converted to salicylic acid by the body after ingestion. Both willow bark and aspirin are salicylates, a class of compounds that work by virtue of their salicylic acid content. Aspirin (acetylsalicylic acid) is also converted to salicylic acid after ingestion.

All salicylates share substantially the same side effects. The major adverse effects include irritation of the stomach lining, adverse effects when used during pregnancy (including stillbirth, bleeding, prolonged gestation and labor, and low-birth-weight infants), stroke, and adverse effects in children with fever and dehydration. Children with influenza or chickenpox should avoid salicylates because their use, even in small doses, is associated with development of Reye syndrome, which is characterized by severe, sometimes fatal, liver injury. Salicylate intoxication (headache, dizziness, ringing in ears, difficulty hearing, dimness of vision, confusion, lassitude, drowsiness, sweating, hyperventilation, nausea, vomiting, and central nervous system disturbances in severe cases) may occur as the result of over-medication, or kidney or liver insufficiency. Hypersensitivity, manifested by itching, bronchospasm and localized swelling (which may be life-threatening), can occur with very small doses of salicylates, and may occur even in those without a prior history of sensitivity to salicylates. Approximately 5 percent of the population is hypersensitive to salicylates.

Ma Huang

Ma huang is one of several names for herbal products containing members of the genus *Ephedra*. There are many common names for these evergreen plants, including squaw tea and Mormon tea. Serious adverse effects, including hypertension (high blood pressure), palpitation (rapid heart rate), neuropathy (nerve damage), myopathy (muscle injury), psychosis, stroke, and memory loss, have been reported to FDA with products containing Ma huang as ingredients.

> **✔ Quick Tip**
>
> If you have been injured or suffered an adverse effect after taking a dietary supplement or any product containing an ephedrine alkaloid, call 1-800-FDA-4010.

The *Ephedras* have been shown to contain various chemical stimulants, including the alkaloids ephedrine, pseudoephedrine, and norpseudoephedrine, as well as various tannins and related chemicals. The concentrations of these alkaloids depends upon the particular species of *Ephedra* used. Ephedrine and pseudoephedrine are amphetamine-like chemicals used in over-the-counter (OTC) and prescription drugs. Many of these stimulants have known serious side effects.

Ma huang is sold in products for weight control, as well as in products that boost energy levels. These products often contain other stimulants, such as caffeine, which when combined may intensify the effects leading to a greater chance for harm.

✤ It's A Fact!!

The Food and Drug Administration is warning consumers not to purchase or consume ephedrine-containing dietary supplements with labels that often portray the products as apparent alternatives to illegal street drugs such as "ecstasy," because these products pose significant health risks to consumers. These products contain botanical, or so-called "natural," sources of ephedrine. Ephedrine is an amphetamine-like stimulant that can have potentially dangerous effects on the nervous system and heart.

These types of products are marketed under a variety of brand names with labels that claim or imply that they produce such effects as euphoria, increased sexual sensations, heightened awareness, increased energy, and other effects. Possible adverse effects of ephedrine range from clinically significant effects such as heart attack, stroke, seizures, psychosis and death, to clinically less significant effects that may indicate the potential for more serious effects (for example, dizziness, headache, gastrointestinal distress, irregular heartbeat, and heart palpitations).

Ingredient panels on these products may list ma huang, Chinese ephedra, ma huang extract, ephedra, Ephedra sinica, ephedra extract, ephedra herb powder, epitonin or ephedrine. Any one of these ingredients listed on the label indicate the presence of ephedrine in the product.

Many of these ephedrine-containing products bear labels that appear to be targeted at adolescents and young adults and that imply the products can produce a "high." The FDA considers this type of promotion and these claims to violate federal laws that govern the U.S. marketing of dietary supplement products.

The FDA has issued several, increasingly severe warnings regarding the use of Ephedra supplements due to multiple reports of high blood pressure, strokes, heart attacks, and deaths associated with their use. It has also set standards for maximum dosages of Ephedra in supplements, but some pills still contain more than the FDA limits. Adverse events have been reported even with dosages below these limits. Ephedra-containing supplements should be used with great caution, if at all.

Kava Kava

Kava kava is a widely-marketed supplement made from the Kava kava plant. It appears to have some sedative effects. It has been recommended for treating anxiety, sleeplessness, stress, and menopausal symptoms. The FDA has recently issued warnings regarding Kava-containing products. There have been multiple reports of severe liver inflammation, hepatitis, cirrhosis, liver failure, and death in Kava users. Concerns have also been raised about excessive sedation if Kava is taken in combination with alcohol or other drugs that cause drowsiness.

St. John's Wort

St. John's Wort has become a popular herbal supplement in recent years. It has been recommended for treating mild depression and anxiety. Additionally, some have recommended it for treatment of AIDS. Its effectiveness for depression is unclear. Several small studies showed effects similar to some prescription antidepressants. However, newer, large studies have found no effect on depression at all. Studies have failed to find any benefit in improving AIDS patients' health.

It has been known for some time that St. John's Wort can cause photosensitivity (unusual sensitivity to sunlight). People taking St. John's Wort need to be careful about sun exposure, because they will sometimes get severe sunburns from short periods in the sun.

Recently, it has been recognized that St. John's Wort interacts with a large number of prescription medications. If combined with prescription antidepressants, it can cause a serious condition called "serotonin syndrome" which can cause high blood pressure, life-threatening fever, seizures, and death. Additionally, it has been reported to decrease the effectiveness of many prescription drugs. It interferes with several drugs used to treat AIDS, causing them not to work properly. It also interferes with cyclosporine, a drug used to treat patients with organ transplants and certain diseases of the immune system. Several cases of organ rejection in heart transplant patients have been reported. The list of drugs known to have interactions with St. John's Wort is growing rapidly, with new ones discovered every month.

If you take any kind of prescription drug, you should ask your doctor first whether it is safe to use St. John's Wort. Keep in mind that this drug, like many herbal products, may have interactions with other drugs that have not been discovered yet.

Amino Acids

Amino acids are the individual parts that make up proteins. There are nine amino acids needed for growth and development in children and to maintain health in adults. Most people who eat food containing protein get enough of these essential amino acids in their diets.

When amino acids are marketed as dietary supplements they are sold as single compounds, in combinations of two or more amino acids, as components of protein powders, as chelated single compounds, or in chelated mixtures. Amino acids are promoted for a variety of uses, including body-building.

The Federation of American Societies for Experimental Biology (FASEB) conducted an exhaustive search of available data on amino acids and concluded that there was insufficient information to establish a safe intake level for any amino acids in dietary supplements, and that their safety should not be assumed. FASEB warned that consuming amino acids in dietary supplement form posed potential risks for several groups of people, including women of childbearing age (especially if pregnant or nursing), infants, children, adolescents, the elderly, individuals with inherited disorders of amino acid metabolism, and individuals with certain diseases. At least two of the amino acids consumed in dietary supplements have also been associated with serious injuries in healthy adults.

L-Tryptophan

L-tryptophan is associated with the most serious outbreak of illness and death known to be due to consumption of dietary supplements. In 1989, public health officials realized that an epidemic of eosinophilia-myalgia syndrome (EMS) was associated with the ingestion of L-tryptophan in a dietary supplement. EMS is a systemic connective tissue disease characterized by severe muscle pain, an increase in white blood cells, and certain skin and neuromuscular manifestations.

More than 1,500 cases of L-tryptophan-related EMS have been reported to the national Centers for Disease Control and Prevention (CDC). At least 38 patients are known to have died. The true incidence of L-tryptophan-related EMS is thought to be much higher. Some of the individuals suffering from L-tryptophan-related EMS have recovered, while other individuals' illnesses have persisted or worsened over time.

Phenylalanine

A number of illnesses, including those similar to the eosinophilia myalgia syndrome (EMS) associated with L-tryptophan consumption, have been reported to FDA in individuals using dietary supplements containing phenylalanine. There are also published reports of scleroderma/scleroderma-like illnesses, which have symptoms similar to EMS, occurring in children with poorly controlled blood phenylalanine levels, as well as in those with phenylketonuria (PKU), a genetic disorder characterized by the inability to metabolize phenylalanine.

Vitamins And Minerals

Vitamin and mineral dietary supplements have a long history of use at levels consistent with the Recommended Dietary Allowances (RDA's) or at low multiples of the RDA's, and are generally considered safe at these levels for most people. Intakes above the RDA, however, vary widely in their potential for adverse effects. Certain vitamins and minerals that are safe when consumed at low levels are toxic at higher doses. The difference between a safe low dose and a toxic higher dose is quite large for some vitamins and minerals and quite small for others.

Vitamin A

Vitamin A is found in several forms in dietary supplements. Preformed vitamin A (vitamin A acetate and vitamin A palmitate) has well-recognized toxicity when consumed at levels of 25,000 International Units (IU) per day, or higher. (Beta-carotene does not have the potential for adverse effects that the other forms of vitamin A do, because high intakes of beta-carotene are converted to vitamin A in the body at much lower levels). The RDA for vitamin A is 1,000 retinol equivalents (RE) for men, which is equivalent to 3,300 IU of preformed vitamin A, and 80 percent of these amounts for women.

The adverse effects associated with consumption of vitamin A at 25,000+ IU include severe liver injury (including cirrhosis), bone and cartilage diseases, elevated pressure in the brain, and birth defects in infants whose mothers consumed vitamin A during pregnancy. Groups especially vulnerable to vitamin A toxicity are children, pregnant women, and people with liver disease caused by a variety of factors, including alcohol, viral hepatitis, and severe protein-energy malnutrition.

There are some studies that suggest vitamin A toxicity has occurred at levels of ingestion below 25,000 IU. In addition, because the injuries that occur at 25,000 IU are so high, there may be substantial, but less severe and less readily recognized, injuries occurring at lower intakes. Most experts recommend that vitamin A intake not exceed 10,000 IU for most adults or 8,000 IU for pregnant and nursing women.

Vitamin B_6

Neurologic toxicity, including ataxia (alteration in balance) and sensory neuropathy (changes in sensations due to nerve injury), is associated with intake of vitamin B_6 (pyridoxine) supplements at levels above 100 milligrams per day. As

Remember!!

Some herbal and other "natural" products sold as dietary supplements have been associated with serious safety problems. In addition, they may have interactions with medications. Use caution and talk with your doctor whenever you take any substance—even if it is labeled "natural."

little as 50 milligrams per day has caused symptoms to resume in an individual previously injured by higher intakes. The RDA for vitamin B_6 is 2 milligrams. Vitamin B_6 is marketed in capsules containing dosages in the 100-, 200-, and 500-milligrams range.

Niacin (Nicotinic Acid And Nicotinamide)

Niacin taken in high doses is known to cause a wide range of adverse effects. The RDA for niacin is 20 milligrams. Niacin is marketed in dietary supplements at potencies of 250 mg, 400 mg, and 500 mg, in both immediate and slow-release formulations. Daily doses of 500 mg from slow-release formulations, and 750 mg of immediate-release niacin, have been associated with severe adverse reactions, including gastrointestinal distress (burning pain, nausea, vomiting, bloating, cramping, and diarrhea) and mild to severe liver damage. Less common, but more serious (in some cases life-threatening), reactions include liver injury, myopathy (muscle disease), maculopathy of the eyes (injury to the eyes resulting in decreased vision), coagulopathy (increased bleeding problems), cytopenia (decreases in cell types in the blood), hypotensive myocardial ischemia (heart injury caused by too low blood pressure), and metabolic acidosis (increases in the acidity of the blood and urine).

Niacin (nicotinic acid) is approved as a prescription drug to lower cholesterol. Many of the observed adverse reactions have occurred when patients have switched to OTC formulations of niacin, and particularly when they have switched from immediate-release formulations to dietary supplements containing slow-release niacin formulations without the knowledge of their physicians.

Selenium

Selenium is a mineral found in dietary supplement products. At high doses (approximately 800 to 1,000 micrograms per day), selenium can cause tissue damage, especially in tissues or organs that concentrate the element. The toxicity of selenium depends upon the chemical form of selenium in the ingested supplement and upon the selenium levels in the foods consumed. Human injuries have occurred following ingestion of high doses over a few weeks.

Chapter 29

Heroin

Heroin is a highly addictive drug, and its use is a serious problem in America. Recent studies suggest a shift from injecting heroin to snorting or smoking because of increased purity and the misconception that these forms of use will not lead to addiction.

Heroin is processed from morphine, a naturally occurring substance extracted from the seedpod of the Asian poppy plant. Heroin usually appears as a white or brown powder. Street names for heroin include "smack," "H," "skag," and "junk." Other names may refer to types of heroin produced in a specific geographical area, such as "Mexican black tar."

Pure heroin is a white powder with a bitter taste. Most illicit heroin is distributed in powder form and may vary in color from white to dark brown because of impurities left from the manufacturing process or the presence of additives. During the last decade, the purity of street heroin ranged from one to ten percent; more recently, the purity of heroin, especially that from South America, has skyrocketed to rates as high as 98 percent, with the national purity average at 41 percent.

Black tar heroin, which is produced in Mexico, may be sticky like roofing tar or hard like coal, and its color may vary from dark brown to black. The

About This Chapter: This chapter includes excerpts from "Heroin," National Institute on Drug Abuse (NIDA), Infofax No. 13548, October 2001; "Heroin," Drug Enforcement Administration (DEA); and "Heroin Information for Adolescents," Center for Substance Abuse and Prevention.

color and consistency of black tar heroin result from the crude processing methods used to illicitly manufacture heroin in Mexico. Black tar heroin is often sold on the street in its tar-like state at purities ranging from 20 to 80 percent. It is most frequently dissolved, diluted, and injected.

The effects that heroin may have on users include euphoria, drowsiness, respiratory depression, constricted pupils, and nausea. Effects of heroin overdose include slow and shallow breathing, clammy skin, convulsions, coma, and possible death.

✤ It's A Fact!!

Heroin is so addictive because it activates many regions of the brain, particularly the regions that are responsible for producing both the pleasurable sensation of "reward" and physical dependence. Together, these actions account for the user's loss of control and the drug's habit-forming action.

Health Hazards

Heroin abuse is associated with serious health conditions, including fatal overdose, spontaneous abortion, collapsed veins, and infectious diseases, including HIV/AIDS and hepatitis.

The short-term effects of heroin abuse appear soon after a single dose and disappear in a few hours. After an injection of heroin, the user reports feeling a surge of euphoria ("rush") accompanied by a warm flushing of the skin, a dry mouth, and heavy extremities. Following this initial euphoria, the user goes "on the nod," an alternately wakeful and drowsy state. Mental functioning becomes clouded due to the depression of the central nervous system. Long-term effects of heroin appear after repeated use for some period of time. Chronic users may develop collapsed veins, infection of the heart lining and valves, abscesses, cellulitis, and liver disease. Breathing complications, including various types of pneumonia, may result from the poor health condition of the abuser, as well as from heroin's depressing effects on respiration.

In addition to the effects of the drug itself, street heroin may have additives that do not readily dissolve and result in clogging the blood vessels that lead to the lungs, liver, kidneys, or brain. This can cause infection or even death of small patches of cells in vital organs.

Reports from the Substance Abuse and Mental Health Services Administration (SAMHSA)'s 1995 Drug Abuse Warning Network (DAWN), which collects data on drug-related hospital emergency room episodes and drug-related deaths from 21 metropolitan areas, rank heroin second as the most frequently mentioned drug in overall drug-related deaths. From 1990 through 1995, the number of heroin-related episodes doubled. Between 1994 and 1995, there was a 19 percent increase in heroin-related emergency department episodes.

✤ It's A Fact!!

What other problems are related to heroin use?

AIDS: Needle sharing by IV drug users is fast becoming the leading cause of new AIDS cases. The AIDS virus is carried in contaminated blood left in the needle, syringe, or other drug-related implements and is injected into the new user when he or she uses this equipment to inject heroin or other drugs. There is no cure for AIDS and no proven vaccine to prevent it.

Infants: Heroin use during pregnancy is associated with stillbirths and miscarriages. Babies born addicted to heroin must undergo withdrawal after birth, and these babies show a number of developmental problems.

Tolerance, Addiction, And Withdrawal

With regular heroin use, tolerance develops. This means the abuser must use more heroin to achieve the same intensity or effect. As higher doses are used over time, physical dependence and addiction develop. With physical dependence, the body has adapted to the presence of the drug and withdrawal symptoms may occur if use is reduced or stopped.

Withdrawal, which in regular abusers may occur as early as a few hours after the last administration, produces drug craving, restlessness, muscle and bone pain, insomnia, diarrhea and vomiting, cold flashes with goose bumps ("cold turkey"), kicking movements ("kicking the habit"), and other symptoms. Major withdrawal symptoms peak between 48 and 72 hours after the last dose and subside after about a week. Sudden withdrawal by heavily dependent users who are in poor health is occasionally fatal, although heroin withdrawal is considered much less dangerous than alcohol or barbiturate withdrawal.

✔ Quick Tip

How can you tell if someone is using heroin?

The signs and symptoms of heroin use include euphoria, drowsiness, respiratory depression (which can progress until breathing stops), constricted pupils, and nausea. Withdrawal symptoms include watery eyes, runny nose, yawning, loss of appetite, tremors, panic, chills, sweating, nausea, muscle cramps, and insomnia. Elevations in blood pressure, pulse, respiratory rate, and temperature occur as withdrawal progresses. Symptoms of a heroin overdose include shallow breathing, pinpoint pupils, clammy skin, convulsion, and coma.

Treatment

There is a broad range of treatment options for heroin addiction, including medications as well as behavioral therapies. Science has taught us that when medication treatment is integrated with other supportive services, patients are often able to stop heroin (or other opiate) use and return to more stable and productive lives.

In November 1997, the National Institutes of Health (NIH) convened a Consensus Panel on Effective Medical Treatment of Heroin Addiction. The panel of national experts concluded that opiate drug addictions are diseases of the brain and medical disorders that indeed can be treated effectively. The panel strongly recommended (1) broader access to methadone maintenance treatment programs for people who are addicted to heroin or other opiate drugs; and (2) the Federal and State regulations and other barriers impeding this access be eliminated. This panel also stressed the importance of providing substance abuse counseling, psychosocial therapies, and other supportive services to enhance retention and successful outcomes in methadone maintenance treatment programs.

Methadone, a synthetic opiate medication that blocks the effects of heroin for about 24 hours, has a proven record of success when prescribed at a high enough dosage level for people addicted to heroin. LAAM, also a synthetic opiate medication for treating heroin addiction, can block the effects of heroin for up to 72 hours. Other approved medications are naloxone, which is used to treat cases of overdose, and naltrexone, both of which block the effects of morphine, heroin, and other opiates. Several other medications for use in heroin treatment programs are also under study.

There are many effective behavioral treatments available for heroin addiction. These can include residential and outpatient approaches. Several new behavioral therapies are showing particular promise for heroin addiction. Contingency management therapy uses a voucher-based system, where patients earn "points" based on negative drug tests, which they can exchange for items that encourage healthful living. Cognitive-behavioral interventions are designed to help modify the patient's thinking, expectancies, and behaviors and to increase skills in coping with various life stressors.

Extent Of Use

Monitoring The Future Study

The Monitoring the Future (MTF) survey is conducted by the University of Michigan's Institute for Social Research and is funded by National Institute on Drug Abuse, National Institutes of Health; it has tracked 12th graders' illicit drug use and related attitudes since 1975. In 1991, 8th and 10th graders were added to the study. For the 1998 study, 49,866 students were surveyed from a representative sample of 422 public and private schools nationwide. Copies of the latest survey are available from the National Clearinghouse for Alcohol and Drug Information at 1-800-729-6686.

According to the 1999 MTF, rates of heroin use remained relatively stable and low since the late 1970s. After 1991, however, use began to rise among 10th- and 12th-graders, and after 1993, among 8th-graders. In 1999, prevalence of heroin use was comparable for all three grade levels. Although past year prevalence rates for heroin use remained relatively low in 1999, these rates are about two to three times higher than those reported in 1991.

Community Epidemiology Work Group

The Community Epidemiology Work Group (CEWG) is a NIDA-sponsored network of researchers from 20 major U.S. metropolitan areas and selected foreign countries who meet semiannually to discuss the current epidemiology of drug abuse.

In June 2000, CEWG members reported that heroin indicators showed mixed trends. Mortality figures were mixed, with deaths increasing notably in Austin, Detroit, Minneapolis/St. Paul, and Phoenix, and declining in Miami, Philadelphia, St. Louis, San Diego, and Seattle. Emergency room admissions were also mixed, with 10 cities showing decreases (significant in San Francisco and Washington, D.C.), and 10 showing increases (particularly Baltimore and Miami). Heroin continues to account for a substantial proportion of treatment admissions in some CEWG areas (for example, 47.8 percent in Baltimore, 43 percent in New York City, and 32 percent in Detroit). Heroin injection characterizes a large proportion of primary heroin treatment admissions (for example, 90 percent in Texas). During the second quarter of 1999, the highest purity levels were found in Philadelphia (71 percent); New York (63.6 percent); Boston (61.4 percent); Newark (60.7 percent); Atlanta (57.8 percent); and San Diego (57.6 percent). Purity levels in other CEWG areas ranged from 11.8 percent in Dallas to 46.7 percent in Detroit. Injecting is on an upward trend among younger users in Baltimore, Boston, Minneapolis/St. Paul, Newark, New York City, and Seattle. In Boston, Chicago, Denver, Miami, and Washington, D.C., snorting seems to be increasing and is often the starting route for new users.

National Household Survey On Drug Abuse

The National Household Survey on Drug Abuse (NHSDA) is an annual survey conducted by the Substance Abuse and Mental Health Services administration. Copies of the latest survey are available from the National Clearinghouse for Alcohol and Drug Information at 1-800-729-6686.

✤ It's A Fact!!

Heroin Use Among Teens

Rates of heroin use among teenagers rose significantly in eighth, tenth, and twelfth grades during the 1990s. In addition, regular users of heroin started using the drug at an earlier age. The 1999 NHSDA found that the mean age of initiation for heroin declined from 26 years in 1992 to 21.3 in 1998. However, there are some indications that heroin use among youth may have begun to level-off or decline in the later part of this decade. The 1999 Monitoring the Future survey found little change between 1996 and 1999 in annual use among tenth and twelfth graders, and concluded that use in the eighth grade has leveled-off and may have declined. Also, the report discovered that more young people perceive heroin as dangerous; 73.7 percent of tenth graders thought that trying heroin was a "great risk"—the highest percentage recorded in five years.

The 1999 NHSDA study reports the use of illicit drugs by those people age 12 and older. The lifetime prevalence (at least one use in a persons lifetime) for heroin for those people age 12 and older was 1.4 percent. By age category, 0.4 percent were in the 12-17 range; 1.8 percent were 18-25; and 1.4 percent were users age 26 and older.

How Does Heroin Get Into The U.S.?

The sources and types of heroin available in parts of the United States vary from region to region. Most of the heroin found in the eastern United States is from South America, while heroin found in the West is usually black tar heroin from Mexico.

Most of the heroin seized by the DEA now comes from Colombia and Mexico. Previously, Southeast and Southwest Asian heroin dominated the U.S. market, but these types are no longer available in sizable quantities in cities along the East Coast, where, historically, there had been the greatest demand for heroin. In 1998, the DEA Heroin Signature Program indicated that 65 percent of the heroin seized in the United States originated in South America and another 17 percent came from Mexico. Further evidence of increasing amounts of Mexican heroin was substantiated in a 1998 independent study that indicated that 29 percent of the heroin used in the United States comes from Mexico.

Remember!!

Heroin is an illegal opiate drug. It is highly addictive as users find that they have a need for persistent, repeated use of the drug (known as craving) and that their attempts to stop using the drug lead to significant and painful physical withdrawal symptoms. Use of heroin causes physical and psychological problems such as shallow breathing, nausea, panic, insomnia, and a need for increasingly higher doses of the drug to get the same effect.

Chapter 30

Inhalants

Inhalants are breathable chemical vapors that produce psychoactive (mind-altering) effects. Although people are exposed to volatile solvents and other inhalants in the home and in the workplace, many do not think of inhalable substances as drugs because most of them were never meant to be used in that way.

Young people are likely to abuse inhalants, in part because inhalants are readily available and inexpensive.

Types Of Inhalants

Although other abused substances can be inhaled, the term "inhalants" is used to describe a variety of substances whose main common characteristic is that they are rarely, if ever, taken by any route other than inhalation. This definition encompasses a broad range of chemicals found in hundreds of different products that may have different effects on the body. As a result, precise categorization of inhalants is difficult. One classification system lists four general categories of inhalants—volatile solvents, aerosols, gases, and nitrites—based on the form in which they are often found in household, industrial, and medical products.

About This Chapter: This chapter includes text from "Inhalant Abuse," *Research Report Series*, National Institute on Drug Abuse (NIDA), NIH Pub. No. 00-3810, revised July 2000; "Inhalants," NIDA, Infofax No. 13549, October 2001; and "Tips for Teens: The Truth About Inhalants," National Clearinghouse for Alcohol and Drug Information, 1998.

- **Volatile solvents** are liquids that vaporize at room temperatures. They are found in a multitude of inexpensive, easily available products used for common household and industrial purposes.
- **Aerosols** are sprays that contain propellants and solvents.
- **Gases** include medical anesthetics as well as gases used in household or commercial products. Medical anesthetic gases include ether, chloroform, halothane, and nitrous oxide, commonly called "laughing gas. Nitrous oxide is the most abused of these gases.
- **Nitrites** often are considered a special class of inhalants. Unlike most other inhalants, which act directly on the central nervous system (CNS), nitrites act primarily to dilate blood vessels and relax the muscles. And while other inhalants are used to alter mood, nitrites are used primarily as sexual enhancers. Nitrites include cyclohexyl nitrite, isoamyl (amyl) nitrite, and isobutyl (butyl) nitrite.

What Are The Patterns Of Inhalant Abuse?

Inhalants—particularly volatile solvents, gases, and aerosols—are often among the first drugs that young people use. One national survey indicates about 6 percent of U.S. children have tried inhalants by the time they reach fourth grade. Inhalants also are one of the few substances abused more by younger children than by older ones. Nevertheless, inhalant abuse can become

✎ Weird Words

Terms Related To Inhalant Abuse

Anesthetic: An agent that causes loss of sensation.

Central Nervous System: The brain and spinal cord.

Dementia: A condition of deteriorated mentality.

Dopamine: A neurotransmitter present in regions of the brain that regulate movement, emotion, motivation, and feeling of pleasure.

Epidemiology: The sum of the factors controlling the presence or absence of a disease or condition.

Toxic: Causing temporary or permanent effects that are detrimental to the functioning of a body organ or group of organs.

Withdrawal: A variety of symptoms that occur after use of an addictive drug is reduced or stopped.

chronic and extend into adulthood. Generally, inhalant abusers will abuse any available substance. However, effects produced by individual inhalants vary, and some individuals will go out of their way to obtain their favorite inhalant.

Data from national and state surveys suggest inhalant abuse reaches its peak at some point during the seventh through ninth grades. For example,

✎ Weird Words

Chemicals Found In Commonly Abused Inhalants

Amyl Nitrite, Butyl Nitrite (also called "poppers," "video head cleaner"): Can cause sudden sniffing death syndrome, suppressed immunologic function, and injury to red blood cells (interfering with oxygen supply to vital tissues).

Benzene: Found in gasoline; can cause bone marrow injury, impaired immunologic function, increased risk of leukemia, and reproductive system toxicity.

Butane, Propane: Found in lighter fluid, hair and paint sprays; can cause sudden sniffing death syndrome via cardiac effects and serious burn injuries (because of flammability).

Freon: Used as a refrigerant and aerosol propellant; can cause sudden sniffing death syndrome, respiratory obstruction and death (from sudden cooling/cold injury to airways), and liver damage.

Methylene Chloride: Found in paint thinners and removers and degreasers; can cause reduction of oxygen-carrying capacity of blood, changes to the heart muscle and heartbeat.

Nitrous Oxide (also called "laughing gas") and Hexane: Can cause death from lack of oxygen to the brain, altered perception and motor coordination, loss of sensation, limb spasms, blackouts caused by blood pressure changes, and depression of heart muscle functioning.

Toluene: Found in gasoline, paint thinners and removers, and correction fluid; can cause brain damage (loss of brain tissue mass, impaired cognition, gait disturbance, loss of coordination, loss of equilibrium, limb spasms, hearing and vision loss), and liver and kidney damage.

Trichloroethylene: Found in spot removers and degreasers; can cause sudden sniffing death syndrome, cirrhosis of the liver, reproductive complications, and hearing and vision damage.

the American Drug and Alcohol Survey of children in the 4th through 12th grades indicates that the percentage of children who have ever used inhalants peaks in the 8th grade. In the Monitoring the Future (MTF) study, an annual survey supported by the National Institute of Drug Abuse (NIDA) of the Nation's secondary school students, 8th-graders also regularly report the highest rate of current, past year, and lifetime inhalant abuse; 10th- and 12th-graders report less abuse.

Gender differences in inhalant abuse have been identified at different points in childhood. One study indicates inhalant abuse is higher for boys than girls in grades 4 through 6, occurs at similar rates in grades 7 through 9—when overall use is highest—and becomes more prevalent again among boys in grades 10 through 12. The National Household Survey on Drug Abuse (NHSDA), an annual survey of drug use among the Nation's noninstitutionalized civilians, reports that similar percentages of 12- to 17-year-old boys and girls abused inhalants in 1998. However, the percentage of 18- to 25-year-old males who abused inhalants was more than twice that of females in that age group, suggesting that sustained abuse of inhalants is more common among males.

✤ It's A Fact!!

Inhalants affect your brain. Inhalants are substances or fumes from products such as glue or paint thinner that are sniffed or "huffed" to cause an immediate high. Because they affect your brain with much greater speed and force than many other substances, they can cause irreversible physical and mental damage before you know what's happened.

Inhalants affect your heart. Inhalants starve the body of oxygen and force the heart to beat irregularly and more rapidly—that can be dangerous for your body.

Inhalants damage other parts of your body. People who use inhalants can lose their sense of smell; experience nausea and nosebleeds; and develop liver, lung, and kidney problems. Chronic use can lead to muscle wasting and reduced muscle tone and strength.

Inhalants can cause sudden death. Inhalants can kill you instantly. Inhalant users can die by suffocation, choking on their vomit, or having a heart attack.

People who abuse inhalants are found in both urban and rural settings. Research on factors contributing to inhalant abuse suggests that adverse socioeconomic conditions, rather than racial or cultural factors per se, may account for most reported racial and ethnic differences in rates of inhalant abuse. Poverty, a history of childhood abuse, poor grades, and dropping out of school all are associated with inhalant abuse. Native American youths who live on reservations, where socioeconomic distress and school dropout rates are high, typically have higher rates of inhalant abuse than both the general population of young people and those Native American youths who do not live on reservations.

What Is The Scope Of Inhalant Abuse?

Inhalant abuse among the nation's 8th-, 10th-, and 12th-graders declined in 1999, continuing an apparent gradual decline that began in 1996, according to MTF data. For example:

- The percentage of high school seniors who abused any inhalants declined to 5.6 percent in 1999 from a peak of 8 percent in 1995. Abuse of nitrites, specifically, also declined to less than 1 percent (0.9) among seniors in 1999.
- Abuse of all inhalants by 10th-graders declined to 7.2 percent in 1999, from 9.6 percent in 1995.
- Among eighth-graders, abuse declined to 10.3 percent in 1999 from 12.8 percent in 1995.

Despite the declines in abuse among schoolchildren in recent years, inhalants are still being abused at higher rates than they were a decade ago, according to the NHSDA. The 1998 survey indicates that the rate of first use among 12- to 17-year-olds rose significantly from 8.4 to 18.8 per 1,000 potential new users from 1989 to 1995 and remained at those levels through 1997. The rate of first use of inhalants for young adults aged 18 to 25 also rose, from 3.7 to 10.7 per 1,000 potential new users between 1989 and 1996, before leveling off in 1997.

MTF's lifetime prevalence figures also indicate that the percentages of students who have tried inhalants remain at high levels. In 1999, 19.7 percent of

8th-graders, 17.0 percent of 10th-graders, and 15. 4 percent of 12th-graders said they had abused inhalants at least once in their lives. These data raise a question: How can fewer 12th-graders than 8th-graders consistently report they have ever abused inhalants? Possibly, many 12th-graders fail to recall their much earlier use of inhalants or, more troubling, many 8th-grade inhalant abusers may have dropped out of school by the 12th grade and are no longer included in the survey population. The latter explanation is supported by research that shows higher rates of inhalant abuse among children who have poor grades or have dropped out of school than among their classmates who remain in good standing in school.

Inhalants Cause Toxic Effects

Inhaled chemicals are rapidly absorbed through the lungs into the bloodstream and quickly distributed to the brain and other organs. Within minutes of inhalation, the user experiences intoxication along with other effects similar to those produced by alcohol. Alcohol-like effects may include slurred speech, an inability to coordinate movements, euphoria, and dizziness. In addition, users may experience lightheadedness, hallucinations, and delusions, such as thinking they can fly.

Because intoxication lasts only a few minutes, abusers frequently seek to prolong the high by continuing to inhale repeatedly over the course of several hours, a very dangerous practice. With successive inhalations, abusers can suffer loss of consciousness and death. At the least, they will feel less inhibited and less in control. After heavy use of inhalants, abusers may feel drowsy for several hours and experience a lingering headache.

Many brain systems may be involved in the anesthetic, intoxicating, and reinforcing effects of different inhalants. Nearly all abused inhalants (other than nitrites) produce an effect by depressing the CNS. A recent study indicates that toluene, a solvent found in many commonly abused inhalants, activates the brain's dopamine system. The dopamine system has been shown to play a role in how the use of many other drugs of abuse can lead to addiction. Nitrites, in contrast, dilate and relax blood vessels rather than acting as anesthetic agents.

Health Hazards

Although different in makeup, nearly all abused inhalants produce effects similar to anesthetics, which act to slow down the body's functions. When inhaled via the nose or mouth into the lungs in sufficient concentrations, inhalants can cause intoxicating effects. Intoxication can last only a few minutes or several hours if inhalants are taken repeatedly. Initially, users may feel slightly stimulated; with successive inhalations, they may feel less inhibited and less in control; finally, a user can lose consciousness.

✔ Quick Tip

How can you tell if a friend is using inhalants? Sometimes it's tough to tell. But there are signs you can look for. If your friend has one or more of the following warning signs, he or she may be using inhalants:

- Slurred speech
- Drunk, dizzy, or dazed appearance
- Unusual breath odor
- Chemical smell on clothing
- Paint stains on body or face
- Red eyes
- Runny nose

What can you do to help someone who is using inhalants? Be a real friend. Save a life. Encourage your friend to seek professional help. For information and referrals, call the National Clearinghouse for Alcohol and Drug Information at 800-729-6686.

Sniffing highly concentrated amounts of the chemicals in solvents or aerosol sprays can directly induce heart failure and death. This is especially common from the abuse of fluorocarbons and butane-type gases. High concentrations of inhalants also cause death from suffocation by displacing oxygen in the lungs and then in the central nervous system so that breathing ceases. Other irreversible effects caused by inhaling specific solvents are as follows:

- Hearing loss: from toluene (paint sprays, glues, dewaxers) and trichloroethylene (cleaning fluids, correction fluids)
- Peripheral neuropathies or limb spasms: from hexane (glues, gasoline) and nitrous oxide (whipping cream, gas cylinders)
- Central nervous system or brain damage: from toluene (paint sprays, glues, dewaxers)
- Bone marrow damage: from benzene (gasoline).

Serious but potentially reversible effects include:

- Liver and kidney damage: from toluene-containing substances and chlorinated hydrocarbons (correction fluids, dry-cleaning fluids)
- Blood oxygen depletion: from organic nitrites ("poppers," "bold," and "rush") and methylene chloride (varnish removers, paint thinners).

Death from inhalants usually is caused by a very high concentration of fumes. Deliberately inhaling from an attached paper or plastic bag or in a closed area greatly increases the chances of suffocation. Even when using aerosols or volatile products for their legitimate purposes (that is, painting, cleaning, etc.), it is wise to do so in a well-ventilated room or outdoors.

Amyl and butyl nitrites have been associated with Kaposi's sarcoma (KS), the most common cancer reported among AIDS patients. Early studies of KS showed that many people with KS had used volatile nitrites. Researchers are continuing to explore the hypothesis of nitrites as a factor contributing to the development of KS in HIV-infected people.

✤ It's A Fact!!

Inhalant abusers risk devastating medical consequences. Prolonged sniffing of the highly concentrated chemicals in solvents or aerosol sprays can induce irregular and rapid heart rhythms and lead to heart failure and death within minutes of a session of prolonged sniffing. This syndrome, known as "sudden sniffing death," can result from a single session of inhalant use by an otherwise healthy young person. Sudden sniffing death is particularly associated with the abuse of butane, propane, and chemicals in aerosols. Inhalant abuse also can cause death by:

- *Asphyxiation*: From repeated inhalations, which lead to high concentrations of inhaled fumes displacing the available oxygen in the lungs;
- *Suffocation*: From blocking air from entering the lungs when inhaling fumes from a plastic bag placed over the head;
- *Choking*: From inhalation of vomit after inhalant use; or
- *Fatal injury*: From accidents, including motor vehicle fatalities, suffered while intoxicated.

Special Risks For Nitrite Abusers

Nitrites are abused mainly by older adolescents and adults. Typically, individuals who abuse nitrites are seeking to enhance sexual function and pleasure. Research shows that abuse of these drugs in this context is associated with unsafe sexual practices that greatly increase the risk of contracting and spreading such infectious diseases as HIV/AIDS and hepatitis.

✔ Quick Tip

Fact sheets on the health effects of inhalants and other abused drugs and other drug abuse topics can be ordered free of charge, in English and Spanish, from NIDA Infofax at 1-888-NIH-NIDA (1-888-644-6432) or, for deaf persons, 1-888-TTY-NIDA (1-888-889-6432).

Information is available also on the NIDA Web site (www.drugabuse.gov) or the NCADI Web site (www.health.org).

Recent animal research raises the possibility that there may be a link between abuse of nitrite inhalants and the development and progression of infectious diseases and tumors. The research indicates that inhaling nitrites depletes many cells in the immune system and impairs immune system mechanisms that fight infectious diseases. A recent study found that even a relatively small number of exposures to butyl nitrite can produce dramatic increases in tumor incidence and growth rates in animals.

Questions And Answers About Inhalants

Since inhalants are found in household products, aren't they safe?

No. Even though household products have legal, useful purposes, when they are used as inhalants they are harmful and dangerous. These products are not intended to be inhaled.

Doesn't it take many "huffs" before you're in danger?

No. One "huff" of an inhalant can kill you. Or the 10th. Or the 100th. Every huff can be dangerous. Even if you have huffed before without experiencing a problem, there's no way of knowing how the next huff will affect you.

Can inhalants make me lose control?

Yes. Inhalants affect your brain and can cause you to suddenly engage in violent, or even deadly, behavior. You could hurt yourself or the people you love.

Where can I get further scientific information about inhalant abuse?

To learn more about inhalants and other drugs of abuse, contact the National Clearinghouse for Alcohol and Drug Information (NCADI) at 1-800-729-6686. Information specialists are available to help you locate information and resources.

Remember!!

Inhalants include a large group of chemicals that are found in such household products as aerosol sprays, cleaning fluids, glue, paint, paint thinner, gasoline, propane, nail polish remover, correction fluid, and marker pens. None of these are safe to inhale—they all can kill you. Inhalants can kill you the very first time you use them.

If you know someone who uses inhalants, urge him or her to stop or get help. If you're using inhalants—stop. The longer you ignore the real facts, the more chances you take with your life.

Chapter 31

Marijuana

Marijuana is a green or gray mixture of dried, shredded flowers and leaves of the hemp plant *Cannabis sativa*. There are over 200 slang terms for marijuana including "pot," "herb," "weed," "boom," "Mary Jane," "gangster," and "chronic." It is usually smoked as a cigarette (called a joint or a nail) or in a pipe or bong. In recent years, marijuana has appeared in blunts, which are cigars that have been emptied of tobacco and refilled with marijuana, often in combination with another drug, such as crack. Some users also mix marijuana into foods or use it to brew tea.

The main active chemical in marijuana is THC (delta-9-tetrahydrocannabinol). In 1988, it was discovered that the membranes of certain nerve cells contain protein receptors that bind THC. Once securely in place, THC kicks off a series of cellular reactions that ultimately lead to the high that users experience when they smoke marijuana. The short term effects of marijuana use include problems with memory and learning; distorted perception; difficulty in thinking and problem-solving; loss of coordination; and increased heart rate, anxiety, and panic attacks.

Scientists have found that whether an individual has positive or negative sensations after smoking marijuana can be influenced by heredity. A recent

About This Chapter: This chapter includes text from "Marijuana," National Institute on Drug Abuse (NIDA), Infofax No. 13551, October 2001; "Marijuana: Facts for Teens," NIDA, updated March 2001; and "Tips for Teens: The Truth About Marijuana," National Clearinghouse for Alcohol and Drug Information, 1998.

study demonstrated that identical male twins were more likely than non-identical male twins to report similar responses to marijuana use, indicating a genetic basis for their sensations. Identical twins share all of their genes, and fraternal twins share about half.

Environmental factors such as the availability of marijuana, expectations about how the drug would affect them, the influence of friends and social contacts, and other factors that differentiate identical twins' experiences also were found to have an important effect; however, it also was discovered that the twins' shared or family environment before age 18 had no detectable influence on their response to marijuana.

Health Hazards

Effects Of Marijuana On The Brain

Researchers have found that THC changes the way in which sensory information gets into and is processed by the hippocampus. The hippocampus is a component of the brain's limbic system that is crucial for learning, memory, and the integration of sensory experiences with emotions and motivations. Investigations have shown that neurons in the information processing system of the hippocampus and the activity of the nerve fibers in this region are suppressed by THC. In addition, researchers have discovered that learned behaviors, which depend on the hippocampus, also deteriorate via this mechanism.

✎ Weird Words

Slang Terms for Marijuana Include: Weed, Pot, Grass, Reefer, Ganja, Mary Jane, Blunt, Joint, Roach, Nail, Herb, Boom, Gangster, and Chronic

Recent research findings also indicate that long-term use of marijuana produces changes in the brain similar to those seen after long-term use of other major drugs of abuse.

Effects On The Lungs

Someone who smokes marijuana regularly may have many of the same respiratory problems as tobacco smokers. These individuals may have daily cough and phlegm, symptoms of chronic bronchitis, and more frequent chest colds. Continuing to smoke marijuana can lead to abnormal functioning of lung tissue injured or destroyed by marijuana smoke.

Regardless of the THC content, the amount of tar inhaled by marijuana smokers and the level of carbon monoxide absorbed are three to five times greater than among tobacco smokers. This may be due to the marijuana users' inhaling more deeply and holding the smoke in the lungs and because marijuana smoke is unfiltered.

Effects On Heart Rate And Blood Pressure

Recent findings indicate that smoking marijuana while shooting up cocaine has the potential to cause severe increases in heart rate and blood pressure. In one study, experienced marijuana and cocaine users were given marijuana alone, cocaine alone, and then a combination of both. Each drug alone produced cardiovascular effects; when they were combined, the effects were greater and lasted longer. The heart rate of the subjects in the study increased 29 beats per minute with marijuana alone and 32 beats per minute with cocaine alone. When the drugs were given together, the heart rate increased by 49 beats per minute, and the increased rate persisted for a longer time. The drugs were given with the subjects sitting quietly. In normal circumstances, an individual may smoke marijuana and inject cocaine and then do something physically stressful that may significantly increase the risk of overloading the cardiovascular system.

Effects Of Marijuana Use On Learning And Social Behavior

A study of college students has shown that critical skills related to attention, memory, and learning are impaired among people who use marijuana heavily, even after discontinuing its use for at least 24 hours. Researchers compared 65 "heavy users," who had smoked marijuana a median of 29 of the past 30 days, and 64 "light users," who had smoked a median of 1 of the past 30 days. After a closely monitored 19- to 24-hour period of abstinence from marijuana and other illicit drugs and alcohol, the undergraduates were given several standard tests measuring aspects of attention, memory, and learning. Compared to the light users, heavy marijuana users made more errors and had more difficulty sustaining attention, shifting attention to meet the demands of changes in the environment, and in registering, processing, and using information. These findings suggest that the greater impairment among heavy users is likely due to an alteration of brain activity produced by marijuana.

Other research on marijuana use among young people below college age indicates those who used marijuana have lower achievement than the non-users,

♣ It's A Fact!!

Marijuana affects your brain. THC (the active ingredient in marijuana) affects damages the nerve cells in the part of the brain where memories are formed, making it hard to remember things.

Marijuana affects your self-control. Marijuana can seriously affect your sense of time and your ability to do things that require coordination—like driving. In 1998, nearly 77,000 people were admitted to emergency rooms suffering from marijuana-related problems. This was an increase of more than 373 percent since 1991.

Marijuana affects your lungs. There are more than 400 known chemicals in marijuana. A single joint contains four times as much cancer-causing tar as a filtered cigarette.

Marijuana affects other aspects of your health. Marijuana can limit your body's ability to fight off infection. It can increase your heart rate and lead to frequent chest colds. Some research even shows that long-term marijuana use can increase the risk of developing certain mental illnesses.

Marijuana is not always what it seems. Before it is sold, marijuana can be laced with other dangerous drugs without your knowledge. "Blunts" —hollowed-out cigars filled with marijuana—sometimes have substances such as crack cocaine, PCP, or embalming fluid added to them.

Marijuana can be addictive. As with alcohol and many other drugs, not everyone who uses marijuana becomes addicted, but some users do develop signs of dependence on the drug. They may experience such withdrawal symptoms as loss of appetite, sleep problems, weight loss, and shaky hands. In 1995, 165,000 people entered drug treatment programs to kick their marijuana habit.

more acceptance of deviant behavior, more delinquent behavior and aggression, greater rebelliousness, poorer relationships with parents, and more associations with delinquent and drug-using friends.

Research also shows more anger and more regressive behavior (thumb sucking, temper tantrums) in toddlers whose parents use marijuana than among the toddlers of non-using parents.

Effects On Pregnancy

Any drug of abuse can affect a mother's health during pregnancy, making it a time when expectant mothers should take special care of themselves. Drugs of abuse may interfere with proper nutrition and rest, which can affect good functioning of the immune system. Some studies have found that babies born to mothers who used marijuana during pregnancy were smaller than those born to mothers who did not use the drug. In general, smaller babies are more likely to develop health problems.

A nursing mother who uses marijuana passes some of the THC to the baby in her breast milk. Research indicates that the use of marijuana by a mother during the first month of breast-feeding can impair the infant's motor development (control of muscle movement).

Addictive Potential

A drug is addicting if it causes compulsive, often uncontrollable drug craving, seeking, and use, even in the face of negative health and social consequences. Marijuana meets this criterion. More than 120,000 people enter treatment per year for their primary marijuana addiction. In addition, animal studies suggest marijuana causes physical dependence, and some people report withdrawal symptoms.

Extent Of Use

Monitoring The Future Study

Monitoring the Future (MTF) is an annual survey on drug use and related attitudes of America's adolescents that began in 1975. The survey is conducted by the University of Michigan's Institute for Social Research and is funded by NIDA. Copies of the latest survey are available from the National Clearinghouse for Alcohol and Drug Information at 1-800-729-6686.

MTF provides an annual assessment of drug use among 12th, 10th, and 8th grade students and young adults nationwide. After decreasing for over a decade, marijuana use among students began to increase in the early 1990s. From 1998 to 1999, use of marijuana at least once (lifetime use) increased among 12th- and 10th-graders, continuing the trend seen in recent years. The seniors' rate of lifetime marijuana use is higher than any year since 1987, but all rates remain well below those seen in the late 1970s and early 1980s. Past year and past month marijuana use did not change significantly from 1998 to 1999 in any of the three grades, suggesting the sharp increases of recent years may be slowing. Daily marijuana use in the past month increased slightly among all three grades as well.

Community Epidemiology Work Group

CEWG is a NIDA-sponsored network of researchers from 20 major U.S. metropolitan areas and selected foreign countries who meet semiannually to discuss the current epidemiology of drug abuse. CEWG's most recent reports are available on the CEWG web site (www.nida.nih.gov/CEWG/CEWGHome.html).

✔ Quick Tip

How can you tell if a friend is using marijuana?

Sometimes it's tough to tell. But there are signs you can look for. If your friend has one or more of the following warning signs, he or she may be using marijuana:

- Seeming dizzy and having trouble walking
- Having red, bloodshot eyes
- Having a hard time remembering things that just happened
- Acting disinterested in school, family, or activities he or she used to enjoy
- Acting silly for no apparent reason

What can you do to help someone who is using marijuana or other drugs? Be a real friend. Encourage your friend to seek professional help. For information and referrals, call the National Clearinghouse for Alcohol and Drug Information at (800) 729-6686.

In 1998, marijuana indicators continued an upward trend in most of the 20 CEWG metropolitan areas. Rates of emergency department mentions of marijuana increased significantly in seven sites, with the largest increases occurring in Dallas (emergency room mentions increased to 63.9 percent), Boston (to 44.1 percent), Denver (to 40 percent), San Diego (to 35.1 percent), and Atlanta (to 31.7 percent). The highest percent increase in emergency room mentions comparing the first half of 1997 and the first half of 1998 was among 12- to 17-year olds.

Treatment data for primary abuse of marijuana increased in six CEWG sites and remained stable elsewhere. Marijuana treatment admissions were highest in Denver (41 percent of all admissions), Miami (30 percent), New Orleans (22 percent), and Minneapolis/St. Paul (20 percent). Half of the treatment admissions for marijuana in Minneapolis/St. Paul were under age 18.

In six of the CEWG sites, juvenile arrestees testing positive for marijuana ranged from a low of 40.3 percent in St. Louis to a high of 63.7 percent in Phoenix. More than 50 percent of juvenile arrestees in Los Angeles, Denver, and Washington, D.C. tested positive for marijuana, and 48.9 percent in San Diego. Among all arrestees, Seattle was the only site where women were more likely than men (37.9 percent vs. 35.4 percent) to test positive for marijuana.

National Household Survey On Drug Abuse

The National Household Survey on Drug Abuse (NHSDA) is an annual survey conducted by the Substance Abuse and Mental Health Services Administration. Copies of the latest survey are available from the National Clearinghouse for Alcohol and Drug Information at 800-729-6686.

Marijuana remains the most commonly used illicit drug in the United States. There were an estimated 2.1 million people who started using marijuana in 1998. According to data from the 1998 NHSDA, more than 72.0 million Americans (33 percent) 12 years of age and older have tried marijuana at least once in their lifetimes, and almost 18.7 million (8.6 percent) had used marijuana in the past year. In 1985, 56.5 million Americans (29.4 percent) had tried marijuana at least once in their lifetimes, and 26.1 million (13.6 percent) had used marijuana within the past year.

Questions And Answers About Marijuana

> **✤ It's A Fact!!**
> Most teenagers do not use marijuana. Fewer than one in four high school seniors is a current marijuana user.

What is marijuana? Aren't there different kinds?

Marijuana is a green, brown, or gray mixture of dried, shredded leaves, stems, seeds, and flowers of the hemp plant. You may hear marijuana called by street names such as pot, herb, weed, grass, boom, Mary Jane, gangster, or chronic. There are more than 200 slang terms for marijuana.

Sinsemilla (pronounced "sin-seh-me-yah"; it's a Spanish word), hashish ("hash" for short), and hash oil are stronger forms of marijuana.

All forms of marijuana are mind-altering. In other words, they change how the brain works. They all contain THC (delta-9-tetrahydrocannabinol), the main active chemical in marijuana. They also contain more than 400 other chemicals. Marijuana's effects on the user depend on the strength or potency of the THC it contains. THC potency of marijuana has increased since the 1970s but has been about the same since the mid-1980s.

How is marijuana used?

Marijuana is usually smoked as a cigarette (called a joint or a nail) or in a pipe or a bong. Recently, it has appeared in cigars called blunts.

How long does marijuana stay in the user's body?

THC in marijuana is strongly absorbed by fatty tissues in various organs. Generally, traces (metabolites) of THC can be detected by standard urine testing methods several days after a smoking session. However, in heavy chronic users, traces can sometimes be detected for weeks after they have stopped using marijuana.

How many teens smoke marijuana?

Contrary to popular belief most teenagers have not used marijuana and never will. Among students surveyed in a yearly national survey, only about one in five 10th graders report they are current marijuana users (that is, used marijuana within the past month). Fewer than one in four high school seniors is a current marijuana user.

Why do young people use marijuana?

There are many reasons why some children and young teens start smoking marijuana. Most young people smoke marijuana because their friends or brothers and sisters use marijuana and pressure them to try it. Some young people use it because they see older people in the family using it.

Others may think it's cool to use marijuana because they hear songs about it and see it on TV and in movies. Some teens may feel they need marijuana and other drugs to help them escape from problems at home, at school, or with friends.

No matter how many shirts and caps you see printed with the marijuana leaf, or how many groups sing about it, remember this: You don't have to use marijuana just because you think everybody else is doing it. Most teens do not use marijuana.

What happens if you smoke marijuana?

The effects of the drug on each person depend on the user's experience, as well as:

- how strong the marijuana is (how much THC it has);
- what the user expects to happen;
- where (the place) the drug is used;
- how it is taken; and
- whether the user is drinking alcohol or using other drugs.

Some people feel nothing at all when they smoke marijuana. Others may feel relaxed or high. Sometimes marijuana makes users feel thirsty and very hungry—an effect called "the munchies."

Some users can get bad effects from marijuana. They may suffer sudden feelings of anxiety and have paranoid thoughts. This is more likely to happen when a more potent variety of marijuana is used.

What are the short-term effects of marijuana use?

The short-term effects of marijuana include:

- problems with memory and learning;
- distorted perception (sights, sounds, time, touch);
- trouble with thinking and problem-solving;
- loss of coordination; and
- increased heart rate, anxiety.

✤ It's A Fact!!

Using marijuana or other drugs increases your risk of injury from car crashes, falls, burns, drowning, and other accidents.

These effects are even greater when other drugs are mixed with the marijuana; and users do not always know what drugs are given to them.

Does marijuana affect school, sports, or other activities?

It can. Marijuana affects memory, judgment and perception. The drug can make you mess up in school, in sports or clubs, or with your friends. If you're high on marijuana, you are more likely to make stupid mistakes that could embarrass or even hurt you. If you use marijuana a lot, you could start to lose interest in how you look and how you're getting along at school or work.

Athletes could find their performance is off; timing, movements, and coordination are all affected by THC. Also, since marijuana use can affect thinking and judgment, users can possibly expose themselves to HIV, the virus that causes AIDS.

What are the long-term effects of marijuana use?

Findings so far show that regular use of marijuana or THC may play a role in some kinds of cancer and in problems with the respiratory and immune systems.

- *Cancer:* It's hard to know for sure whether regular marijuana use causes cancer. But it is known that marijuana contains some of the same, and sometimes even more, of the cancer-causing chemicals found in tobacco smoke. Studies show that someone who smokes five joints per week may be taking in as many cancer-causing chemicals as someone who smokes a full pack of cigarettes every day.

- *Lungs and airways*: People who smoke marijuana often develop the same kinds of breathing problems that cigarette smokers have: coughing and wheezing. They tend to have more chest colds than nonusers. They are also at greater risk of getting lung infections like pneumonia.
- *Immune system*: Animal studies have found that THC can damage the cells and tissues in the body that help protect people from disease. When the immune cells are weakened, you are more likely to get sick.

Does marijuana lead to the use of other drugs?

It could. Long-term studies of high school students and their patterns of drug use show that very few young people use other illegal drugs without first trying marijuana. For example, the risk of using cocaine is 104 times greater for those who have tried marijuana than for those who have never tried it. Using marijuana puts children and teens in contact with people who are users and sellers of other drugs. So there is more of a risk that a marijuana user will be exposed to and urged to try more drugs.

To better determine this risk, scientists are examining the possibility that long-term marijuana use may create changes in the brain that make a person more at risk of becoming addicted to other drugs, such as alcohol or cocaine. While not all young people who use marijuana go on to use other drugs, further research is needed to predict who will be at greatest risk.

How can you tell if someone has been using marijuana?

If someone is high on marijuana, he or she might:

- seem dizzy and have trouble walking;
- seem silly and giggly for no reason;
- have very red, bloodshot eyes; and
- have a hard time remembering things that just happened.

When the early effects fade, over a few hours, the user can become very sleepy.

Is marijuana sometimes used as a medicine?

There has been much talk about the possible medical use of marijuana. Under U.S. law since 1970, marijuana has been a Schedule I controlled substance. This means that the drug, at least in its smoked form, has no commonly accepted medical use.

THC, the active chemical in marijuana, is manufactured into a pill available by prescription that can be used to treat the nausea and vomiting that occur with certain cancer treatments and to help AIDS patients eat more to keep up their weight. According to scientists, more research needs to be done on marijuana's side effects and potential benefits before it is used medically with any regularity.

Can marijuana help cure cancer?

No. Some people with cancer, HIV/AIDS, and other diseases claim to experience relief from pain and other symptoms that they attribute to marijuana use. However, scientific research has not yet confirmed these benefits and more research on this topic is being done. What is known is that smoking marijuana can cause lung damage.

How does marijuana affect driving?

Marijuana has serious harmful effects on the skills required to drive safely: alertness, the ability to concentrate, coordination, and the ability to react quickly. These effects can last up to 24 hours after smoking marijuana. Marijuana use can make it difficult to judge distances and react to signals and sounds on the road.

✤ It's A Fact!!

Marijuana and driving do not mix. Users often have delayed responses to sights and sounds drivers need to notice.

Marijuana may play a role in car accidents. In one study conducted in Memphis, TN, researchers found that, of 150 reckless drivers who were tested for drugs at the arrest scene, 33 percent tested positive for marijuana, and 12 percent tested positive for both marijuana and cocaine. Data have also shown that while smoking marijuana, people show the same lack of coordination on standard "drunk driver" tests as do people who have had too much to drink.

If a woman is pregnant and smokes marijuana, will it hurt the baby?

Doctors advise pregnant women not to use any drugs because they could harm the growing fetus. One animal study has linked marijuana use to loss of the fetus very early in pregnancy.

Some scientific studies have found that babies born to marijuana users were shorter, weighed less, and had smaller head sizes than those born to mothers who did not use the drug. Smaller babies are more likely to develop health problems. There are also research data showing nervous system problems in children of mothers who smoked marijuana.

Researchers are not certain whether a newborn baby's health problems, if they are caused by marijuana, will continue as the child grows. Preliminary research shows that children born to mothers who used marijuana regularly during pregnancy may have trouble concentrating.

What does marijuana do to the brain?

Some studies show that when people have smoked large amounts of marijuana for years, the drug takes its toll on mental functions. Heavy or daily use of marijuana affects the parts of the brain that control memory, attention, and learning. A working short-term memory is needed to learn and perform tasks that call for more than one or two steps.

Smoking marijuana causes some changes in the brain that are like those caused by cocaine, heroin, and alcohol. Some researchers believe that these changes may put a person more at risk of becoming addicted to other drugs, such as cocaine or heroin. Scientists are still learning about the many ways that marijuana could affect the brain.

Can people become addicted to marijuana?

Yes. While not everyone who uses marijuana becomes addicted, when a user begins to seek out and take the drug compulsively, that person is said to be dependent or addicted to the drug. In 1995, 165,000 people entering drug treatment programs reported marijuana as their primary drug of abuse, showing they need help to stop using the drug.

According to one study, marijuana use by teenagers who have prior serious antisocial problems can quickly lead to dependence on the drug.

Some frequent, heavy users of marijuana develop a tolerance for it. "Tolerance" means that the user needs larger doses of the drug to get the same desired results that he or she used to get from smaller amounts.

✤ It's A Fact!!

It has not yet been proven that using marijuana leads to using other drugs. But, the fact is very few people use other drugs without first using marijuana. Teens who smoke marijuana are more likely to try other drugs, in part because they have more contact with people who use and sell them.

What if a person wants to quit using the drug?

Up until a few years ago, it was hard to find treatment programs specifically for marijuana users. Now researchers are testing different ways to help marijuana users abstain from drug use. There are currently no medications for treating marijuana addiction. Treatment programs focus on counseling and group support systems. There are also a number of programs designed especially to help teenagers who are abusers. Family doctors are also a good source for information and help in dealing with adolescent marijuana problems.

Chapter 32

Methamphetamine

Methamphetamine is an addictive stimulant drug that strongly activates certain systems in the brain. Methamphetamine is closely related chemically to amphetamine, but the central nervous system effects of methamphetamine are greater. Both drugs have some medical uses, primarily in the treatment of obesity, but their therapeutic use is limited.

Methamphetamine is made in illegal laboratories and has a high potential for abuse and dependence. Street methamphetamine is referred to by many names, such as "speed," "meth," and "chalk." Methamphetamine hydrochloride—clear chunky crystals resembling ice, which can be inhaled by smoking—is referred to as "ice," "crystal," and "glass."

Health Effects

Methamphetamine releases high levels of the neurotransmitter dopamine, which stimulates brain cells, enhancing mood and body movement. It also appears to have a neurotoxic effect, damaging brain cells that contain dopamine and serotonin, another neurotransmitter. Over time, methamphetamine appears to cause reduced levels of dopamine, which can result in symptoms like those of Parkinson's disease, a severe movement disorder.

About This Chapter: Text in this chapter includes text from "Methamphetamine," National Institute on Drug Abuse (NIDA), Infofax #13552, October 2001; "Tips for Teens: The Truth About Methamphetamine," National Clearinghouse for Alcohol and Drug Information, 1999; and "Brain Imaging Studies Show Long-Term Damage From Methamphetamine Abuse," by Patrick Zickler, in *NIDA Notes*, Vol. 15, No. 3, August 2000.

Methamphetamine is taken orally or intranasally (snorting the powder), by intravenous injection, and by smoking. Immediately after smoking or intravenous injection, the methamphetamine user experiences an intense sensation, called a "rush" or "flash," that lasts only a few minutes and is described as extremely pleasurable. Oral or intranasal use produces euphoria—a high, but not a rush. Users may become addicted quickly, and use it with increasing frequency and in increasing doses.

✎ Weird Words
Slang terms used for methamphetamine include: Speed, Meth, Crystal, Crank, Tweak, Go-fast, Ice, Glass, Uppers, and Black Beauties

Animal research going back more than 20 years shows that high doses of methamphetamine damage neuron cell-endings. Dopamine- and serotonin-containing neurons do not die after methamphetamine use, but their nerve endings ("terminals") are cut back and re-growth appears to be limited.

The central nervous system (CNS) actions that result from taking even small amounts of methamphetamine include increased wakefulness, increased physical activity, decreased appetite, increased respiration, hyperthermia, and euphoria. Other CNS effects include irritability, insomnia, confusion, tremors, convulsions, anxiety, paranoia, and aggressiveness. Hyperthermia and convulsions can result in death.

Methamphetamine causes increased heart rate and blood pressure and can cause irreversible damage to blood vessels in the brain, producing strokes. Other effects of methamphetamine include respiratory problems, irregular heartbeat, and extreme anorexia. Its use can result in cardiovascular collapse and death.

Extent Of Use

Monitoring The Future Study

Monitoring the Future (MTF) is an annual survey on drug use and related attitudes of America's adolescents that began in 1975. The survey is conducted by the University of Michigan's Institute for Social Research and is funded by NIDA. Copies of the latest survey are available from the National Clearinghouse for Alcohol and Drug Information at 1-800-729-6686.

MTF assesses the extent of drug use among adolescents (8th-, 10th-, and 12th-graders) and young adults across the country. Recent data from the survey:

- In 1997, 4.4 percent of high school seniors had used crystal methamphetamine at least once in their lifetimes—an increase from 2.7 percent in 1990.
- Data show that 2.3 percent of seniors reported past year use of crystal methamphetamine in 1997—an increase from 1.3 percent in 1990.

Community Epidemiology Work Group

Community Epidemiology Work Group (CEWG) is a NIDA-sponsored network of researchers from 20 major U.S. metropolitan areas and selected foreign countries who meet semiannually to discuss the current epidemiology of drug abuse. CEWG's most recent reports are available on the CEWG web site (www.nida.nih.gov/CEWG/CEWGHome.html).

Methamphetamine is the dominant illicit drug problem in San Diego. San Francisco and Honolulu also have substantial methamphetamine-using populations. Patterns of increasing use have been seen in Denver, Los Angeles, Minneapolis, Phoenix, Seattle, and Tucson. New trafficking patterns have increased availability of the drug in Missouri, Nebraska, and Iowa.

National Household Survey On Drug Abuse

National Household Survey on Drug Abuse (NHSDA) is an annual survey conducted by the Substance Abuse and Mental Health Services Administration. Copies of the latest survey are available from the National Clearinghouse for Alcohol and Drug Information at 1-800-729-6686.

According to the 1996 NHSDA, 4.9 million people (aged 12 and older) had tried methamphetamine at least once in their lifetimes (2.3 percent of population). This is not a statistically significant increase from 4.7 million people (2.2 percent) who reported using methamphetamine at least once in their lifetime in the 1995 NHSDA.

Questions And Answers About Methamphetamine

Isn't methamphetamine less harmful than crack, cocaine, or heroin?

Some users get hooked the first time they snort, smoke, or inject meth. Because it can be made from lethal ingredients like battery acid, drain cleaner, lantern fuel, and antifreeze, there is a greater chance of suffering a heart attack, stroke, or serious brain damage with this drug than with other drugs.

Isn't using methamphetamine like using diet pills?

No. Though it is easily attainable, methamphetamine is dangerous and addictive. Between 1993 and 1995, deaths due to meth rose 125 percent.

✤ It's A Fact!!

Methamphetamine affects your brain. In the short term, meth causes mind and mood changes such as anxiety, euphoria, and depression. Long-term effects can include chronic fatigue, paranoid or delusional thinking, and permanent psychological damage.

Methamphetamine affects your body. Over "amping" on any type of speed is pretty risky. Creating a false sense of energy, these drugs push the body faster and further than it's meant to go. It increases the heart rate, blood pressure, and risk of stroke.

Methamphetamine affects your self-control. Meth may be as addictive as crack and more powerful.

Methamphetamine is not what it seems. Speed drugs are not always safe. Even jolts of the well-known stimulants caffeine or ephedrine can cause stroke or cardiac arrest when overused or used by people with a sensitivity to them.

Methamphetamine can kill you. An overdose of meth can result in heart failure. Long-term physical effects such as liver, kidney, and lung damage may also kill you.

> ✔ Quick Tip
>
> **How can you tell if a friend is using meth?**
>
> It may not be easy to tell. But there are signs you can look for. Symptoms of methamphetamine use may include:
>
> - Inability to sleep
> - Increased sensitivity to noise
> - Nervous physical activity, like scratching
> - Irritability, dizziness, or confusion
> - Extreme anorexia
> - Tremors or even convulsions
> - Increased heart rate, blood pressure, and risk of stroke
> - Presence of inhaling paraphernalia, such as razor blades, mirrors, and straws
> - Presence of injecting paraphernalia, such as syringes, heated spoons, or surgical tubing
>
> **What can you do to help someone who is using meth?**
>
> Be a real friend. You might even save a life. Encourage your friend to stop or seek professional help. For information and referrals, call the National Clearinghouse for Alcohol and Drug Information at (800) 729-6686.

Between 1996 and 1997, meth-related emergency room visits doubled. Use by 12- to 17-year-olds has increased dramatically in the past few years.

Brain Imaging Studies Show Long-Term Damage From Methamphetamine Abuse

NIDA-supported research has demonstrated that methamphetamine abusers risk long-term brain damage.

Dr. Thomas Ernst and Dr. Linda Chang at the Harbor-UCLA Medical Center in Torrance, California, used a noninvasive brain imaging technique called magnetic resonance spectroscopy (MRS) to measure levels of brain chemicals that indicate whether brain cells are healthy or are diseased or damaged. "We found abnormal brain chemistry in methamphetamine users in all the brain regions we studied. In one of the regions, the amount of damage was also related to the history of drug use—those abusers who had the greatest cumulative lifetime methamphetamine use had the strongest indications of cell damage," Dr. Chang says.

Dr. Chang and Dr. Ernst measured levels of chemical markers in the brains of 26 participants who had a history of methamphetamine abuse but had not used the drug for periods ranging from 2 weeks to 21 months with a median of 4.25 months since last use. They compared the results to measurements of 24 participants who had no history of methamphetamine use.

"Methamphetamine may be substantially toxic to the cells we use in thinking," Dr. Ernst says. "This long-term, and perhaps permanent, alteration in basic brain chemistry is additional evidence that methamphetamine abuse, like abuse of other drugs, should be considered a brain disease and treated accordingly."

☞ **Remember!!**

Methamphetamine is a powerfully addictive stimulant that acts on the central nervous system to produce increased wakefulness and physical activity as well as irritability, insomnia, confusion, tremors, convulsions, anxiety, paranoia, and aggresiveness. The drug increases heart rate and blood pressure and can irreversibly damage blood vessels in the brain.

Chapter 33

Concerns About Prescription And Over-the-Counter Drugs

Over $78 billion in prescription and over-the-counter (OTC) drugs are produced each year in the United States. Although most people use these medications properly, a significant number do not. They might take them without a doctor's prescription, use more than prescribed, or take them for reasons other than those for which that the drugs were prescribed. In 1998, the Substance Abuse and Mental Health Services Administration's (SAMHSA) National Household Survey on Drug Abuse showed that more than 20 million people over the age of 12 reported having used one or more psychotherapeutic drugs (stimulants, sedatives, tranquilizers, and analgesics available through prescription) for non-medical purposes at some time in their lives. Stimulants, analgesics, and tranquilizers were the most widely used drugs of abuse that fit this category. Psychotherapeutic drugs are abused because they directly affect the brain and central nervous system (CNS).

About This Chapter: This chapter includes text from "Give 'Em the Facts: Prescription and Over-the-Counter Drug Abuse," National Clearinghouse for Alcohol and Drug Information, Substance Abuse and Mental Health Services Administration, 1998; "Pain Medications and Other Prescription Drugs," National Institute on Drug Abuse (NIDA), Infofax No. 13553, October 2001; "Methylphenidate (Ritalin)," NIDA, Infofax No. 13555, November 1999; "Hydrocodone, Dihydrocodeinone (Vicodin, Lortab)," *Drugs and Chemicals of Concern*, Drug Enforcement Administration (DEA), August 2001; "Dextromethorphan (DXM, DM, Robo, Velvet, Rojo)," *Drugs and Chemicals of Concern*, DEA, August 2001; and "Oxycodone (Trade Names: Dylox, Percodan, OxyContin)," *Drugs and Chemicals of Concern*, DEA, August 2001.

Trends In Prescription Drug Abuse

In 1999, an estimated 4 million people, about 2 percent of the population age 12 and older, were currently (use in past month) using prescription drugs non-medically. Of these, 2.6 million misused pain relievers, 1.3 million misused sedatives and tranquilizers, and 0.9 million misused stimulants. While prescription drug abuse affects many Americans, some trends of particular concern can be seen among older adults, adolescents, and women.

The misuse of prescribed medications may be the most common form of drug abuse among the elderly. Older people are prescribed medications about three times more frequently than the general population, and have poorer compliance with directions for use.

The National Household Survey on Drug Abuse numbers indicate that the sharpest increases in new users of prescription drugs for non-medical purposes occur in 12 to 17 and 18 to 25 year-olds. Among 12 to 14 year-olds, psychotherapeutics (for example, pain killers, tranquilizers, sedatives, and stimulants) were reported to be one of two primary drugs used.

The 1999 Monitoring the Future Survey of 8th, 10th, and 12th graders nationwide, showed that for barbiturates, tranquilizers, and narcotics other than heroin, general long-term declines in use in the 1980s leveled off in the early 1990s, with modest increases again in the mid-1990s.

Overall, men and women have roughly similar rates of nonmedical use of prescription drugs, with the exception of 12 to 17 year olds. In this age group, young women are more likely than young men to use psychotherapeutic drugs nonmedically. Also, among women and men who use either a sedative, anti-anxiety drug, or hypnotic (medicine for sleeping), women are almost twice as likely to become addicted.

The Drug Abuse Warning Network, which collects data on drug-related hospital emergency room episodes, reported that mentions of hydrocodone as a cause for visiting an emergency room increased 37 percent among all age groups from 1997 to 1999. Also, mentions of clonazepam increased 102 percent since 1992.

✤ It's A Fact!!

Misuse of some common over-the-counter pain killers (analgesics) can lead to serious side effects.

- **Aspirin:** The most common analgesic used today to treat fever, arthritis and pain; possible side effects can include nausea, heartburn or development of bleeding ulcers. Reye's syndrome may develop if aspirin is given to children with the flu or chicken pox. This disease is characterized by vomiting, swelling of the brain and liver, difficulty with mental functioning, and can often lead to death. People with liver damage should also avoid using aspirin.

- **Acetaminophen (Tylenol):** Is used to treat aches, pains, and fevers and is generally free from side effects. Large doses or overuse of this drug may cause rashes, fevers or changes in blood composition. People with kidney or liver problems should consult a doctor before using acetaminophen.

- **Ibuprofen (Motrin, Advil, Nuprin):** Is used to relieve pain associated with arthritis, menstrual cramping and discomfort, fever, and muscle strains. Possible side effects might include upset stomach, dizziness, drowsiness, headache, or ringing in the ears. Overuse of this drug may lead to confusion, tingling in hands and feet, and vomiting.

Common Medications: Their Uses And Side Effects

Antidepressants

These are prescription medications used to treat depression, a disease affecting over 15 million Americans. Some of the original drugs of this group were Nardil, Tofranil and Elavil. Although not technically an antidepressant, lithium, which used to treat manic depression, is often in this group. The side effects of prolonged and excessive use of these drugs are excessive urination or thirst, diarrhea, vomiting, drowsiness, dizziness or muscle weakness. Some newer antidepressants that show great promise in treating this disease are Wellbutrin, Prozac and Zoloft. The incidence of side effects with these seem to be less than with the previously used medications.

Sedative-Hypnotics And Tranquilizers

Benzodiazepines are the most widely prescribed tranquilizers and sleep-inducing medications. Drugs used to treat anxiety and tension are Valium, Xanax, Ativan, and Tranxene. Drugs used for sleeping are Dalmane, Restoril and Halcion. Possible side effects include drowsiness, poor coordination or light-headedness. Overuse of these drugs can lead to respiratory difficulties, sleeplessness, coma and even death.

✤ It's A Fact!!

Misuse of prescription and OTC drugs can often lead to psychological and physical dependence. People use increased amounts of drugs to ensure a sense of well-being while treating unrelated illnesses or health problems, or for non-medical purposes. Many medications contain alcohol and narcotics such as codeine, which can be addictive and life-threatening. Use of alcohol, a depressant, with some prescription and over-the-counter drugs may inhibit or increase the drug's effectiveness and cause a loss of coordination. Combining OTC drugs with some prescription drugs can cause the similar effects, or even more harmful types of reactions.

Barbiturates

Barbiturates are less commonly prescribed medications used to treat anxiety and insomnia. Some examples are Seconal, Phenobarbital and Nembutal. If improperly used, these drugs can cause an individual to feel depressed or experience respiratory difficulties.

Cough And Cold Preparations

Colds are caused by viruses and typically last 7 to 10 days. Most cold preparations are designed to treat specific cold symptoms and provide temporary relief from discomfort. Most widely used cold remedies include the following:

- *Antihistamines and Decongestants*: These medications are typically used to relieve the itchy, watery eyes and reduce congestion due to allergies, colds and flu. They can cause drowsiness or excitability.
- *Antitussives and Expectorants*: Antitussives are cough suppressants used to treat painful, persistent coughs. Expectorants are used to help clear mucous from the respiratory system. Both medications may contain alcohol and some may contain narcotics, such as codeine, to relieve pain and induce sleep. Some may be addictive.

Laxatives

Laxatives are among the most widely misused and abused over the counter medications. Use of laxatives should be restricted to short term-use for constipation, since chronic use leads to dependency.

Classes Of Commonly Abused Drugs

While many prescription drugs can be abused or misused, these three classes are most commonly abused:

- *Opioids:* Often prescribed to treat pain.
- *CNS Depressants:* Used to treat anxiety and sleep disorders.
- *Stimulants:* Prescribed to treat narcolepsy and attention deficit/hyperactivity disorder.

Opioids

Opioids are commonly prescribed because of their effective analgesic or pain relieving properties. Many studies have shown that properly managed medical use of opioid analgesic drugs is safe and rarely causes clinical addiction, which is defined as compulsive, often uncontrollable use. Taken exactly as prescribed, opioids can be used to manage pain effectively.

Among the drugs that fall within this class—sometimes referred to as narcotics—are morphine, codeine, and related drugs. Morphine is often used before or after surgery to alleviate severe pain. Codeine is used for milder pain. Other examples of opioids that can be prescribed to alleviate pain include oxycodone (OxyContin—an oral, controlled release form of the drug); propoxyphene (Darvon); hydrocodone (Vicodin); hydromorphone (Dilaudid); and meperidine (Demerol), which is used less often because of its side effects. In addition to their effective pain relieving properties, some of these drugs can be used to relieve severe diarrhea (Lomotil, for example, which is diphenoxylate) or severe coughs (codeine).

Opioids act by attaching to specific proteins called opioid receptors, which are found in the brain, spinal cord, and gastrointestinal tract. When these drugs attach to certain opioid receptors in the brain and spinal cord they can effectively block the transmission of pain messages to the brain.

In addition to relieving pain, opioid drugs can affect regions of the brain that mediate what we perceive as pleasure, resulting in the initial euphoria that many opioids produce. They can also produce drowsiness, cause constipation, and, depending upon the amount of drug taken, depress breathing. Taking a large single dose could cause severe respiratory depression or be fatal.

Opioids may interact with other drugs and are only safe to use with other drugs under a physician's supervision. Typically, they should not be used with substances such as alcohol, antihistamines, barbiturates, or benzodiazepines. These drugs slow down breathing, and their combined effects could risk life-threatening respiratory depression.

Chronic use of opioids can result in tolerance to the drugs so that higher doses must be taken to obtain the same initial effects. Long-term use also can lead to physical dependence—the body adapts to the presence of the drug and withdrawal symptoms occur if use is reduced abruptly.

Symptoms of withdrawal can include restlessness, muscle and bone pain, insomnia, diarrhea, vomiting, cold flashes with goose bumps ("cold turkey"), and involuntary leg movements.

Options for effectively treating addiction to prescription opioids are drawn from experience and research on treating heroin addiction. Some examples follow.

Methadone, a synthetic opioid that blocks the effects of heroin and other opioids, eliminates withdrawal symptoms, and relieves drug craving. It has been used for over 30 years to successfully treat people addicted to opioids.

Other medications include LAAM (levo-alpha-acetyl-methadol), an alternative to methadone that blocks the effects of opioids for up to 72 hours. Naltrexone is a long acting opioid blocker often used with highly motivated individuals in treatment programs promoting complete abstinence, and also to prevent relapse.

Buprenorphine, another synthetic opioid, will soon be available. Also, naloxone counteracts the effects of opioids and is used to treat overdoses.

CNS Depressants

CNS depressants slow down normal brain function. In higher doses, some CNS depressants can become general anesthetics.

CNS depressants can be divided into two groups, based on their chemistry and pharmacology:

- Barbiturates, such as mephobarbital (Mebaral) and pentobarbital sodium (Nembutal), which are used to treat anxiety, tension, and sleep disorders.
- Benzodiazepines, such as diazepam (Valium), chlordiazepoxide HCl (Librium), and alprazolam (Xanax), which can be prescribed to treat anxiety, acute stress reactions, and panic attacks. Benzodiazepines that have a more sedating effect, such as triazolam (Halcion) and estazolam (ProSom) can be prescribed for short-term treatment of sleep disorders.

There are many CNS depressants, and most act on the brain similarly—they affect the neurotransmitter gamma-aminobutyric acid (GABA). Neurotransmitters are brain chemicals that facilitate communication between brain cells. GABA works by decreasing brain activity. Although different classes of CNS depressants work in unique ways, ultimately it is their ability to increase GABA activity that produces a drowsy or calming effect. Despite these beneficial effects for people suffering from anxiety or sleeping disorders, barbiturates and benzodiazepines can be addictive and should be used only as prescribed.

CNS depressants should not be combined with any medication or substance that causes sleepiness, including prescription pain medicines, certain over-the-counter cold and allergy medications, or alcohol. The effects of the drugs can combine to slow breathing, or slow both the heart and respiration, which can be fatal.

Discontinuing prolonged use of high doses of CNS depressants can lead to withdrawal. Because they work by slowing the brain's activity, a potential consequence of abuse is that when one stops taking a CNS depressant the brain's activity can rebound to the point that seizures can occur. Someone thinking about ending their use of a CNS depressant, or who has stopped and is suffering withdrawal, should speak with a physician and seek medical treatment.

In addition to medical supervision, counseling in an in-patient or outpatient setting can help people who are overcoming addiction to CNS depressants. For example, cognitive-behavioral therapy has been used successfully to help individuals in treatment for abuse of benzodiazepines. This type of therapy focuses on modifying a patient's thinking, expectations, and behaviors while simultaneously increasing their skills for coping with various life stressors.

Often the abuse of CNS depressants occurs in conjunction with the abuse of another substance or drug, such as alcohol or cocaine. In these cases of polydrug abuse, the treatment approach needs to address the multiple addictions.

Stimulants

Stimulants are a class of drugs that enhance brain activity—they cause an increase in alertness, attention, and energy that is accompanied by increases in blood pressure, heart rate, and respiration.

Historically, stimulants were used to treat asthma and other respiratory problems, obesity, neurological disorders, and a variety of other ailments. As their potential for abuse and addiction became apparent, the use of stimulants began to wane. Now, stimulants are prescribed for treating only a few health conditions, including narcolepsy, attention deficit hyperactivity disorder (AD/HD), and depression that has not responded to other treatments. Stimulants may also be used for short-term treatment of obesity, and for patients with asthma.

Stimulants such as dextroamphetamine (Dexedrine) and methylphenidate (Ritalin) have chemical structures that are similar to key brain neurotransmitters called monoamines, which include norepinephrine and dopamine. Stimulants increase the levels of these chemicals in the brain and body. This, in turn, increases blood pressure and heart rate, constricts blood vessels, increases blood glucose, and opens up the pathways of the respiratory system. In addition, the increase in dopamine is associated with a sense of euphoria that can accompany the use of these drugs.

Research indicates that people with AD/HD do not become addicted to stimulant medications, such as Ritalin, when taken in the form prescribed and at treatment dosages. However, when misused, stimulants can be addictive.

The consequences of stimulant abuse can be extremely dangerous. Taking high doses of a stimulant can result in an irregular heartbeat, dangerously high body temperatures, and/or the potential for cardiovascular failure or lethal seizures. Taking high doses of some stimulants repeatedly over a short period of time can lead to hostility or feelings of paranoia in some individuals.

Stimulants should not be mixed with antidepressants or over-the-counter cold medicines containing decongestants. Anti-depressants may enhance the effects of a stimulant, and stimulants in combination with decongestants may cause blood pressure to become dangerously high or lead to irregular heart rhythms.

Treatment of addiction to prescription stimulants, such as methylphenidate and amphetamines, is based on behavioral therapies proven effective for treating cocaine or methamphetamine addiction. At this time, there are no proven medications for the treatment of stimulant addiction. Antidepressants, however, may be used to manage the symptoms of depression that can accompany early abstinence from stimulants.

Depending on the patient's situation, the first step in treating prescription stimulant addiction may be to slowly decrease the drug's dose and attempting to treat withdrawal symptoms. This process of detoxification could then be followed with one of many behavioral therapies. Contingency management, for example, uses a system that enables patients to earn vouchers for drug-free urine tests; the vouchers can be exchanged for items that promote healthy living. Cognitive-behavioral therapies are proving beneficial, and recovery support groups may also be effective in conjunction with a behavioral therapy.

Specific Drugs Of Concern

Dextromethorphan (DXM, DM, Robo, Velvet, Rojo)

Dextromethorphan has the useful property of cough suppression without the traditional opiate central nervous system effects. It does not produce analgesia or an intense "rush" of well-being after administration. Additionally, DXM does not produce respiratory depression at therapeutic drug doses. Dextromethorphan, when taken in therapeutic doses, does not produce many side-effects and has a long history of safety and effectiveness. It is one of the active ingredients in many over-the-counter cough syrups.

There have been reports of sporadic abuse of dextromethorphan (DXM), with isolated case reports of overdose and death. Many users of DXM have opted for a powdered form of the drug because of the large volumes of cough syrup which need to be ingested in order to achieve intoxication. DXM-intoxication is typically referred to as "Robo-ing." Recent adverse event reports to the DEA have led to monitoring of the drug.

Abuse: The abuse of DXM by teenagers and young adults seems related to its over-the-counter availability and more recently to the sale of the powdered form. The abusers report a heightened sense of perceptual awareness, altered time perception, and visual hallucinations. Vomiting will occur as a result of the ingestion of the large volume of syrup required for intoxication.

The typical clinical presentation of DXM intoxication involves hyperexcitability, lethargy, ataxia, slurred speech, sweating, hypertension, and/or nystagmus. The majority of abuse occurs among teenagers and young adults.

Methylphenidate (Ritalin)

Methylphenidate is a medication prescribed for individuals (usually children) who have an abnormally high level of activity or attention deficit hyperactivity disorder (AD/HD). According to the National Institute of Mental Health, about 3 to 5 percent of the general population has the disorder, which is characterized by agitated behavior and an inability to focus on tasks. Methylphenidate also is occasionally prescribed for treating narcolepsy.

Health Effects: Methylphenidate is a central nervous system (CNS) stimulant. It has effects similar to, but more potent than, caffeine and less potent than amphetamines. It has a notably calming effect on hyperactive children and a "focusing" effect on those with AD/HD.

Research at Brookhaven National Laboratory may begin to explain how methylphenidate helps people with AD/HD. The researchers used positron emission tomography (PET—a noninvasive brain scan) to confirm that administering normal therapeutic doses of methylphenidate to healthy, adult men increased their dopamine levels. The researchers speculate that methylphenidate amplifies the release of dopamine, a neurotransmitter, thereby improving attention and focus in individuals who have dopamine signals that are weak, such as individuals with AD/HD.

When taken as prescribed, methylphenidate is a valuable medicine. Research shows that people with AD/HD do not become addicted to stimulant medications when taken in the form prescribed and at treatment dosages. Another study found that AD/HD boys treated with stimulants such as methylphenidate are significantly less likely to abuse drugs and alcohol when they are older than are non-treated AD/HD boys.

Because of its stimulant properties, however, in recent years there have been reports of abuse of methylphenidate by people for whom it is not a medication. Some individuals abuse it for its stimulant effects: appetite suppression, wakefulness, increased focus/attentiveness, and euphoria. When abused, the tablets are either taken orally or crushed and snorted. Some abusers dissolve the tablets in water and inject the mixture—complications can arise from this because insoluble fillers in the tablets can block small blood vessels.

Trends in Ritalin Abuse: At their June 2000 meeting, members of NIDA's Community Epidemiology Work Group shared the following information.

- The abuse of methylphenidate has been reported in Baltimore, mostly among middle and high schools students; Boston, especially among middle and upper-middle class communities; Detroit; Minneapolis/St. Paul; Phoenix; and Texas.
- When abused, methylphenidate tablets are often used orally or crushed and used intranasally.
- In 1999, 165 methylphenidate-related poison calls were made in Detroit; 419 were reported in Texas, with 114 of those involving intentional misuse or abuse.
- On Chicago's South Side, some users inject methylphenidate (this is referred to as "west coast"). Also, some mix it with heroin (a "speedball") or in combination with both cocaine and heroin for a more potent effect.

Because stimulant medicines such as methylphenidate do have potential for abuse, the U.S. Drug Enforcement Administration (DEA) has placed stringent, Schedule II controls on their manufacture, distribution, and prescription. For example, DEA requires special licenses for these activities, and prescription refills are not allowed. States may impose further regulations, such as limiting the number of dosage units per prescription.

Hydrocodone, Dihydrocodeinone (Vicodin, Lortab)

Hydrocodone is an effective antitussive (anti-cough) agent, and as an opiate it is also an effective analgesic for mild to moderate pain control. Five mg of hydrocodone is equivalent to 30 mg of codeine when administered orally. Hydrocodone is considered to be morphine-like.

Hydrocodone abuse has been escalating over the last decade. There has been large scale diversion of hydrocodone. For example, an estimated 7 million dosage units were diverted in 1994 and over 11 million in 1997. In 1998 there were over 56 million new prescriptions written for hydrocodone products and by 2000 there were over 89 million. From 1990 the average consumption nationwide has increased by 300%. In the same period there has been a 500% increase in the number of Emergency Department visits attributed to hydrocodone abuse with 19,221 visits estimated in 2000.

Health Effects: As with most opiates, the adverse effects of hydrocodone abuse are dependence and tolerance development. Its co-formulation with acetaminophen has also increased the likelihood of acetaminophen-induced hepatic (liver) necrosis with high dose acute dosing, but slow escalation of dose over time seems to protect the liver during high dose chronic exposures seen with this drug.

Oxycodone (Trade Names: Tylox, Percodan, OxyContin)

Oxycodone is an effective analgesic for mild to moderate pain control, chronic pain syndromes, and for the treatment of terminal cancer pain. Five mg of oxycodone is equivalent to 30 mg of codeine when administered orally. Oxycodone is considered to be similar to morphine, in all respects, including its abuse and dependence liabilities.

Abuse: Oxycodone abuse has been a continuing problem in the United States since the early 1960s. In passing the Controlled Substances Act of 1970, Congress placed oxycodone in Schedule II (CII). In spite of its CII status, oxycodone continued to be abused. The abuse of a new sustained-release formulation of oxycodone has escalated over the last year. Drug abuse treatment centers, law enforcement personnel, and health care professionals have reported a dramatic increase in the abuse of these sustained release products in Maine, Virginia, West Virginia, Ohio, Kentucky and Maryland. Recently, abuse has spread to other states such as Pennsylvania and Florida. The estimated number of emergency department (ED) episodes involving oxycodone were stable from 1990 through 1996. However, the number of ED episodes more than tripled from 1996 to 2000: 3,190 episodes in 1996 to 10,825 in 2000.

As with most opiates, the adverse effects of oxycodone abuse are dependence and tolerance development. Oxycodone's co-formulation with acetaminophen has also increased the likelihood of acetaminophen-induced hepatic necrosis with chronic dosing. Its availability in sustained release formulations has increased the dosage forms from 10 to 160 mg per tablet making it more attractive than oxycodone to opiate abusers and doctor-shoppers. The original idea of polymer-formulations of oxycodone was to reduce the likelihood of misuse with high dose formulations. Opiate abusers quickly learned the ease of extraction of the molecule from the polymer formula and have been injecting or snorting the crushed and/or dissolved tablets because of its' higher dosage formulations.

Every age-group has been affected by the relative ease of oxycodone availability and the perceived safety of these products by professionals. Sometimes seen as a "white-collar" addiction, oxycodone abuse has increased among all ethnic and economic groups.

For More Information

The National Clearinghouse for
Alcohol and Drug Information
P.O. Box 2345
Rockville, MD 20847-2345
Toll Free: 800-729-6686

Remember!!

Prescription drugs make complex surgery possible, relieve pain for millions of people, and enable many individuals with chronic medical conditions to control their symptoms and lead productive lives. Most people who take prescription medications use them responsibly. However, the non-medical use of prescription drugs is a serious public health concern. Nonmedical use of prescription drugs like opioids, central nervous system (CNS) depressants, and stimulants can lead to abuse and addiction, characterized by compulsive drug seeking and use.

Addiction rarely occurs among people who use a pain reliever, CNS depressant, or stimulant as prescribed; however, inappropriate use of prescription drugs can lead to addiction in some cases. Patients, healthcare professionals, and pharmacists all have roles in preventing misuse and addiction. For example, if a doctor prescribes a pain medication, CNS depressant, or stimulant, the patient should follow the directions for use carefully, and also learn what effects the drug could have and potential interactions with other drugs by reading all information provided by the pharmacist.

Part 5

Other Drug-Related Health Concerns

Chapter 34

Drug-Facilitated Rape

More than 430,000 sexual assaults occur annually in the United States, according to victimization surveys. Many of these assaults involve alcohol and drugs, which are often used voluntarily by both victim and offender. But in the mid- and late 1990's, rape crisis centers began hearing reports of drugs, often referred to as "roofies" and "liquid ecstasy," being used to immobilize victims, impair their memory, and thus facilitate rape. Two drugs in particular were mentioned in these reports: Rohypnol (the pharmaceutical trade name for flunitrazepam) and GHB (gamma-hydroxybutyrate).

These drugs can produce loss of consciousness and the inability to recall recent events. Victims may not be aware that they have taken drugs or that they have been raped while under the influence of drugs.

What Are Rape-Facilitating Drugs?

The most commonly implicated drugs are Rohypnol and GHB. Rohypnol, or flunitrazepam, belongs to a class of drugs called benzodiazepines and is approved for use in 80 countries, but not in the United States or Canada. It is available only in pill form, is tasteless, odorless, and colorless, and dissolves to some degree in liquid.

About This Chapter: Text in this chapter is excerpted from "Drug-Facilitated Rape: Looking for the Missing Pieces," by Nora Fitzgerald and K. Jack Riley, National Institute of Justice, NCJ No. 181731, April 2000.

Rohypnol mentally and physically incapacitates an individual, particularly when used in combination with alcohol, and is capable of producing anterograde amnesia. *Anterograde* amnesia is a condition in which events that occurred during the time the drug was in effect are forgotten, in contrast to *retrograde* amnesia, in which events prior to the intervening agent are forgotten.

GHB, a drug first synthesized in the 1920's, occurs naturally in the human body in minute amounts. It was under development as an anesthetic agent in the late 1950's and early 1960's, but no commercial products were developed from these efforts. Until the FDA banned the drug in 1990, it was available through health food stores and marketed as both a sleep aid and as a body-building supplement. Several vendors distributed products containing GHB under trade names such as "Gamma Hydrate" and "Somatomax PM."

✤ It's A Fact!!

Sexual assault victims who believe drugs were given to them without their knowledge typically report remembering sensations of drunkenness that do not correspond with the amounts of alcohol consumed, unexplained gaps in memory, altered levels of consciousness, and unexplainable signs of physical trauma.

GHB is marketed in some European countries as an adjunct to anesthesia and currently is being tested for treatment of narcolepsy as well as alcohol addiction and withdrawal (with mixed results) in Europe and the United States.

How Common Is Drug-Facilitated Rape?

No one really knows how common drug-facilitated rape is because today's research tools do not offer a means of measuring the number of incidents.

Another factor complicating science's ability to measure the incidence and prevalence of these drugs is the lack of law enforcement evidence. Investigations of suspected drug-facilitated assaults often turn out to be inconclusive because many victims do not seek assistance until hours or days later. By the time they do report a suspected assault, conclusive forensic evidence may have been lost. Even when victims do suspect a drug-facilitated rape and seek help immediately, law enforcement agencies may not know how to collect evidence appropriately or how to test urine using the sensitive method required.

To add more complexity to the puzzle, school-based surveys seem to suggest that Rohypnol and GHB are consumed voluntarily, perhaps increasingly so, because these drugs are cheap, easy to share, and easy to hide. Use appears to be concentrated among populations that also are at the highest risk of sexual assault, including middle school, high school, and college age students.

The good news is that public awareness about the drugs and their effects appears to be increasing.

Learning From Victims

Information in this section was written by Gail Abarbanel, LCSW, director of the Rape Treatment Center (RTC) at Santa Monica–UCLA Medical Center.

In late 1995, the Rape Treatment Center at Santa Monica–UCLA Medical Center began to see a new pattern in sexual assault cases. Victims were coming in who believed someone slipped a drug into their drink. As they consumed the drink, they began to feel disoriented or sick. The next thing they remembered was waking up hours later, sometimes in a different location.

When they regained consciousness, some victims were unsure if they had been sexually assaulted. Others found signs that they had been: They were undressed; they had semen stains on their bodies and/or clothing; they had vaginal or anal trauma, such as soreness and/or lacerations. All of these victims reported significant memory impairment. Most could not recall what was done to them, who participated, or how many people were present while they were unconscious. Some could remember brief, intermittent periods of awakening, during which they were aware of their surroundings but were unable to move or speak. They felt "paralyzed."

When victims began to report these crimes to the authorities, their cases often were dismissed. One victim was told, "He has his memory, you don't have yours. There's no evidence. The case is closed."

When these cases initially appeared, there was little information about rape drugs or drug-facilitated sexual assaults. Victims were a crucial source of information. Their reports helped define this emerging crime pattern by identifying the characteristics of these crimes that distinguished them from other sexual assaults.

> **✎ Weird Words**
>
> Anterograde Amnesia: Amnesia in reference to events occurring after the trauma or disease that caused the condition.
>
> Forensic: Pertaining or applicable to personal injury, murder, and other legal proceedings
>
> Retrograde Amnesia: Amnesia in reference to events that occurred before the trauma or disease that caused the condition.
>
> Source: From *Stedman's Medical Dictionary, 27th Edition*,

What Victims Have Taught Us

How Rape Drugs Facilitate Sexual Assaults. Rape drugs make it relatively easy for rapists to gain control of their victims. Perpetrators do not have to overcome any form of resistance. They do not have to use physical force. They do not have to threaten to harm the victim to get compliance. Nor do they have to be concerned about a victim's screams attracting attention. The drugs they administer immobilize and silence the victim.

How Victims Are Prevented From Detecting Threats to Their Safety. Victims of these crimes do not sense any threat to their safety when the assailant is incapacitating them. The "weapon" used to overpower and disable them is invisible. It is hidden in a drink.

How Victims Are Inhibited From Exercising Self-Defense. The ability to sense danger is critical to a person's ability to implement self-defense strategies. When faced with the threat of being raped, most people employ one or more protective measures, such as talking with the assailant, thinking about their options, screaming, stalling, attempting to escape, and/or physically resisting. If these efforts fail to prevent the rape, victims may "fight back" in other ways. They may memorize details about the assailant's physical characteristics, the location of the crime, and other factors that can later be used to aid authorities in apprehending and prosecuting the offender. The incapacitating effects of rape drugs rob victims of their ability to use these coping strategies.

How Rapists Can Appear To Be Rescuers. When victims are drugged in places where other people are present, such as restaurants, clubs, bars, and parties, the rapist may appear to bystanders and witnesses to be a rescuer. The behavioral effects of rape drugs look very much like the effects of voluntary alcohol consumption. To onlookers, the victim may seem drunk. When the rapist carries or leads the victim to another location where the sexual assault will be committed, he may be viewed as "helping" or transporting a vulnerable person to a safe place.

How Rape Drugs Affect Reporting Patterns. Victimization surveys consistently indicate very low reporting rates among rape victims. Delayed reports also are common, particularly in acquaintance rapes. In drug-facilitated rapes, additional factors may account for low and delayed reporting, including the immediate and residual effects of the drugs (the victim may be unconscious for several hours after the assault and may have hangover effects after regaining consciousness); feelings of guilt or self-blame because of prior voluntary ingestion of alcohol and/or drugs; confusion and uncertainty about what happened; and reluctance to make an accusation without personal knowledge or memory of the assault circumstances.

How Victims' Inability To Recall What Happened Affects The System's Response. Many aspects of a rape investigation are facilitated by a victim's ability to describe what happened. When victims of drug-facilitated rapes cannot give a complete narrative, they often encounter suspicion, disbelief, and/or frustration. Their inability to supply information that could assist the investigation and/or prosecution compounds their sense of helplessness.

How People Misjudge And Minimize Victims' Trauma. Because most victims of drug-facilitated rapes have no memory of the sexual assault, people may mistakenly minimize the trauma they suffered. For all rape victims, the loss of control experienced during an assault is profoundly traumatic. In drug-facilitated rapes, the additional experiences of being unable to think about options and safety during the assault and anterograde amnesia afterwards subject the victim to an extreme form of powerlessness.

How Drugging Is A Unique Form Of Trauma. Many of the difficulties victims face in the aftermath of these assaults are due to the effects of the drugs given by offenders. The drugging of a victim is, in and of itself, a cruel and criminal violation of the person. Some victims describe this aspect of the trauma as "mind rape." The drugging should be recognized as a separate and distinct act of victimization in addition to any other acts of abuse and degradation to which the victim was subjected.

How Being Unable To Forget Compares With Being Unable To Remember. In the aftermath of rape, most victims suffer acute stress disorder and post-traumatic stress disorder symptoms. One of the most disturbing symptoms is their inability to *forget* what happened. The trauma is re-experienced repeatedly. Victims commonly have recurrent, intrusive recollections of the rape, including thoughts, flashbacks, and nightmares. For victims of drug-facilitated rapes, this aspect of the aftermath may be experienced differently. Because they cannot *recall* what happened during a significant time period, they have to cope with a gap in their memory. They experience the horror, powerlessness, and humiliation of not knowing what was done to them. They can only imagine what happened.

For More Information

Print Resources

Anglin, D., K.L. Spears, and H. Range Hutson, "Flunitrazepam and Its Involvement in Date or Acquaintance Rape," *Journal of Academic Emergency Medicine* 4(4) (1997).

Calhoun, S.R., D.R. Wesson, G.P. Galloway, and D.E. Smith, "Abuse of Flunitrazepam (Rohypnol) and Other Benzodiazepines in Austin and South Texas," *Journal of Psychoactive Drugs* 28(2) (April–June 1996).

Fitzgerald, N., K.J. Riley, T. Alston, C. Mamalian, M. Mendez, A. Resnick, B. Taylor, and J. Wiseman, *Report to the Attorney General From the Drug-Facilitated Rape Working Group*, Washington, D.C.: U.S. Department of Justice, National Institute of Justice, 1998 (NCJ 181396). To obtain a copy, contact the National Criminal Justice Reference Service at P.O. Box 6000, Rockville, MD 20849-6000, 1-800-851-3420.

Inciardi, J.A., and C.A. Saum, "Rohypnol Misuse in the United States," *Journal of Substance Use and Misuse* 32(6):723 (1997).

Woods, J.H., and Gail Winger, "Abuse Liability of Flunitrazepam," *Journal of Clinical Psychopharmacology* 17,(3) (June 1997), Supp. 2.

Available Online

The National Institute on Drug Abuse's party drugs Web site: http://www.clubdrugs.org.

☞ Remember!!

Drug-facilitated rape may be initiated in social settings, like parties and clubs, not traditionally considered high-risk environments. Drugs can produce loss of consciousness and the inability to recall recent events. Victims may not be aware that they have taken drugs or that they have been raped while under the influence of drugs.

Chapter 35

Sex Under The Influence Of Alcohol And Other Drugs

Alcohol and other drug use is linked to risky sexual behavior and poses significant threats to the health of adolescents. Substance abuse may impair adolescents' ability to make judgments about sex and contraception, placing them at increased risk for unplanned pregnancy, sexual assault, or becoming infected with a sexually transmitted disease (STD), including HIV/AIDS.

We know the AIDS virus can be transmitted through sharing hypodermic needles. Less is known about the dangerous role of alcohol and other drugs in sexual behavior that may lead to STDs and to HIV/AIDS. To compound matters, there is also considerable evidence that alcohol and other drugs weaken the immune system, thereby increasing susceptibility to infection and disease.

Make Your Decision About Sex With a Clear Head, Without Drugs

Sometimes you can feel pressured to have sex when you may not want to, and drugs make it harder to say no. Pressure about sex can be hard to deal

About This Chapter: This chapter is taken from "Sex Under the Influence of Alcohol and Other Drugs," National Clearinghouse for Alcohol and Drug Information, NCADI Inventory Number ML005, Spring 1995, and excerpts from "How Getting High Can Get You AIDS," National Clearinghouse for Alcohol and Drug Information (NCADI), ADM 92-1826, 1994. Despite the age of these documents, the concerns highlighted are still valid.

with—it can come from your boyfriend or girlfriend, from the crowd you hang out with, or even from your own feelings.

> ✤ **It's A Fact!!**
>
> Teens who use condoms during sex tend to use them less if they've been drinking or using other drugs.

The first thing to remember is you're charge of your body and what you choose to do with it. The second thing to remember is there is a lot at stake—a decision about sex can have consequences that last a lifetime.

It helps to make a plan and stick to it. Then if someone offers you drugs or suggests sex, you'll know what to do. Plan not to use drugs so you can keep a clear head. Plan how to say no, to be careful, and to think about what to do. The time to make your plan is when you have a clear head.

Making Your Plan

Think about who you are and what's important to you, think about how using drugs and having sex could affect that. When you have a plan it's easier to handle situations where you want to have fun with friends but don't want to use drugs or have sex.

If someone pressures you about drugs you can say nicely but firmly, "I'm not interested," or, "I don't use drugs."

If someone pressures you about sex you could let them know where you stand by saying: I'm not ready for it yet," or, "Maybe it feels right for you, but it's not for me."

Sex And Drugs: Know The Risks

Consider the following statistics:

- The use of alcohol and other drugs can affect judgment and lead to taking serious sexual risks. There were 18,540 cases of AIDS among 13- to 24-year-olds reported to the Centers for Disease Control and Prevention by the end of 1994. (Source: Centers for Disease Control and Prevention, *HIV/AIDS Surveillance Report, 1994*, Vol. 6., No. 2, Summary of Findings, 1994.)

- About 75 percent of high school seniors have had sexual intercourse at least once in their lives; about 20 percent have had more than four sexual partners by their senior year. (Source: Centers for Disease Control and Prevention, HIV/AIDS Prevention, "Facts About: Adolescents and HIV/AIDS," December 1994.)

- Studies show that adolescents are less likely to use condoms when having sex after drinking alcohol than when sober. This places them at even higher risk for HIV infection, STDs, and unwanted pregnancy. (Source: Strunin, L., and Hingson, R. Alcohol Use and Risk for HIV Infection, *Alcohol and Health Research World*, Vol. 17, No. 1, National Institute on Alcohol Abuse and Alcoholism.)

- A survey of high school students found that 18 percent of females and 39 percent of males say it is acceptable for a boy to force sex if the girl is stoned or drunk. (Source: Inspector General, U.S. Department of Health and Human Services, *Youth and Alcohol: Dangerous and Deadly Consequences: Report to the Surgeon General*, April 1992.)

- According to the Centers for Disease Control and Prevention, HIV/AIDS has been the sixth leading cause of death among 15- to 20-year-olds in the United States for over three years. One in five of the new AIDS cases diagnosed is in the 20 to 29 year age group, meaning that HIV transmission occurred during the teen years. Additionally, more than half of new cases of HIV infection in 1994 were related to drug use. (Source: Centers for Disease Control and Prevention, HIV/AIDS Prevention, "Facts About: Adolescents and HIV/AIDS," December 1994.)

It's A Fact!

"These findings suggest a direct association between alcohol and other drug use and unsafe sexual behavior." (Quote from *Eighth Special Report to the U.S. Congress on Alcohol and Health*, Secretary of Health and Human Services, October 1993.)

Additional Information

For more information, call the National Clearinghouse for Alcohol and Drug Information at 1-800-729-6686.

☞ Remember!!

There is still much to be learned about the relationship between alcohol and other drugs and sexual behavior. During the past decade, teens reported higher levels of sexual activity at earlier ages, experienced more unplanned pregnancies, and suffered higher rates of sexually transmitted diseases. To reduce the incidence of these problems in the future, prevention of alcohol and other drug abuse must be a top priority.

Chapter 36

Drug Abuse And AIDS

AIDS—acquired immunodeficiency syndrome—is caused by HIV, the human immunodeficiency virus. HIV impairs your immune system, making it less resistant to diseases and infections. HIV is transmitted through exposure to the bodily fluids of someone infected with HIV. This exposure most commonly occurs during unprotected sex, by sharing needles, through blood transfusions, or by contact with open wounds. Babies born to women with HIV can also become infected.

Alcohol and other drugs affect your self-control. Alcohol and illicit drugs lower your inhibitions and impair your judgment. Drinking and drug use can lead to risky behaviors you're less likely to do if sober, including having unprotected sex. This increases your risk for exposure to HIV/AIDS and other sexually transmitted diseases (STDs).

Any drug use increases the risks for HIV/AIDS. Non-injection drugs also contribute to the spread of HIV/AIDS when users trade sex for drugs or money or when their judgment and decision-making skills are impaired.

About This Chapter: Information in this chapter is excerpted from "Drug Abuse and AIDS," National Institute on Drug Abuse (NIDA), Infofax No. 13558, November 1999, updated October 2001; "How Getting High Can Get You AIDS," National Clearinghouse for Alcohol and Drug Information (NCADI), ADM 92-1826, 1994; and "Tips for Teens: The Truth About AIDS," NCADI, undated. Despite the age of these documents, the concerns are still valid.

Getting High Makes You Forget

Being a teen is exciting. Being a teen in a world with drugs, sex, and AIDS, is hard. You might not know all the ways drugs and AIDS are connected. This information will help you understand the dangers and how to avoid them. Drugs, like alcohol, marijuana, and cocaine can cloud your judgment, make it hard to know right from wrong, they distract you from reality.

Drugs make you forget what's important so you care less about yourself or your friends. When you get high you may mistakenly believe nothing bad could happen to you. Drugs can make you do things you may wish you never did, like:

- act reckless and foolish
- get romantic with someone you don't really like
- have sex without planning
- have sex without thinking of the consequences
- forget to use a condom or forget to have your partner use a condom

When drugs make you forget, you may take risks, like having sex. Teen years are a time of making all kinds of new decisions. One of those decisions is when to have sex. It's important to make that decision with a clear head because sex today is far riskier than ever before. Drugs, like alcohol, marijuana, and cocaine can get in the way of making clear decisions.

✤ It's A Fact!!

Sex is risky. You should know ...

- Unprotected sex with an infected partner and sharing needles to inject drugs are the most common ways HIV, the virus that causes AIDS, is spread.
- Your sex partner may have had sex with someone who shared a needle to inject drugs with an HIV infected person.
- The more sex partners you have, the more chance you have of getting AIDS.
- Two sure ways to avoid the AIDS virus are: not having sex and not sharing needles.
- If you choose to have sex, always use a condom to help reduce the risk of getting AIDS.

Drugs And AIDS: What's The Connection

Behavior associated with drug abuse is now the single largest factor in the spread of HIV infection in the United States. HIV is the human immunodeficiency virus, which causes acquired immunodeficiency syndrome, known as AIDS. AIDS is a condition characterized by a defect in the body's natural immunity to diseases, and individuals who suffer from it are at risk for severe illnesses that are usually not a threat to anyone whose immune system is working properly. Although many individuals who have AIDS or carry HIV may live for many years with treatment, there is no known cure or vaccine.

✔ Quick Tip

To learn more about resources for HIV/AIDS information or HIV testing in your area, call the National AIDS Hotline at 1-800-342-2437 (in Spanish, 1-800-344-7432; deaf, 1-800-243-7889), or the National AIDS Clearinghouse at 1-800-458-5231, or write P.O. Box 6003, Rockville, MD 20849-6003.

Using or sharing unsterile needles, cotton swabs, rinse water, and cookers, such as when injecting heroin, cocaine, or other drugs, leaves a drug abuser vulnerable to contracting or transmitting HIV. Another way people may be at risk for contracting HIV is simply by using drugs of abuse, regardless of whether a needle and syringe are involved. Research sponsored by the National Institute on Drug Abuse (NIDA) and the National Institute on Alcohol Abuse and Alcoholism (NIAAA) has shown that drug and alcohol use interfere with judgment about sexual (and other) behavior, making it more likely that users have unplanned and unprotected sex. This places them at increased risk for contracting HIV from infected sex partners.

Prevention Of HIV Among Injecting Drug Users

It is clear from research that drug abuse treatment is a proven means of preventing the spread of HIV and AIDS, especially when combined with prevention and community-based outreach programs for at-risk people. These efforts can reduce or eliminate drug use and drug-related HIV risk behaviors such as needle sharing and unsafe sex practices. One study comparing HIV infection rates among drug abusers enrolled in methadone treatment programs to rates among those not in treatment found that those not in treatment were nearly seven times more likely to have become infected with HIV during the first 18 months. The study also found that the longer drug abusers remained in treatment, the less likely they were to become infected.

In addition, drug treatment programs help reduce the spread of other blood-borne infections, including hepatitis B and C viruses. Adequate medical care for HIV or AIDS and any related illnesses is also critical to reducing spread.

✤ It's A Fact!!

- More than 20 percent of the people who have AIDS are in their 20's. Since it can take up to 10 years or more for symptoms to start, many got infected in their teens.
- The number of reported AIDS cases among teenagers increased 96% between 1988 and 1990.
- You cannot tell someone has the HIV virus by looking at them. A blood test is the only way to be sure.

Symptoms Of HIV/AIDS

How can you tell if you or someone else may already have HIV? If you have not shared a needle or had unprotected sex, it is very unlikely that you have HIV. The only way to be certain is to be tested. Most people with HIV do not have any visible symptoms for many years. Once symptoms do begin to show, some of the more common ones include:

- Rapid weight loss
- Profuse night sweats

- Ongoing, unexplained fatigue
- Swollen lymph glands
- Diarrhea that lasts longer than a week
- White spots or blemishes in the mouth or throat
- Pneumonia

Do not assume you are infected if you have any of these symptoms. Each of these symptoms can easily be related to other illnesses. Again, the only way to determine for sure whether you are infected with HIV is to be tested.

✔ Quick Tip

What can you do to help someone whose substance abuse problem is putting them at risk for HIV/AIDS? Be a real friend. You might even save a life. Encourage your friend to stop using substances or seek professional help. For information and referrals, call the National Clearinghouse for Alcohol and Drug Information at 800-729-6686. For more information go to http://www.health.org.

Questions And Answers About HIV/AIDS

Can you get HIV/AIDS from deep kissing or from someone's sweat?

No. There are no known cases of HIV transmission through sweat or saliva. HIV is primarily transmitted in blood, semen, or vaginal fluid during unprotected sex or from sharing needles.

If you already have the HIV virus, does it really matter whether you drink and use drugs?

Yes. Being smoke-free, clean, and sober improves your chances of staying healthy longer.

Who is most likely to get HIV/AIDS?

Anyone who has unprotected sex, shares needles, or exchanges bodily fluids or blood with an infected person is at risk. HIV is a virus. AIDS is a disease. Viruses do not care about age, race, or sexual orientation.

☞ **Remember!!**

If you know someone who is risking exposure to HIV/AIDS, urge him or her to stop or get more information. If your behavior places you at risk for exposure to HIV/AIDS—stop. If you have already possibly been exposed to HIV/AIDS, get tested and follow your doctor's instructions. The longer you ignore the real facts, the more chances you take with your life.

Chapter 37

Hepatitis C: A Silent Epidemic For Injection Drug Users

This virus is the most common blood-borne illness in the United States. It is the most common cause of liver transplants and it kills up to 10,000 Americans each year.

This virus is not HIV. Rather, it is the hepatitis C virus, also called HCV. The National Institute on Drug Abuse (NIDA) reports that about four million Americans are infected with HCV. That's less than 2 percent of the country's population. But among people who start injecting illegal drugs, 50 to 80 percent get infected with HCV within one year. Injection drug use accounts for at least 60 percent of the HCV infection in the United States. Most of the injection drug users will not know they are infected, because symptoms can go undetected for 10 to 20 years.

Among people who contract HCV, about 15 percent are able to rid the virus naturally from the bloodstream, according to NIDA. The rest live with hepatitis C as a chronic illness—one that increases their risk of liver damage, including cirrhosis and liver cancer.

Other viruses, including hepatitis A and B, can also damage the liver. Yet these viruses rarely lead to long-term infection. While we have vaccines to prevent hepatitis A and B, no vaccine exists for HCV and none is expected soon. Current treatments for HCV include the drugs interferon and ribavirin. But these drugs can have serious side effects, including fatigue, and not everyone is a candidate for treatment.

The only way that people can prevent HCV infection is through their behavior. Most importantly, they need to:

- Avoid shooting drugs—or, get into treatment if they do inject drugs.
- Avoid sharing toothbrushes, razors, and other personal care items that could have blood on them.
- Have sex only with one uninfected partner.
- Consider the health risks of body piercing and tattooing, which can spread infection when done by people who don't wash their hands, use disposable gloves, or clean their tools well.

People who've injected illegal drugs at any time should get a blood test for hepatitis C. Others who should be screened include people who got blood transfusions or organ transplants before 1992 (when blood supplies began being tested for HCV), people born to an HCV-positive mother, and those with HIV.

HCV is not spread by casual contact, including coughing and sneezing. Yet the infection triggers fears. People living with HCV may find that friends stop hugging them and that spouses stop sleeping with them.

✎ Weird Words

Hepatitis: Inflammation of the liver, due usually to viral infection but sometimes to toxic agents. Hepatitis ranks as a major public health problem in industrialized nations. The 3 most common types of viral hepatitis (A, B, and C) afflict millions worldwide

Source: From *Stedman's Medical Dictionary, 27th Edition*, Copyright © 2000 Lippincott Williams & Wilkins. All rights reserved.

"Some individuals experience grief and loss, not only related to HCV diagnosis but to the physical limitations of the illness," said Sue Hoisington, executive director of Hazelden Mental Health Centers. Many with HCV suffer loss of energy and have to make lifestyle changes that require curtailing physical activities that they truly enjoy. Another common response is anger, especially among people in recovery from addiction who've abstained from drugs for years and are diagnosed with HCV, yet another chronic illness.

Even so, people who entered recovery via the Twelve Steps of Alcoholics Anonymous have tools for living well with this virus. One is the Serenity Prayer that is often quoted at AA meetings, "God grant me the serenity to accept the things I cannot change, courage to change the things I can, and wisdom to know the difference."

"What works well with addiction and alcoholism certainly works with this chronic illness too in terms of powerlessness and acceptance," said Bob, who lives with HCV. "I try to focus on the glass being half full instead of half empty. At the same time, I can take action steps, including carrying the message that having hepatitis C is not a death sentence and that you can achieve quality life with the illness."

For More Information

To learn more about hepatitis C, contact:

- Hepatitis Foundation International, 1-800-891-0707, http://www.hepfi.org
- American Liver Foundation, 1-800-465-4837, http://www.liverfoundation.org
- National Institute on Drug Abuse, 301-443-1124, http://www.drugabuse.gov/
- Hazelden Foundation, 1-800-257-7810, http://www.hazelden.org

Chapter 38

Impaired Driving Among Youth

Despite the fact that it is illegal for youth under 21 to purchase alcohol, they still drink and they still die.

Impaired driving is a preventable social problem that costs Americans billions of dollars each year. While the Nation has witnessed considerable reductions in impaired driving among all residents in recent years, almost 37 percent of youth traffic crash fatalities in the United States in 1996 were alcohol related.

The personal and societal costs associated with impaired driving are staggering. The annual cost of alcohol-related crashes has been estimated at $148 billion. Though much less well studied, it is likely that driver impairment from drugs adds to these costs. The groups most affected are teenagers and young adults.

Drivers 15 to 20 years old have a higher rate of fatal alcohol-related motor vehicle crashes than older drivers. A recurring result in impaired driving research has been that young drivers more frequently crash at lower blood

About This Chapter: Text in this chapter was excerpted from *Technical Report: Impaired Driving Among Youth*, Substance Abuse and Mental Health Services Administration, Center for Substance Abuse Prevention, DHHS Publication No. (SMA) 99-3364, 1999. For single copies of this document, contact SAMHSA's National Clearinghouse for Alcohol and Drug Information (NCADI), P.O. Box 2345, Rockville, MD 20847-2345; 1-800-729-6686, 301-468-2600, or TDD 1-800-487-4889; or visit the website at http://www.health.org.

alcohol concentrations (BACs) than do older drivers, perhaps because of the former's inexperience with drinking, with driving, or both.

Many strategies have been shown to prevent alcohol-related crashes among youth, including those designed as deterrence and those designed to affect alcohol consumption. Three of these youth-oriented deterrence and alcohol policy strategies, are:

- **Age 21 Laws:** Minimum age 21 alcohol purchase laws are now in place in all 50 states and the District of Columbia. The National Highway Traffic Safety Administration (NHTSA) estimates that more than 16,500 traffic deaths have been averted since states started raising the minimum drinking age. The laws are not well enforced, however. A number of strategies have been developed to improve enforcement and decrease youth access to alcohol. These strategies include decoy or sting programs, responsible beverage service training, and the development of driver's licenses that are more difficult to alter or counterfeit.
- **Zero Tolerance:** Many states have enacted BAC limits of 0.02 percent or less for drivers under age 21. These limits reflect the facts that drinking is illegal for anyone under 21 and that young drivers are particularly vulnerable to impairment at low BACs. These laws have been found to reduce alcohol-related crashes in the affected age group by as much as 50 percent in some states and by between 17 and 22 percent consistently. The effectiveness of the laws increases when they are combined with a public awareness campaign.
- **Graduated Licensing:** Graduated licensing is a process by which learning drivers can be gradually granted driving privileges. When young people drink and drive, they experience far more trouble—with less alcohol—than older drivers. Reductions in traffic crashes, both alcohol related and not alcohol related, have been measured as a result of nighttime driving curfews, increased age of licensure, and graduated driving privileges (in which a variety of driving restrictions are gradually lifted as the driver gains experience and maturity). Such licensing systems have been found to be very effective in New Zealand and Australia and are supported by both parents and young people.

Trends In Impaired Driving

Impaired driving is a preventable social problem that costs Americans billions of dollars each year. In 1996, more than 21 percent of drivers between 15 and 20 years of age involved in fatal crashes had blood alcohol concentrations (BACs) between 0.01 and 0.10. Examining trends in impaired driving provides answers to many questions concerning the nature and extent of this problem, such as who drives impaired and how impaired driving rates vary over time and by state.

✤ It's A Fact!!

When young drivers combine alcohol and driving, they experience more trouble with less alcohol than older drivers. The problem is related to both their immaturity and their lack of driving experience. The estimated medical, monetary, and lost quality-of-life costs associated with injuries in crashes of young-drivers are staggering.

How is impaired driving defined?

Impaired driving is the joint occurrence of (1) driving a vehicle and (2) having a BAC of 0.01 or greater or being under the influence of some other psychoactive substance. NHTSA defines a fatal crash as "alcohol-related" if either a driver or a nonoccupant (for example, a pedestrian) has a BAC greater than or equal to 0.01 in a police-reported traffic crash. Those with a BAC of 0.10 or greater are considered "intoxicated."

What is the magnitude of the problems caused by impaired driving?

During 1996, alcohol-related motor vehicle crashes in the United States caused more than 17,000 deaths and more than 321,000 injuries. In 1996, alcohol-related fatalities for youth ages 15 to 20 increased by nearly 5 percent. More than 2,300 youth died in alcohol-related crashes (36.6 percent of their total traffic fatalities). Moreover, NHTSA reported that high BACs (in excess of 0.10 percent) accounted for all of the increase in alcohol-related fatalities among youth in 1996.

Does the area of the country make a difference?

✤ It's A Fact!!

It is unlawful in all states for any person who is under the influence of any alcoholic beverage or any drug to drive a vehicle.

Substantial regional differences exist in the incidence of alcohol-related motor vehicle fatalities. The lowest rates for all alcohol-related motor vehicle fatalities are found in the northeastern states, such as New York, Massachusetts, and Rhode Island. Rates three, four, and five times higher, respectively, are found in the South, Southwest, and Mountain states. In 1996, the states with the highest rates were New Mexico, Mississippi, Wyoming, and Alabama. Among youth, lowest percentages are in Utah, Virginia, and Georgia. States with the highest percentages of youth alcohol-related fatalities are Vermont, North Dakota, and Montana.

Why are there such significant differences among states' rates?

A variety of factors interact to influence the rate of alcohol-related motor vehicle fatalities. These factors include population density, population composition (regarding age and sex), cultural differences, law enforcement techniques, and the like. States with large populations of young drivers and lenient drinking and driving policies are likely to have higher rates of alcohol-related motor vehicle fatalities.

How do we know that driving under the influence of alcohol causes crashes?

The largest case-control study of drinking and driving ever conducted was completed in Grand Rapids, Michigan, during the early 1960's (see: Hyman, M. M. "Accident vulnerability and blood alcohol concentrations of drivers by demographic characteristics," *Quarterly Journal of Studies on Alcohol*

(Suppl. 4), 34-57, 1968). The results for the 13,485 crash-involved and comparison drivers studied indicated that the risk of becoming involved in a crash increased after just a few drinks and increased exponentially with the number of drinks consumed.

The results indicate that crash risk increases gradually up to a BAC of about 0.10 percent (about four to five drinks in 1 to 2 hours for a 160-pound person). Then, crash risk increases exponentially with increasing amounts of alcohol. When compared with drivers who had not been drinking, drivers with BACs from 0.10 percent to 0.25 percent were 6 to 32 times more likely to become involved in a crash.

What special attention have underage drinking drivers received?

Drinking and driving by youth has been a major focus of preventionists for most of the past 15 years. In 1984, President Reagan signed legislation to withhold highway safety funds from states that did not set 21 as the minimum purchasing age for alcohol. By July 1988, all 50 states had set that minimum purchasing age. It is estimated that these laws have saved approximately 16,500 lives since 1975. Many states also adopted low or zero tolerance presumptive BAC limits for drivers under the age of 21 and "use and lose" laws, which link drug and alcohol convictions, irrespective of motor vehicle involvement, to loss of the driver's license.

Can convicted drinking drivers be successfully rehabilitated?

Impaired driving is often symptomatic of some degree of an underlying substance abuse problem. BACs of 0.20 percent at the time of arrest are not uncommon; BACs of 0.15 percent are typical. Persons who do not have alcohol problems rarely reach such levels. Therefore, alcohol or drug assessment, education, and treatment have traditionally been part of the sanctioning and relicensing process for convicted drinking drivers.

Evaluations of such treatment programs in terms of subsequent crashes and violations have been mixed. Results were negative when treatment was applied in lieu of traditional license withdrawal; they were positive when added to license withdrawal and for drivers whose substance abuse problems were less severe.

Are crashes being prevented?

Yes. The numbers of vehicles, drivers, road miles, and miles driven have increased steadily throughout the 1980's and 1990's. Yet the numbers of alcohol-related fatalities, drinking drivers involved in fatal crashes, and drinking drivers randomly sampled in roadside surveys have declined.

In 1983, there were 23,646 alcohol-related fatalities in motor vehicle crashes (or 55 percent of all motor vehicle fatalities during that year). In 1996, there were 17,126 alcohol-related fatalities in motor vehicle crashes (or 41 percent of all motor vehicle fatalities in that year). Thus, for the period 1982 through 1995, both the absolute number of alcohol-related fatalities and the percentage of alcohol-related fatalities among all motor vehicle fatalities declined.

A similar method of assessing the decline in fatal crashes is to examine the BACs of drivers involved in these crashes. In 1982, approximately 9 percent of all drivers involved in fatal crashes had BACs between 0.01 percent and 0.09 percent at the time of the crash, and 30 percent had BACs of 0.10 percent or higher. By 1996, these percentages had declined to 6 percent and 19 percent, respectively.

Who is still drinking and driving?

Despite progress, many people, especially males under age 25, continue to drink and drive. In 1996, 21 percent of all male drivers involved in fatal crashes had a BAC of 0.10 percent or greater, compared with only 11 percent of all female drivers involved in fatal crashes.

Most drinking drivers of passenger vehicles (including light trucks and vans) who were involved in fatal crashes were 25 to 34, followed by drivers under the age of 25. When looking only at drivers whose BAC was between 0.01 percent and 0.09 percent, the age group with the highest rate of impaired drivers was under 25 years. Young drivers (15 to 20 years old) have a higher rate of fatal alcohol-related motor vehicle crashes than older drivers.

Who is being killed in alcohol-related crashes?

In 1996, most of the 17,126 fatalities in alcohol-related crashes were drivers (60 percent), most of whom were between ages 16 and 44 (47 percent). The remainder were passengers (22 percent), pedestrians (15 percent), and others, including bicyclists (2 percent). Many of the passengers were children or teenagers. The fatally injured pedestrians in alcohol-related crashes tended to be older than either the fatally injured drivers or the fatally injured passengers. While some children age 15 or younger and some persons age 65 or older die in these crashes, it is teenagers and young adults, followed by middle-aged adults, who suffer by far the greatest losses.

When do alcohol-related crashes occur?

The month with the largest number of alcohol-related motor vehicle deaths during 1996 was August (9.7 percent). June was second (9.3 percent), followed by September (9.0 percent), November (8.8 percent), and October (8.6 percent). December ranked seventh (8.3 percent). The months with the fewest deaths were January (6.8 percent) and February (6.8 percent).

Consistent with popular belief, most deaths that resulted from alcohol-related crashes occurred on a Saturday (24 percent), followed by Sunday (20 percent) and Friday (16 percent). The day with the fewest alcohol-related crash deaths was Tuesday (9 percent).

The results for time of day confirm that most alcohol-related deaths resulted from crashes at night. The time of the crash for approximately two of every three alcohol-related deaths was between 8 p.m. and 5:59 a.m. (65 percent). Approximately 1 in 5 deaths occurred between 4 p.m. and 7:59 p.m. (20 percent), and approximately 1 in 10 occurred between 11 a.m. and 3:59 p.m. (9 percent).

Are drugs a problem?

Available evidence concerning drugs suggests that they have a small, yet measurable, association with impaired driving and the occurrence of impaired driving crashes.

Of 1,882 fatally injured drivers sampled in seven states during 1991 and 1992, postmortem blood samples showed alcohol in 51.5 percent of the drivers. Of the 43 other drugs for which tests were conducted, the most prevalent were cannabis (6.7 percent), cocaine (5.3 percent), benzodiazepine tranquilizers

(2.9 percent), and amphetamines (1.9 percent). Analysis of the circumstances surrounding each of these fatal crashes suggested that they were caused by impairment effects associated with alcohol (alone), alcohol-drug combinations, and drug-drug combinations (see Terhune, K. W., Ippolito, C. A., Hendricks, D. L., Michalovic, J. G., Bogema, S. C., Santinga, P., Blomberg, R., & Preusser, D. F. *The incidence and role of drugs in fatally injured drivers: Final report*. Washington, DC: National Highway Traffic Safety Administration, NTIS No. PB 94-151768, 1992).

Another study examined 10 police agencies in which officers were specifically trained to identify drivers impaired by drugs. Of 1,469 drivers arrested under suspicion of drug intoxication, 50 percent had BACs of 0.00, and 40 percent had BACs of less than 0.10 percent. Laboratory results indicated that 46.5 percent of these suspects tested positive for cannabis. Other drugs found were central nervous system (CNS) stimulants including cocaine (29.6 percent), CNS depressants (23.3 percent), narcotic analgesics (15.5 percent), phencyclidine, known as "PCP" (5.9 percent), inhalants (1.4 percent), and hallucinogens (0.8 percent). Between 1 and 4 percent of all persons arrested for impaired driving during this study were found to be under the influence of drugs. This finding is consistent with the conclusion that drugs are a small, yet measurable, part of the total impaired driving problem (see Preusser, D. F., Ulmer, R. G., and Preusser, C. W. Evaluation of the impact of the drug evaluation and classification program on enforcement and adjudication. Washington, DC: National Highway Traffic Safety Administration, NTIS No. PB 94-143 302-WTS, 1992a).

What works to prevent impaired driving among youth?

Overall, impaired driving has declined nearly every year since 1982. The reasons for the decline likely have involved the interaction of several factors, including the general deterrents described above, changing social attitudes fostered by citizen pressure, and generally lower levels of alcohol consumption.

✤ It's A Fact!!

Impaired driving among youth is one negative consequence of the abuse of alcohol and other drugs, but it can be prevented.

In 1996, however, alcohol-related fatalities for youth ages 15 to 20 increased by almost 5 percent.

Minimum Age 21 Alcohol Purchase Laws

Drinking alcohol is a particularly risky activity for young people, who lack experience and judgment. The risks of alcohol use by youth include traumatic injury, perpetrating or being the victim of crime or violence, and the possibility of developing chronic alcohol abuse. Minimum age 21 alcohol purchase laws are an important and effective countermeasure to address these problems. They have been particularly successful in reducing alcohol-related crashes among young drivers. NHTSA estimates that these laws have reduced traffic fatalities involving 18- to 20- year-old drivers by 13 percent and have saved more than 16,500 lives since 1975.

Have minimum drinking age laws contributed to a reduction in underage drinking?

Historically, there has been a trend toward lower alcohol use, particularly among high school students. This trend apparently began in the 1980's as states were passing minimum age 21 purchase laws. Monthly use of alcohol among high school seniors declined from 72 percent in 1980 to 51 percent in 1993. Drinking five or more drinks in a row on at least one occasion during the past 2 weeks (binge drinking) declined from 41 percent in 1983 to 28 percent in 1993. However, there are signs that this trend may have ended.

Has there been a reduction in alcohol-related traffic crashes?

Historically, the trend in motor vehicle fatalities for persons 21 or older was similar to the trend for those under 21. After 1988, the year in which the last state passed the minimum age 21 purchase regulations, both groups' trendlines continued to decline; however, the fatality rate for those ages 15 to 20 declined faster than the rate for older drivers, representing a significant minimum age effect.

Why and when did states adopt the minimum age 21 purchase laws?

Twenty-nine states lowered their minimum alcohol purchase age from 21 to 18, 19, or 20 during the early 1970's—the same period during which minimum age limits for activities such as voting were also being lowered. The result was a substantial increase in alcohol-related crashes involving young persons. After researchers documented these increases and brought them to the attention of activists and policy-makers, states began to return to an age 21 purchasing requirement in the late 1970's and early 1980's, with a subsequent decrease in alcohol-related crashes.

By 1984, 23 states had a minimum age 21 purchasing law, and federal legislation was passed that would have withheld highway funds from the remaining 27 states. As of July 1988, it was illegal in all 50 states and the District of Columbia to sell alcohol to anyone under the age of 21.

> **✤ It's A Fact!!**
>
> Minimum purchase age laws have been successful in reducing alcohol use and related problems among our country's youth. They have prevented thousands of alcohol-related traffic deaths. Still, underage drinking has not been eliminated, and many existing state laws are not comprehensive.

What is "use and lose"?

One penalty that may be especially meaningful and threatening to young people is the loss of their driver's license. Laws that allow for the suspension of the driver's license following a conviction for any alcohol or drug violation are often referred to as "use-and-lose" laws. In most cases, the alcohol or drug violation need not be associated with driving or riding in a car. The violation could be alcohol or drug consumption, possession, or attempt to purchase with or without the use of false ID. The license suspension could be for a certain period of time or until some specified age is reached. Persons who are not yet licensed could have their licensure delayed.

Zero Tolerance: A Strategy For Preventing Impaired Driving Among Youth

Almost all states (plus the District of Columbia) have enacted a law to prohibit underage drivers from operating a motor vehicle after drinking. The details of the laws, such as the precise permissible BAC, vary from state to state. Zero tolerance laws, when properly implemented and enforced, can be effective in sending a no-use message to young people and preventing alcohol-related crashes among young drivers.

What is zero tolerance?

Zero tolerance laws prohibit young persons from driving a vehicle while they have a BAC greater than 0.00 percent, 0.01 percent, or 0.02 percent (depending on the state). The BAC depends on a person's body weight, the number of drinks consumed, and the length of time over which the drinks were consumed. If a police officer has probable cause to believe that a driver has been drinking, the officer administers a breath test. In most states with zero tolerance laws, any amount of alcohol in the body of a driver under 21 is an offense for which the driver's license may be suspended. Because of the high value young drivers place on their licenses, the threat of revocation has proven to be an especially effective sanction—for both its punitive and its deterrent effect.

The most commonly specified BAC for drivers under 21 is 0.02 percent, which is approximately equal to one drink for the average person (34 states). Ten states and the District of Columbia have adopted the 0.00-percent level, and two states, 0.01 percent. states that set levels lower than the adult level, yet higher than 0.02 percent, are not considered to have zero tolerance for alcohol.

Are zero tolerance laws effective in reducing traffic crashes involving youth who have been drinking?

The first four states to reduce the legal BAC limit for young drivers were Maine, North Carolina, Wisconsin, and New Mexico. These states experienced a 34-percent decline in nighttime fatal crashes among adolescents targeted by the lower BAC levels. This decline was approximately one-third greater than a similar decline observed in four nearby states selected for comparison.

By the end of 1990, 12 states had lowered BAC levels for youth. These states experienced a 16-percent overall decline in nighttime single-vehicle fatal crashes among young drivers targeted by the new laws, compared with a 1-percent rise among drivers of the same age in selected comparison states. Of the 12 states, four had adopted a BAC level of 0.00 percent, four had a level of 0.02 percent, and four had levels ranging from 0.04 percent to 0.06 percent. Measured crash reductions were statistically significant for the 0.00—percent states (22-percent reduction) and the 0.02-percent states (17 percent) but not for the 0.04-percent to 0.06-percent states (7 percent).

✤ It's A Fact!!

Teenage drivers increase their risk of crashes after only one or two drinks. The goal of zero tolerance is to eliminate driving by young persons who have consumed any alcohol. Beginning with Maine in 1983, most states have now adopted zero tolerance laws. Substantial crash reductions have been documented, particularly in places where the law has been well publicized.

What penalties are appropriate for zero tolerance violations?

All states have laws against driving while intoxicated (DWI) or operating a motor vehicle while under the influence of alcohol. These laws carry severe penalties, including a possible jail sentence, loss of license, and a substantial fine. A second or third impaired-driving arrest can lead to a felony conviction. Under zero tolerance laws, however, lesser charges are typically brought against young drivers; the strategy is not intended to send young persons to jail or to produce a criminal record.

The penalties for a zero tolerance violation vary widely among the states, but they nearly always involve the suspension or revocation of the driver's license. In some states, the term of the license suspension can be equal to or greater than the term of suspension for a DWI conviction. Penalties may also involve alcohol or drug assessment, some form of alcohol or drug education or treatment, and a fine.

Why 0.02 percent rather than zero?

States adopting 0.02 percent as the zero tolerance threshold have argued that alcohol levels between 0.00 percent and 0.01 percent can occur from the use of over-the-counter medications and some food preparations and thus would not necessarily constitute underage drinking. Also, the 0.02-percent level allows for some variability in measurement. Nevertheless, the clear intent of these laws, regardless of BAC, is to prohibit drinking among drivers under 21.

Graduated Licensing: A Strategy For Preventing Impaired Driving Among Youth

Driver licensing systems have been developed that can protect young people as they gain maturity and experience behind the wheel. These systems—usually referred to as graduated licensing—are especially valuable in improving traffic safety. They are also an important strategy to prevent substance abuse.

What is graduated licensing?

According to NHTSA, graduated licensing is "a system designed to ease beginning drivers into the traffic environment under controlled exposure to progressively more difficult driving experiences." A licensing system is considered to be graduated if it contains at least three distinct steps or stages:

- **Learning:** The young person is required to undergo a period of practice driving under the supervision of an experienced licensed driver.
- **Restricted:** The young person can engage in unsupervised driving subject to certain restrictions. A key restriction is a prohibition against driving after drinking any alcohol. Restrictions on night driving may also reduce the probability that the young driver will drive after using harmful psychoactive substances. Other possible restrictions include added requirements for seatbelt use, limitations on passengers, and limitations on the types of vehicles that can be driven. During the restricted stage, license actions and suspensions are often rendered for fewer and less serious traffic violations. Often there are very serious penalties for driving under the influence of any amount of alcohol.
- **Full:** The young person is issued a full-privilege (drive anywhere at any time) license.

To enter the learning stage in a typical graduated licensing system, the young person needs to have attained the minimum age (typically 15 or 16) and pass vision and rules-of-the-road tests. Entry into the restricted stage requires completing a minimum period of violation-free driving as a learner and passing a road test. Full licensure requires reaching some minimum age, typically 17 or 18, and completing the restricted stage with few or no violations or at-fault crashes. The required learning period and the required restricted period distinguish graduated licensing systems from traditional systems, in which the young person need only attain a certain age and pass rules, vision, and road tests before receiving a full-privilege license.

Does night driving increase the risk of crashes?

Yes, young drivers have much higher crash rates during the night than during the day. In fact, while drivers ages 16 to 17 accumulate only 14 percent of their miles driven between the hours of 9 p.m. and 6 a.m., they experience 39 percent of their fatal crashes during that time period. It is highly likely that some of the increased risk at night is due to the consumption of alcohol or drugs.

An integral element in any graduated licensing system is a restriction on night driving—other than for work or school or when accompanied by a parent or guardian—during the intermediate or restricted phase of the system. This night driving restriction may be in place for some period of time (for example, the first year of driving in Maryland), until reaching some specified age (typically 17 or 18), or until the young person has reached some specified age and has completed a driver education course (for example, in New York and Pennsylvania).

Night driving restrictions have been shown to be highly effective in reducing teen driver crashes. Reductions in fatal crashes have been demonstrated nationally by comparing states with and without such restrictions and studying selected cities. Reductions in night crashes associated with night driving restrictions can be dramatic—as much as 69 percent—despite the fact that night driving with a parent or guardian, or to or from work or school, is typically allowed.

Are teen passengers a problem for teen drivers?

Several studies have shown that teen drivers are more likely to crash when carrying only teen passengers than when traveling alone or with other passenger

> **☞ Remember!!**
>
> Youth between the ages of 15 and 20 are more likely to die in traffic crashes than from any other cause. On a per-mile-driven basis, the risk of a crash is four to eight times higher for teenage drivers than for older drivers. When alcohol or drugs are added to the mix, the combination is often deadly.

combinations. New Zealand's graduated licensing system and the system recently adopted in Georgia restrict unsupervised teen drivers from transporting teen passengers. Evaluation of the New Zealand law has shown a reduction in the number of teenagers injured as passengers in cars driven by teens.

Does gender make a difference?

Licensing data indicate that males and females become licensed at approximately the same rate once they turn 16. Data have indicated, however, that proportionately more females among 16-year-old drivers are involved in crashes than male teenagers and older drivers. There is some indication that females enter the licensing process with somewhat less learning-driving experience than males. This fact may account for the somewhat higher crash rate of 16-year-old females, which dissipates by age 17 or 18. Accumulating driving experience under supervised and controlled situations prior to full-privilege licensure would seem to be important for both males and females.

At what age should teens begin learning to drive?

Most states that recently changed their licensing laws to resemble graduated licensing more closely have left unchanged the age at which learning driving can begin. They have extended their required learning period and often added an intermediate or restricted-driving period before full-privilege licensure. The effect of these changes has been to delay the time when a young person can obtain a license to drive anywhere at any time.

Two states, Michigan and Virginia, lowered the age at which learning driving may begin. On the one hand, lowering the learning age should allow for the accumulation of more supervised driving experience prior to full-privilege licensure. On the other hand, if people enter the licensing process at an earlier age, they may qualify for a license when they are younger. More practice is consistent with the goals of graduated licensing; younger licensing is not. Allowing younger people to learn to drive may give them access to vehicles and driving knowledge at an even younger age, thereby contributing to more unlicensed and unsupervised operation of motor vehicles.

Does graduated licensing reduce crashes?

Yes. Maryland implemented a graduated—then called provisional—licensing system with a night driving restriction in 1979. A 5-percent reduction in the number of teen drivers involved in crashes and a 10-percent reduction in traffic law violations and convictions were found for 16- and 17-year-old drivers. New Zealand implemented a graduated licensing system, including a night driving restriction, in 1987. An 8-percent reduction in crashes was found for drivers ages 15 to 19.

Upstate New York and Pennsylvania have had a key component of graduated licensing—a night driving restriction for 16-year-olds and some 17-year-olds—for several years. These two states were compared with Connecticut and Delaware, which licensed 16-year-olds at the time of the study but did not have graduated systems, and with New Jersey and Long Island, which did not license until age 17. The results indicated that New Jersey and Long Island, with no licensing until age 17, had a huge advantage over Delaware and Connecticut for 16-year-olds. However, crash rates were higher in New Jersey and on Long Island for the remaining teen years. New York and Pennsylvania, with the night-driving restriction, had rates lower than Delaware and Connecticut for 16-year-olds and somewhat lower rates for 17-year-olds, followed by rates comparable to Connecticut and Delaware for the remaining teen years. Researchers argued that New York and Pennsylvania were better able to ease young drivers into the traffic stream by allowing them to accumulate driving experience during the less hazardous daylight hours.

✤ It's A Fact!!

The goal of graduated licensing is to phase in exposure to increasingly complex driving tasks and environments as young people mature and develop their driving skills. During this process, alcohol is subject to a zero tolerance restriction. Unsupervised night driving is also restricted. Both these restrictions should limit the extent to which alcohol and other drugs contribute to the crash injury and fatality of young drivers.

Chapter 39

Youth Violence Linked To Substance Use

National Household Survey On Drug Abuse And Reports Of Violence

The National Household Survey on Drug Abuse (NHSDA) is an annual survey sponsored by the Substance Abuse and Mental Health Services Administration (SAMHSA). The 1999 data are based on information obtained from nearly 70,000 persons aged 12 or older. The survey collects data by administering questionnaires to a representative sample of the population through face-to-face interviews at their place of residence.

The 1999 National Household Survey on Drug Abuse (NHSDA) asked youths aged 12 to 17 to report on their participation in violent behavior during the year before the survey, including serious fighting at school or work, group-against-group fighting, and attacking others with the intent to seriously hurt them. Youths were also asked about their use of alcohol and illicit drugs during the month before the survey. Illicit drug use was defined as use at least once of marijuana/hashish, cocaine (including crack), inhalants, hallucinogens (including PCP and LSD), heroin, or any prescription-type psychotherapeutic used non-medically.

About This Chapter: Text in this chapter is from "Youth Violence Linked to Substance Use," *The NHSDA Report*, October 12, 2001. The full document, including references and statistical tables, is available online at: http://www.samhsa.gov/oas/facts/Violence.htm.

Prevalence Of Youth Violence

> **✎ Weird Words**
>
> Prevalence: The number of cases existing in a given population at a specific period of time (*period prevalence*) or at a particular moment in time (*point prevalence*).
>
> Source: From *Stedman's Medical Dictionary, 27th Edition*,

Violence among young people has increased during the past 15 years. Of the estimated 23 million youths in the United States aged 12 to 17, the 1999 NHSDA showed that more than 5 million reported participating in serious fighting at school or work, almost 4 million took part in a group-against-group fight, and almost 2 million attacked others with the intent of seriously hurting them during the past year.

Youths aged 14 or 15 were more likely than 16 or 17 year olds to report being involved in serious fighting at school or work during the past year, and youths aged 14 to 17 were more likely than 12 or 13 year olds to report attacking others with the intent to seriously hurt them in the past year. There were no significant differences between age groups in reporting group-against-group fighting.

> **✤ It's A Fact!!**
>
> - Among youths aged 12 to 17, males were more likely than females to participate in violent behaviors.
> - Asian youths were less likely than youths from other racial/ethnic groups to engage in serious fighting at school or work and attacking others with the intent to seriously hurt them during the past year.
> - Youths who reported participating in violence during the past year were more likely to use alcohol and illicit drugs during the past month than youths who did not report past year violence.

Males were more likely than females to participate in these violent behaviors. Asian youths (13 percent) were less likely than youths from other racial/ethnic groups (white 21 percent; American Indian/Alaska Native 21 percent; Hispanic 25 percent; and black 26 percent) to participate in serious fighting at school or work during the past year and attacking others with the intent to seriously hurt them during the past year (Asian 4 percent, compared with white 7 percent; Hispanic 9 percent; American Indian/Alaska native 9 percent; and black 13 percent). There were no clear differences between racial/ethnic groups in reporting past year group-against-group fighting. Also, no clear differences in violent behaviors emerged between youths who lived in metropolitan versus non-metropolitan counties.

Link Between Violent Behaviors And Use Of Alcohol And Illicit Drugs

According to the 1999 NHSDA, youths who participated in violent behaviors during the past year were more likely to use alcohol and illicit drugs than youths who did not participate in violent behaviors during this time period. For example, 26 percent of youths who had participated in a serious fight at school or work during the past year reported past month use of alcohol compared with 14 percent of youths who had not participated in a serious fight at school or work during the past year. Also, 18 percent of youths who had participated in a serious fight at school or work during the past year reported past month use of illicit drugs compared with 7 percent of youths who had not participated in a serious fight at school or work during the past year.

Remember!!

NHSDA findings illustrate the close link between youths' participation in violent behaviors and their use of alcohol and illicit drugs. Youths who engaged in violent behaviors during the past year were more likely to report past month alcohol and illicit drug use than youths who did not engage in violent behaviors during the past year.

Chapter 40

Substance Abuse And Learning Disabilities

Foreword

The relationship between learning disabilities and substance abuse is a subject about which we know very little. We do know that there is a great deal of stigma attached to both drug abuse and addiction and learning disabilities. This problem of stigma may help explain why it has not yet been well researched.

The subject, however, demands attention because the implications are tremendous. As many as 20 percent of school age children may suffer from a learning disability. A large number of these children also suffer from a behavioral disorder. If there is reason to believe that these children may be more likely to take drugs, we need to know and we need to understand the relationship as thoroughly as possible.

Understanding the relationship may help us better understand the motivation of a very large number of drug users. People use drugs for two basic reasons. Some use them simply to seek novelty. Others use them to alleviate the pain and stress of a difficult life situation, to self-medicate. Some children

About This Chapter: This chapter contains excerpts from *Substance Abuse and Learning Disabilities: Peas in a Pod or Apples and Oranges?* The National Center on Addiction and Substance Abuse at Columbia University (CASA), © September 2000 CASA; reprinted with permission. The full text of this report, including references and notes, can be found on CASA's website at http://www.casacolumbia.org.

and teens may well use drugs to deal with the negative consequences of a learning disability or behavioral disorder. By identifying those who are at risk for using drugs as well as their motivation for doing so, we can develop more effective and appropriate prevention and treatment programs.

The first question that needs to be answered is, Is there actually a relationship between learning disabilities and substance abuse? We can feel pretty confident in saying that there is. What we don't know is the precise relationship.

—Alan I. Leshner, Ph.D., Director
National Institute on Drug Abuse

Learning Disabilities May Increase The Risk For Substance Abuse

The link begins in the womb. Prenatal smoking, drinking and drug use can seriously damage the fetus. A 1996 study showed that children prenatally exposed to cigarettes had lower intelligence scores and more behavioral problems, such as anxiety, disobedience, and difficulty concentrating and relating to other children.

Alcohol use during pregnancy is the leading cause of mental retardation in children. Drinking during pregnancy can produce fetal alcohol syndrome, fetal alcohol effects, low birth weight, learning disabilities, attention deficit disorder (ADD) and attention deficit hyperactivity disorder (ADHD). Some experts believe that alcohol has in some way harmed between one-third and two-thirds of all children in special education.

Children whose mothers drink, use drugs, and smoke during pregnancy are likelier to have learning disabilities, ADD and ADHD. Children of alcoholics and drug addicts are themselves more likely to become alcoholics and drug addicts. Despite the compelling coincidence of learning disabilities and substance abuse, we know remarkably little about the relationship. There are, however, some compelling facts:

- Children with learning disabilities are at greater risk of school failure and often experience difficulty and frustration relating to others. These children are more likely to perceive themselves as poor students and engage in negative and disruptive behavior, and less likely to be involved in extracurricular activities. Academic failure and peer rejection are common risk factors associated with substance abuse, so is the lower self esteem that accompanies social difficulty and academic failure.

- A child with a learning disability is twice as likely as a member of the general population to suffer attention deficit/hyperactivity disorder. ADHD affected individuals have a high incidence of substance abuse, and ADHD is further associated with an earlier onset of substance abuse and a greater difficulty shaking addiction.
- Studies show that as many as half of those suffering ADHD self-medicate with drugs and alcohol. An individual with ADHD is twice as likely as one without ADHD to abuse substances.
- Individuals in substance abuse treatment have a higher incidence of learning disabilities than the general population. One recent study revealed that 40 percent of people in substance abuse treatment have a learning disability, while another indicated that in residential substance abuse treatment programs, the percentage of learning disabled people has been found to be as high as 60 percent. Correlation is not causation, but such a high statistical coincidence raises enough suspicion to warrant further investigation and prudence requires action by parents, teachers and others who care for the nation's children.

✤ It's A Fact!!

Learning disabilities affect up to 20 percent of American school age children—10.8 million of the 54 million such children. The characteristics of learning disabled children—reduced self-esteem, academic difficulty, loneliness, depression and the desire for social acceptance—closely mirror the risk factors for substance abuse.

Is There Cause For Concern?

Learning disabilities affect up to 20 percent of school age children in the United States, some 10.8 million of the 54 million such children. Behavioral disorders also affect up to 20 percent of school age children. The overlap of these two conditions in children is extensive, but estimates vary widely due to imprecise diagnostic criteria and a lack of data. What is clear is that the characteristics of learning disabilities—reduced self-esteem, academic difficulty, loneliness, depression and the desire for social acceptance—mirror the risk factors for substance abuse.

This cluster of conditions—learning disabilities, behavioral disorders and substance abuse—imposes serious costs on society and on individual families. A better understanding of the nature of the links between learning disabilities, behavior disorders and substance abuse is critical if we are to develop strategies for prevention and treatment in order to avoid these costly human and economic consequences.

What are learning disabilities and behavioral disorders?

There are four main categories of learning disabilities: reading disorders, mathematics disorders, disorders of written expression, and learning disorders not otherwise specified. As these definitions suggest, the learning disorders are not precisely identified. Consequently, the learning disabled are a highly heterogeneous group.

Behavioral disorders often appear in combination with these learning disorders. The most common behavioral disorders—and the most thoroughly studied—are attention deficit/hyperactivity disorder (ADHD) and conduct disorder (CD). To be diagnosed with ADHD, a child must exhibit a combination of several symptoms of either inattention or hyperactivity-impulsivity over an extended period of time. ADHD generally involves an unwillingness or inability to sit down, be quiet or pay attention in social situations. Conduct disorder involves a set of more aggressive and destructive behaviors than those exhibited in ADHD; that is, active interference with the rights of others and aggressive or unreliable behavior.

The tendency of these disorders to occur together, known scientifically as comorbidity, has considerable implications for understanding the connection. Studies to date on the link between learning disabilities and substance abuse have not controlled adequately for the effects of behavioral disorders.

As a result, it remains unclear whether results attributed to learning disabilities are instead the result of behavior disorders or of the interaction between the two sets of disorders.

Why do we care?

If we can better understand how substance abuse is related to learning disabilities and behavioral disorders, we can invest more effectively in prevention and sharply limit the greater costs that are sure to appear further down the road. Whether we can control these costs depends, of course, on whether these are preventable conditions.

Substance abuse clearly is preventable. Effective treatment and prevention programs both in the home and at school can lower drug use rates among children and teens. Whether learning disabilities and behavioral disorders can be prevented depends on the relative importance of genetic and environmental factors in causing these disorders. Some evidence suggests that, at a minimum, proper precautions taken during pregnancy—including abstinence from alcohol, tobacco and illegal drugs—can help to prevent these disorders.

Are we compounding the problem?

A further reason for concern relates to the current controversy surrounding the use of prescription medications to treat children for behavioral problems such as ADHD and learning disabilities. Most recently, national attention focused on a study reporting a sharp increase in the use of medication to treat young children before they even enter school.

There can be little doubt that medication is appropriate for many children with these conditions. In fact, as we study the link between behavioral disorders and substance abuse, it is important to note that a child who is successfully treated with medication may never suffer the emotional problems such as shame and low self-esteem that may predispose him to future drug use.

In some quarters, however, the suspicion remains that many children receive medication that they do not need. Unnecessary medication can be harmful because the safety issues and side effects of these medications are often not understood fully, especially as they relate to young children.

Two other possible consequences of unnecessary medication are especially relevant to a discussion of the relationship of these conditions to substance abuse. First, if doctors are truly engaged in the medicalization of normal behaviors, then many normal children will be unfairly diagnosed with behavioral disorders at an early age. This unnecessarily can contribute to low self-esteem, peer rejection, despair and other factors that may make the child more vulnerable to substance abuse. Second, the children receiving the medication may be convinced at an early age that drugs are the primary way to treat all of their problems. This could make them more likely to turn to illegal drugs or alcohol in the future.

What's The Link?

While research has not determined a causal link [a connection suggesting that one thing causes another] between learning disabilities and substance abuse, there is a good deal of evidence that a correlation exists between the two. This link may work in one of three ways:

- learning disabilities and/or behavioral disorders may cause or contribute to substance abuse by either a child or a parent,
- substance abuse may cause or contribute to learning disabilities and/or behavioral disorders among children, or
- both may share a common cause or set of contributing factors.

Deciding which of these three possible explanations actually reflects reality is a complex task, especially with the extraordinarily large number of physiological or environmental factors that may contribute to the development of learning disabilities or behavioral disorders or to substance abuse problems.

Does substance abuse lead to learning disabilities and/or behavioral disorders?

The strongest evidence of a link between learning disabilities and substance abuse comes from studies of prenatal drug exposure. According to the National Institute on Drug Abuse's 1996 National Pregnancy and Health Survey, of the four million women who become pregnant each year, 20.4

percent smoke cigarettes, 18.8 percent drink alcohol, and 13 percent use illicit drugs during pregnancy. Children who are exposed to alcohol, tobacco and illicit drugs in the womb are at higher risk for various developmental disorders including learning disabilities. In addition, one study found that mothers who smoked more than half a pack of cigarettes per day during pregnancy were four times more likely to have a child with conduct disorder than mothers who did not smoke.

While the intergenerational relationship between substance use, learning disabilities and behavioral disorders is well established, a more difficult question is whether a child's own use of drugs or alcohol can lead to the development of a learning disability. One theory suggests that alcohol and/or drug use can cause learning disabilities or psychological disorders because drugs affect brain functioning and metabolism. Although there is no clear evidence to support this model, there is a suggestion that drug use interferes with physiological, psychological, and emotional functioning.

Establishing this link is complicated by the question of whether learning disabilities are always present at birth or very early childhood or whether they may develop later in life.

Drug use also affects peer interactions, which may result in the appearance of a learning disability. Drug users may choose deviant or marginal groups of friends and behave in ways that can be classified as antisocial. Heavy drug use can also impair a child's academic functioning and success. Over time, such school failure may appear to result from a learning disability rather from drug abuse.

Do learning disabilities and/or behavioral disorders lead to substance abuse?

Most research into the relationship between learning and behavioral disorders and substance abuse has not focused on direct, physiological links between the two, but rather on environmental forces that may provide the bridge between these conditions. No significant theory has yet been presented that points to a direct, neurological, or chemical mechanism or common pathway through which learning disabilities cause substance abuse.

However, there are three major theories about how this relationship may work.

> **✤ It's A Fact!!**
>
> Substance abuse is the number one public health care problem in America today costing society $500 billion each year. Sixty-one million Americans are hooked on cigarettes, and fourteen million either abuse, or are addicted to, alcohol. Nearly 14 million use illegal drugs and about five or six million of them abuse or are addicted to drugs such as heroin, cocaine and amphetamines.

Theory 1: Behavioral Effects Of Learning Disabilities Are Also Risk Factors For Substance Abuse

According to several studies, the risk factors for adolescent substance abuse are very similar to the behavioral effects of learning disabilities—reduced self-esteem, academic difficulty, loneliness, depression and the desire for social acceptance. Thus, learning disabilities may indirectly lead to substance abuse by generating the types of behavior that typically lead adolescents to abuse drugs.

There are several ways in which learning disabilities can lead to these risk factors. For example, learning disabilities will clearly lead to academic difficulty. Academic failure is one of the key causes of peer rejection among teens, and academic failure and peer rejection are among the leading causes of low self-esteem. Adolescents might abuse substances to try and fit in and be accepted by peers.

While this theory provides a compelling rationale for further study of a link between learning disabilities and substance abuse, it does not predict any direct link between a learning disability and a heightened risk of substance abuse. In other words, the mere existence of the learning disability does not increase the likelihood that the child will use drugs. It is only through the behavioral effects of the learning disability that an indirect link with heightened substance abuse risk may be established.

Theory 2: Learning Disabled Children Turn To Drugs For Self Medication

This theory suggests that the child uses drugs to directly counteract neurological disturbances or the feelings of despair and loneliness brought on by the learning disability. For example, adolescents with low self-esteem may use drugs for self-medication purposes—to counter negative feelings associated with social rejection and school failure. Some specialists believe that people with ADHD medicate themselves with drugs such as alcohol, marijuana, heroin, pain medication, caffeine, nicotine and cocaine to counter feelings of restlessness.

Theory 3: Children On Psychoactive Medication Are More Likely To Believe In The Positive Effects Of Drugs

A third possible explanation for the heightened risk of substance abuse among children with learning and behavioral disorders is that children who successfully use drugs to treat a learning disability may be more comfortable with, or less troubled by, the idea of drug use in general. In this case, the drug use may not occur simultaneously with the symptoms of the behavioral disorder. Instead, this theory maintains that a child's positive experience with prescription drugs may make it more likely that he will be enticed by the alleged benefits of illegal drugs or alcohol at some future date. Presently, no empirical research supports this theory.

Are learning disabilities and substance abuse the result of a common cause?

The fact that a correlation exists between substance abuse and learning disabilities does not necessarily imply that one causes the other. We must explore the possibility that both the learning disability and the substance abuse are the result of a common cause. Given the large number of potential causes and contributing factors for both learning disabilities and substance abuse, this promises to be a difficult task.

One particular example may be instructive. Substance abuse by the mother during pregnancy can contribute to both physiological and environmental risk factors for learning disabilities and behavioral disorders. Maternal drug use will also affect a child's environment. Growing up in a home with a parent who is a substance abuser will increase the risk that a child will abuse drugs or alcohol himself. In this case, physiological forces cause the learning disability, while the substance abuse is the result of environmental forces. But both are linked to substance abuse by the mother.

However this is only one of many possible common causes. In order to uncover other possible causes, researchers must begin by searching for common factors, both genetic and environmental, that appear in the backgrounds of both substance abusers and those with learning disabilities and behavioral disorders.

☞ Remember!!

Research suggests a strong relationship between learning and behavior disorders and substance abuse, but the precise nature of the link is still unclear.

Chapter 41

Mental Illness And Emotional And Behavioral Problems In Substance Abusers

Dual Diagnosis In Adolescence

Adolescents are often referred for treatment for substance abuse but are not referred to a qualified mental health professional for appropriate diagnosis and treatment of any underlying cause for their drug and alcohol abuse. However, many teens have symptoms of a mood disorder that may in fact lead to self-medicating with street drugs and alcohol.

Families and caregivers know how difficult it is to find treatment for an adolescent who abuses drugs or alcohol but also is diagnosed with a brain disorder (mental illness); for example, attention deficit/hyperactivity disorder (ADHD), depression, or bipolar disorder. Traditionally, programs that treat individuals with brain disorders do not treat individuals with active substance abuse problems, and programs for substance abusers are not geared for people with mental illness. Adolescents are often caught in this treatment or services gap.

About This Chapter: This chapter includes text from "Dual Diagnosis in Adolescence," a document produced by the National Alliance for the Mentally Ill (NAMI), Colonial Place Three, 2107 Wilson Blvd., Suite 300, Arlington, VA 22201-3042; Phone 703/524-7600; Fax 703/524-9094; Web site: www.nami.org; HelpLine: 1-800/950-NAMI (6264). The text was reviewed by Xavier Amador, Ph.D., director of NAMI's Center for Research, Education, and Practice, March 2002. The section "Serious Emotional, Behavioral Problems Linked to Adolescent Substance Abuse," is from the Substance Abuse and Mental Health Services Administration, Press Release, June 23, 1999, updated December 2000.

✎ Weird Words

Bipolar Disorder: An affective (mood) disorder characterized by the occurrence of alternating periods of euphoria (mania) and depression

Mood: The pervasive feeling, tone, and internal emotional state of an individual which, when impaired, can markedly influence virtually all aspects of a person's behavior or his or her perception of external events.

Physiological: Related to how things normally function in the living organism rather than to their anatomical structure, their biochemical composition, or how they are affected by drugs or disease

Is dual diagnosis common?

The combination of mental illness and substance abuse is so common that many clinicians now expect to find it. Studies show that more than half of young persons with a substance abuse diagnosis also have a diagnosable mental illness.

What causes these disorders?

Mental health and addiction counselors increasingly believe that brain disorders and substance abuse disorders are biologically and physiologically based.

What kind of treatment works?

Families and caregivers may feel angry and blame the adolescent for being foolish and weak-willed. They may feel hurt when their child breaks trust by lying and stealing. But it's important to realize that mental illness and often substance abuse are disorders that the adolescent cannot take control of without professional help.

Teens with difficult problems such as concurrent mental illness and substance abuse disorders do not respond to simplistic advice like "just say no" or "snap out of it." Psychotherapy and medication combined with appropriate self-help and other support groups help most, but patients are still highly prone to relapse.

Treatment programs designed primarily for substance abusers are not recommended for individuals who have a diagnosed mental illness. Their reliance on confrontation techniques and discouragement of use of appropriate prescription medications tend to compound the problems of individuals with mental illness. These strategies may produce stress levels that make symptoms worse or cause relapse.

What is a better approach?

Increasingly, the psychiatric and drug counseling communities agree that both disorders must be treated at the same time. Early studies show that when mental illness and substance abuse are treated together, suicide attempts and psychotic episodes decrease rapidly.

Since dually diagnosed clients do not fit well into most traditional 12-step programs, special peer groups based on the principle of treating both disorders together should be developed at the community level. Individuals who develop positive social networking have a much better chance of controlling their illnesses. Healthy recreational activities are extremely important.

What's the first step in treatment?

The presence of both disorders must first be established by careful assessment. This may be difficult because the symptoms of one disorder can mimic the symptoms of the other. Seek referral to a psychologist or psychiatrist. Local affiliates of the National Alliance for the Mentally Ill (NAMI) are happy to refer families to mental health professionals their members recommend. (Call the NAMI HelpLine at 800-950-6264 for a local contact.)

Once a professional assessment has confirmed a dual diagnosis of mental illness and substance abuse, mental health professionals and family members should work together on a strategy for integrating care and motivating the adolescent.

What do model programs for treating mental illness and substance abuse look like?

There are a growing number of model programs. Support groups are an important component of these programs. Adolescents support each other as they learn about the negative role that alcohol and drugs has had on their lives. They learn social skills and how to replace substance use with new thoughts and behaviors. They get help with concrete situations that arise because of their brain disorder (mental illness). Look into programs that have support groups for family members and friends.

Serious Emotional, Behavioral Problems Linked To Adolescent Substance Abuse

Adolescents with emotional and behavioral problems are more likely to abuse alcohol, tobacco and illicit drugs, according to a new study by the Substance Abuse and Mental Health Services Administration (SAMHSA).

One study found that adolescents inclined toward substance abuse admitted to delinquent behaviors such as stealing, cutting classes or skipping school, and hanging around with others who get into trouble. They also reported poor peer and parental relations, and such problems as difficulty concentrating in school, or focusing attention on tasks at home, at part-time work, or even when involved in sports.

Table 41.1. Adolescent Behavior Problems and Substance Use in Past Month

	Adolescents with Low Level Behavior Problems	Adolescents with Serious Behavior Problems
% who used marijuana	3.6	16.6
% who used other illicit drugs	1.9	12.7
% who used alcohol	13.6	38.5
% who used cigarettes	11.5	38.6

Source: Substance Abuse and Mental Health Services Administration, 1999.

✤ It's A Fact!!

According to a study conducted by the Substance Abuse and Mental Health Services Administration, adolescents who identified themselves as having high levels of serious emotional problems were more likely than those with low levels of serious emotional problems to have alcohol and other drug-related experiences. They were:

- four times more likely to be dependent on alcohol or illicit drugs
- two times as likely to have used marijuana in the past month
- nearly four times as likely to have reported use of other illicit drugs in the past month
- nearly two times as likely to have used alcohol or smoked cigarettes in the past month
- four times as likely to report needing treatment for drug abuse

"This study underscores the urgent need to identify and address the emotional and behavioral problems of children early," said SAMHSA Administrator Nelba Chavez, Ph.D. "Because behavioral and emotional problems may be signs of early diagnosable mental illness, we must recognize a new, clear, window of opportunity for intervention before minor problems lead to serious emotional disturbances, substance abuse, school failure, family discord, violence, or even suicide."

When compared to adolescents having fewer, or less serious, behavioral problems, adolescents with behavioral problems such as stealing, showing physical aggression, or running away from home were seven times more likely to be dependent on alcohol or illicit drugs. They were more than four times as likely to have used marijuana in the past month, and seven times more likely to have used other illicit drugs. They were nearly three times as likely to have used alcohol in the past month, three times as likely to have smoked cigarettes in the past month, and nearly nine times as likely to need treatment for drug abuse, according to the study.

"If we reach children early enough, we may be able to delay or even prevent the development of mental illnesses and substance abuse. What makes this situation even more critical is the fact that today nearly two-thirds of young people in this country who already suffer from a diagnosable mental disorder are not receiving the help they need," said Dr. Chavez.

Findings of the study, "The Relationship Between Mental Health and Substance Abuse Among Adolescents," are based on data from the 1994, 1995 and 1996 National Household Survey on Drug Abuse (NHSDA). The NHSDA is conducted annually by SAMHSA and provides estimates of the prevalence of illicit drug, alcohol and tobacco use in the United States. Data from the 1994, 1995 and 1996 NHSDA surveys were used in this study because, in 1994, the NHSDA added the Youth Self-Report checklist which generates data on adolescent emotional and behavioral problems.

☞ Remember!!

When substance abuse occurs along with a diagnosable mental illness, it is important to treat both conditions.

Chapter 42

Drugs And Suicide

Teen Suicide

The teenage years are a period of turmoil for just about everyone. You're learning new social roles, developing new relationships, getting used to the changes in your body, making decisions about your future. And when you're looking for answers to problems, it can seem like no one has them. That can make a person feel quite alone.

Too often, as the daily news tells us, the search for answers to these challenges is complicated by problems outside teens' control, such as divorce, family alcoholism, domestic violence or even sexual abuse. In such an environment, normal problems—tough enough to deal with in a loving family—can seem insurmountable. Many teens who feel they have nowhere to turn will "medicate" their pain with drugs or alcohol. Or they will express their rage and frustration in acts of violence or destruction.

The Role Of Depression

Depression is also a very common illness among teenagers. The feelings of helplessness and worthlessness that can accompany it, along with disturbances

About This Chapter: This chapter includes excerpts from "Teen Suicide," © 1988, 1996 American Psychiatric Association. Despite the date of this document, it contains information that is helpful for understanding teen suicide, and the American Psychiatric Association continues to offer it as current in its "Let's Talk about..." series of publications. And, text from "Drinking, Drug Use Increase Suicide Risk," © 2000 Reuters Health Information; reprinted with permission. Reuters Health Information is available online at www.reutershealth.com.

in sleep or appetite, can fuel a downward spiral of health and grades, further clouding perspective, making even thought seem intolerably difficult.

If you are suffering situations and feelings like these, you may need some extra help to hold on. If you're depressed or angry, if you're abusing substances to hold back the pain or to feel like you fit in, its vital that you try to break through the feeling of isolation you may have and talk your feelings over with someone, preferably a mental health professional.

It's vital that you break through the isolation because studies have shown that teens who are feeling depressed, abusing substances, or acting out their violent feelings are at high risk for suicide.

What To Look For

Everyone has normal mood swings in which he or she occasionally feels sad. But when that depressed mood lingers for more than two weeks, serious depression could be setting in.

If several of the statements below describe you or a friend, it might be appropriate for you to seek help by talking to a mental health professional such as a psychiatrist or other trusted adult, such as a parent or a school counselor, about how you feel.

- I am sleeping much later than I used to.
- I'm not sleeping well and wake up early in the morning.
- I'm beginning to take a lot of naps.
- My appetite has changed, and I've noticeably lost or gained weight.
- I feel restless.
- I have withdrawn from friends and family.
- I can't concentrate very well.
- I've lost interest or pleasure in activities that I once enjoyed.
- I feel hopeless or guilty.
- I've had sudden mood or behavior changes: I used to be quiet and now I am hyperactive; or once I was outgoing and now I'm withdrawn.
- I feel that life isn't worth living.

Adolescents who consider suicide generally feel alone, hopeless and rejected. They are more vulnerable to having these feelings if they have been abused, feel they have been recently humiliated in front of family or friends, have parents with alcohol or drug problems, or have a family life affected by parental discord, disruptions, separation or divorce. However, a teenager may be depressed and/or suicidal without any of these.

Teenagers who are planning to commit suicide might "clean house" by giving away favorite possessions, cleaning their rooms or throwing things away. They may also become suddenly cheerful after a period of depression, because they think they have "found the solution" by deciding to end their lives.

One of the most dangerous times of a teen's life is when he or she has suffered a loss or humiliation of some kind: loss of self-esteem by doing poorly on a test, the breakup with a boyfriend or girlfriend, or the trauma of parents' divorce.

Research Findings

Every day, psychiatric research is finding new clues to the causes of depression and suicide. Among them:

- Depression and the risk for suicide might have biological as well as psychological causes. Studies have found that some people who are depressed have altered levels of certain brain chemicals. Other studies have shown that aggressive and impulsive people who make violent suicide attempts have reduced amounts of serotonin, a key brain chemical.
- A family history of suicide is a significant risk factor in a young person. The family link might be because young people often identify with those closest to them and are likely to repeat their actions. However, there may be a genetic link as well, because biological relatives of a suicidal person are six times more likely to attempt or succeed in suicide than are adoptive relatives.

What You Can Do

Most people who are depressed or who are thinking about suicide don't or won't talk about how they are feeling. They feel worthless. They have no hope. They deny their emotions or think that talking about their emotions will be a "burden" on others because no one cares. Or they are afraid others will make fun of them.

That's understandable, because when someone mentions suicide, others may treat it as a joke or deny it. Those reactions only make the problem worse. So, if a friend or relative brings up the subject, take it seriously and take some time to talk about it.

Reassure that person that he or she does have someone to turn to. Family, friends, school counselors, physicians or teachers are probably very willing to listen. It's just hard to know how to tell them we want to talk about something as serious as our emotions.

Don't lecture or point out all the reasons a person has to live. Instead, listen and reassure the individual that depression and suicidal tendencies can be treated. Depressive disorders respond readily to treatments such as psychotherapy or appropriate medication. Antidepressants can act within two to three weeks and often are used in addition to psychotherapy. Nearly 90 percent of all depressed people respond to these treatments.

You can find help by contacting your local chapter of the American Psychiatric

✔ Quick Tip

Young people who have attempted suicide in the past or who talk about suicide are at greater risk of future attempts. Listen for hints like "I'd be better off dead" or "I won't be a problem for you much longer" or "Nothing matters; it's no use."

If you or a friend have these feelings, take them seriously. Get help. Ask parents, clergy people, school counselors, or teachers for assistance. Other sources of help include your local mental health association, your family physician, a county medical society, a local hospital's department of psychiatry, a community mental health center, a mood disorders program affiliated with a university or medical school, or a family service/social agency.

For immediate assistance, call The National Hopeline Network at 1-800-SUICIDE (7 days a week, 24 hours a day).

Association, which can suggest a psychiatrist. Psychiatrists are physicians who have special training in emotional and mental health. Other sources include your local mental health association, your family physician, a county medical society, a local hospital's department of psychiatry, a community mental health center, a mood disorders program affiliated with a university or medical school, or a family service/social agency.

Drinking And Drug Use Increase Suicide Risk

Alcohol and drug use can lead to suicidal thoughts and even unplanned spur-of-the-moment suicide attempts while under the influence, according to a new report.

"You don't have to be an alcoholic, just the fact that you're uninhibited at the moment is enough—which is bad news," according to study co-author Ronald C. Kessler, professor of healthcare policy at Harvard Medical School in Boston, Massachusetts.

Kessler and his associates analyzed data collected between 1990 and 1992 by the U.S. National Comorbidity Survey—a nationwide sampling of information related to suicide plans, attempts, mental disorders, and substance use and abuse among over 8,000 men and women aged 15 to 54. Combined with two in-person interview sessions, the researchers assessed the nature of any psychiatric disorders the survey respondents may have had. Their report is published in the *American Journal of Epidemiology*.

The investigators found that among the sample, those exhibiting alcohol and substance dependence did exhibit a higher likelihood of attempting suicide. However, the authors note that for those who had underlying mental disorders in addition to such dependence, it was often the use of the alcohol or drugs itself that led directly to such attempts rather than the history of mental problems.

Kessler and his colleagues also note that current use alone, with or without a history of dependence, was associated with impulsive suicide attempts and thoughts of suicide, and that no one type of drug was more associated with suicide than another—with depressants and stimulants equally likely to illicit suicidal thoughts and attempts. In addition, the researchers found that substance disorders are not associated with the planning of a suicide—as has been the traditional assumption—but rather is more closely associated with suicidal thoughts and unplanned attempts.

In an interview with *Reuters Health* Kessler said the ramifications of the study results could be profound. "Basically, the point is that you don't really have to be a big-time problem drinker," he said. "That has important implications for therapists dealing with patients at risk for suicide. Their antennas are already out for substance abusers, but the fact that even occasional users can be at risk is something that therapists and clinicians need to be concerned about."

Kessler added that individuals at risk for suicide learn early on that drugs dull emotional pain, failing to realize that those same drugs may heighten suicidal thoughts. "Among people who are seriously thinking about killing themselves, people who are in that place in their life are vulnerable in a variety of ways," he said. "And when you are on the edge little things can tip you over. A single bout of heavy drinking sometimes can be enough if people are close enough to that edge. And unfortunately alcohol and drugs are so widely available and there's a stigma to getting professional help for emotional problems."

Kessler further suggested that educators get the word out that drinking and drugs are not the way out of depression and anxiety issues. "One important thing to tell people who have emotional problems is that they have to be cautious or realize what they're doing when they use drugs as a crutch, because in the long-run, they're digging themselves into a hole."

☞ Remember!!

Suicide is the third leading cause of death among young people aged 15 to 24. Some teens who abuse alcohol or drugs are more likely to consider, attempt or succeed at suicide than are non-abusers. According to a government report, thirteen percent of people who committed suicide did so because they were abusing alcohol at the time.

Part 6

Treatment for Substance Abusers

Chapter 43

I'm Not That Bad Yet

Larry

Here's Larry, 17 years old, so hung over and bleary-eyed that he mumbles and stumbles through his notes at an important high school debate. His team loses. Larry shrugs it off.

The judges were biased, he says. We weren't that bad. Still, it was a pretty rotten day for Larry. Monday. He has the whole week to look forward to the weekend.

Larry got drunk last weekend, and the weekend before. No big deal. It's a regular thing, a pattern, his style.

Larry's girlfriend worries because he likes to drive while drinking. Last year, while drunk at the wheel, Larry totaled out his dad's car.

Luckily, neither Larry nor his passengers were injured. And somehow in the confusion, the police never got around to giving breath tests, so Larry lucked out and didn't get a ticket. The newspaper reported that he fell asleep at the wheel.

About This Chapter: Text in this chapter is from "I'm Not That Bad Yet! How (and Why) to Get Help Before Things Get That Bad," by Mark Worden, Do It Now Foundation, Catalog No. 802, © November 2000; reprinted with permission.

Larry's parents have known about his drinking for some time, but were clueless about how to deal with it. At least he's not on drugs, his dad shrugged one day, but it didn't give Larry's mom as much comfort as it did his dad.

Finally, his mom asked their minister to talk to Larry. During the conversation, Larry admitted that he drank—but, then, so did most of the guys he ran around with.

When the minister brought up the subject of alcoholism, Larry thought of his Uncle Ross, who died in a veteran's nursing home. Ross couldn't hold a job, lived on a VA pension, and stayed drunk whenever he could—as long as the money lasted.

Larry remembered Ross as a bleary-eyed loser who ripped the heater out of his trailer one winter to hock it for wine. When drunk, Ross sometimes cried and called Larry "a prince." It was embarrassing.

✔ Quick Tip

Are you concerned about a parent's use of alcohol?

The CAGE is perhaps the most widely used screening test for alcoholism. This tool has been adapted to reflect concern for a parent's drinking through the following four questions:

1. Do you think your parent needs to Cut down on his/her drinking?
2. Does your parent get Annoyed at comments about his/her drinking?
3. Does your parent every feel Guilty about his/her drinking?
4. Does your parent ever take a drink early in the morning as an Eye opener?

A "Yes" answer to any of the questions could indicate a problem. Talk about your concerns with your family doctor, clergyperson, teacher, counselor, relative, or other trusted adult. One source for additional information is:

National Association for Children of Alcoholics
11426 Rockville Pike, #100
Rockville, MD 20852
Toll Free: 888-554-2627
Phone: 301-468-0985
Web site: http://www.nacoa.net
E-mail: nacoa@nacoa.org

Other resources are listed in the end section of this book.

Source: "The Family CAGE" is excerpted from "Breaking the Cycle of Addiction: Prevention and Intervention with Children of Alcoholics," by Ann W. Price, M.A., and James G. Emshoff, Ph.D., in *Alcohol Health and Research World*, Summer 1997, Vol., 21, No., 3.

Sure, Larry knew what an alcoholic was. Ross was an alcoholic. He wasn't.

"Sure, I drink," he told the minister. "I drink beer now and then. But I'm no wino. I'm not an alcoholic. I'm not that bad, yet."

Sondra

At 28, Sondra works two jobs. One is the unpaid job of every single mom—raising two kids without a man in the house.

But she does all right. Her kids have enough to eat, and Sondra keeps them in decent clothes. She can't be accused of neglecting her kids.

Her most demanding job is running a training program for welfare mothers. Sondra works long hours, and often has nighttime meetings.

There's a lot of stress, so she feels entitled to let her hair down now and then. When she does, she likes to dance and get a little loaded—and sometimes, completely wiped out.

Sondra would be outraged if you suggested that she might have a drinking problem.

"I don't drink at all during the week," she'd say. "Maybe a few beers with the girls after a committee meeting. But not that much.

"I'm not an alcoholic. I'm not that bad, yet."

Maybe not. But let's take a look at what happens when Sondra drinks.

For one thing, she and a few other drinkers on the committee persuaded the rest of the members to hold meetings at a bar, so they could "relax" during the meetings. Sometimes things get a little loose, after an hour or so, but not too bad.

Still, three times during the past year Sondra blacked out after a meeting. She'd gotten so drunk that the next morning she couldn't remember how she'd gotten home.

On another occasion, Sondra got arrested for drunk driving. "I only had a couple of beers," she insisted. "I wasn't that drunk."

Still, at the time of her arrest, Sondra's breathalyzer reading was .18, almost double the legal limit in her state (.10 percent, but .08 percent in others), which meant that she'd downed more than "a couple of beers."

"I just lost track," Sondra says. "I wasn't paying that much attention. Anyway, I didn't feel that drunk."

The reason Sondra didn't feel that drunk is because she's built up a tolerance for alcohol. Now it takes more alcohol to give her that tipsy feeling.

One thing does bother her, though. A couple of times in the past year she woke up hung over in bed with a man she didn't know. She doesn't remember what happened.

But it's not that big a deal for Sondra. She claims she's never had a really satisfactory sexual experience. "I can take it or leave it," she says.

Does Sondra have a drinking problem?

She doesn't think so.

A lot of her friends drink the same way she does. Besides, she doesn't drink every day. She doesn't drink hard stuff. She doesn't hide her bottles or sneak drinks or neglect her work and family like real alcoholics do.

"Oh, I've had a little trouble because of my drinking," says Sondra. "But I'm not that bad, yet. I can quit any time I want."

How Bad Do You Have To Get?

Think about it. Add up the costs for a DUI charge—not just the fine, but also the time wasted in (and out of) court, the increased insurance rates, legal fees, and often, jail time.

Remember to add in higher health costs, missed work, and decreased efficiency. And don't forget the shattered relationships, lost friends, and broken families due to drinking and alcohol-related arguments.

How bad do you have to get? Is there a magic moment when you suddenly sit up and announce: "By golly, I guess I'm finally that bad."

Do you have to wait until you're as bad as Larry's Uncle Ross? Do you have to wait until you lose everything? Do you have to get "that bad" before you can get better?

Remember: You don't have to be a falling-down drunk, puke-on-the-piano, sneak-a-drink booze hound to have a drinking problem.

Drinking problems—including alcoholism—start small and escalate. The process usually isn't even dramatic. It takes place slowly, one sip at a time.

Don't Wait To Get Bad

You don't have to get "that bad" at all. If drinking causes problems in your life, admit it. Then take the next logical step: Stop.

That may be hard to do. There may be pressures to drink from friends and fellow workers.

If you find it hard to quit, try talking things over with someone who understands drinking and the problems it can cause.

That someone could be a counselor at work or school, your family doctor, or someone you know who's been there—and back again.

Just don't talk it over with drinking buddies. They're almost guaranteed to have an investment in keeping you from making any serious changes. Being straight with you might mean that they'd have to take a hard look at their own drinking.

But do think it over. And if drinking's a problem for you, do something about it.

With a little insight and a lot of courage—and the support of others who've been there and back—you may never have to get "that bad" at all.

Chapter 44

Treatment Methods And Medications

Treatment Methods

Drug addiction is a treatable disorder. Through treatment that is tailored to individual needs, patients can learn to control their condition and live normal, productive lives. Like people with diabetes or heart disease, people in treatment for drug addiction learn behavioral changes and often take medications as part of their treatment regimen.

Behavioral therapies can include counseling, psychotherapy, support groups, or family therapy. Treatment medications offer help in suppressing the withdrawal syndrome and drug craving and in blocking the effects of drugs. In addition, studies show that treatment for heroin addiction using methadone at an adequate dosage level combined with behavioral therapy reduces death rates and many health problems associated with heroin abuse.

In general, the more treatment given, the better the results. Many patients require other services as well, such as medical and mental health services and HIV prevention services. Patients who stay in treatment longer

About This Chapter: This chapter includes excerpts from "Treatment Methods," National Institute on Drug Abuse (NIDA), Infofax No. 13559, September 2001; "Treatment Medications," NIDA, Infofax No. 13560, September 2001; "Behavioral Change Through Treatment," NIDA Infofax No. 13561, October 2001; and "Principles of Effective Treatment," from *Principles of Drug Addiction Treatment: A Research-Based Guide*, NIDA, September 2001.

than 3 months usually have better outcomes than those who stay less time. Patients who go through medically assisted withdrawal to minimize discomfort but do not receive any further treatment, perform about the same in terms of their drug use as those who were never treated. Over the last 25 years, studies have shown that treatment works to reduce drug intake and crimes committed by drug-dependent people. Researchers also have found that drug abusers who have been through treatment are more likely to have jobs.

Types Of Treatment Programs

The ultimate goal of all drug abuse treatment is to enable the patient to achieve lasting abstinence, but the immediate goals are to reduce drug use,

✎ Weird Words

Counseling: A professional relationship and activity in which one person endeavors to help another to understand and to solve his or her adjustment problems; the giving of advice, opinion, and instruction to direct the judgment or conduct of another.

Psychotherapy: Treatment of emotional, behavioral, personality, and psychiatric disorders based primarily upon verbal or nonverbal communication and interventions with the patient, in contrast to treatments utilizing chemical and physical measures.

Family Therapy: a type of group psychotherapy in which a family in conflict meets as a group with the therapist and explores its relationships and processes; focus is on the resolution of current interactions between members rather than on individual members.

Methadone: A synthetic narcotic drug; an orally effective analgesic similar in action to morphine but with slightly greater potency and longer duration. It produces psychic and physical dependence as with morphine, but withdrawal symptoms are somewhat milder; used as a replacement (oral route) for morphine and heroin; also used during withdrawal treatment in morphine and heroin addiction.

Source: From *Stedman's Medical Dictionary, 27th Edition*,

improve the patient's ability to function, and minimize the medical and social complications of drug abuse.

There are several types of drug abuse treatment programs. Short-term methods last less than 6 months and include residential therapy, medication therapy, and drug-free outpatient therapy. Longer term treatment may include, for example, methadone maintenance outpatient treatment for opiate addicts and residential therapeutic community treatment.

In maintenance treatment for heroin addicts, people in treatment are given an oral dose of a synthetic opiate, usually methadone hydrochloride or levo-alpha-acetyl methadol (LAAM), administered at a dosage sufficient to block the effects of heroin and yield a stable, noneuphoric state free from physiological craving for opiates. In this stable state, the patient is able to disengage from drug-seeking and related criminal behavior and, with appropriate counseling and social services, become a productive member of his or her community.

Outpatient drug-free treatment does not include medications and encompasses a wide variety of programs for patients who visit a clinic at regular intervals. Most of the programs involve individual or group counseling. Patients entering these programs are abusers of drugs other than opiates or are opiate abusers for whom maintenance therapy is not recommended, such as those who have stable, well-integrated lives and only brief histories of drug dependence.

Therapeutic communities (TCs) are highly structured programs in which patients stay at a residence, typically for 6 to 12 months. Patients in TCs include those with relatively long histories of drug dependence, involvement in serious criminal activities, and seriously impaired social functioning. The focus of the TC is on the resocialization of the patient to a drug-free, crime-free lifestyle.

Short-term residential programs, often referred to as chemical dependency units, are often based on the "Minnesota Model" of treatment for alcoholism. These programs involve a 3- to 6-week inpatient treatment phase followed by extended outpatient therapy or participation in 12-step self-help groups, such as Narcotics Anonymous or Cocaine Anonymous.

✤ It's A Fact!!

Drug abuse has a great economic impact on society-an estimated $67 billion per year. This figure includes costs related to crime, medical care, drug abuse treatment, social welfare programs, and time lost from work. Treatment of drug abuse can reduce those costs. Studies have shown that from $4 to $7 are saved for every dollar spent on treatment. It costs approximately $3,600 per month to leave a drug abuser untreated in the community, and incarceration costs approximately $3,300 per month. In contrast, methadone maintenance therapy costs about $290 per month.

Treatment Medications

Treatment for people who abuse drugs but are not yet addicted to them most often consists of behavioral therapies, such as psychotherapy, counseling, support groups, or family therapy. But treatment for drug-addicted people often involves a combination of behavioral therapies and medications. Medications, such as methadone or LAAM (levo-alpha-acetyl-methadol), are effective in suppressing the withdrawal symptoms and drug craving associated with narcotic addiction, thus reducing illicit drug use and improving the chances of the individual remaining in treatment.

The primary medically assisted withdrawal method for narcotic addiction is to switch the patient to a comparable drug that produces milder withdrawal symptoms, and then gradually taper off the substitute medication. The medication used most often is methadone, taken by mouth once a day. Patients are started on the lowest dose that prevents the more severe signs of withdrawal and then the dose is gradually reduced. Substitutes can be used also for withdrawal from sedatives. Patients can be switched to long-acting sedatives, such as diazepam or phenobarbital, which are then gradually reduced.

Once a patient goes through withdrawal, there is still considerable risk of relapse. Patients may return to taking drugs even though they no longer have physical withdrawal symptoms. A great deal of research is being done to find medications that can block drug craving and treat other factors that cause a return to drugs.

Patients who cannot continue abstaining from opiates are given maintenance therapy, usually with methadone. The maintenance dose of methadone, usually higher than that used for medically assisted withdrawal, prevents both withdrawal symptoms and heroin craving. It also prevents addicts from getting a high from heroin and, as a result, they stop using it. Research has shown that maintenance therapy reduces the spread of AIDS in the treated population. The overall death rate is also significantly reduced.

Within various methadone programs, those that provide higher doses of methadone (usually a minimum of 60 mg.) have better retention rates. Also, those that provide other services, such as counseling, therapy, and medical care, along with methadone generally get better results than the programs that provide minimal services.

Another drug approved for use in maintenance treatment is LAAM, which is administered three times a week rather than daily, as is the case with methadone. The drug naltrexone is also used to prevent relapse. Like methadone, LAAM and naltrexone prevent addicts from getting high from heroin. However, naltrexone does not eliminate the drug craving, so it has not been popular among addicts. Naltrexone works best with highly motivated patients.

Behavioral Change Through Treatment

Recovery from the disease of drug addiction is often a long-term process, involving multiple relapses before a patient achieves prolonged abstinence. Many behavioral therapies have been shown to help patients achieve initial abstinence and maintain prolonged abstinence. One frequently used therapy is cognitive behavioral relapse prevention in which patients are taught new ways of acting and thinking that will help them stay off drugs. For example, patients are urged to avoid situations that lead to drug use and to practice drug refusal skills. They also are taught to think of the occasional relapse as a "slip" rather than as a failure. Cognitive behavioral relapse prevention has proven to be a useful and lasting therapy for many drug addicted individuals.

One of the more well-developed behavioral techniques in drug abuse treatment is contingency management, a system of rewards and punishments to make abstinence attractive and drug use unattractive. Ultimately, the aim of contingency management programs is to make a drug-free, pro-social lifestyle more rewarding than a drug-using lifestyle.

> **✤ It's A Fact!!**
>
> There are currently no medications approved by the Food and Drug Administration (FDA) for treating addiction to cocaine, LSD, PCP, marijuana, methamphetamine and other stimulants, inhalants, or anabolic steroids. There are medications, however, for treating the adverse health effects of these drugs, such as seizures or psychotic reactions, and for overdoses from opiates.

Once drug use is under control, education and job rehabilitation become crucial. Rewarding lifestyle options must be found for people in drug recovery to prevent their return to the old environment and way of life.

Principles Of Drug Addiction Treatment

1. No single treatment is appropriate for all individuals.
2. Treatment needs to be readily available.
3. Effective treatment attends to multiple needs of the individual, not just his or her drug use.
4. An individual's treatment and services plan must be assessed continually and modified as necessary to ensure that the plan meets the person's changing needs.
5. Remaining in treatment for an adequate period of time is critical for treatment effectiveness.

6. Counseling (individual and/or group) and other behavioral therapies are critical components of effective treatment for addiction.

7. Medications are an important element of treatment for many patients, especially when combined with counseling and other behavioral therapies.

8. Addicted or drug-abusing individuals with coexisting mental disorders should have both disorders treated in an integrated way.

9. Medical detoxification is only the first stage of addiction treatment and by itself does little to change long-term drug use.

10. Treatment does not need to be voluntary to be effective.

11. Possible drug use during treatment must be monitored continuously.

12. Treatment programs should provide assessment for HIV/AIDS, hepatitis B and C, tuberculosis and other infectious diseases, and counseling to help patients modify or change behaviors that place themselves or others at risk of infection.

13. Recovery from drug addiction can be a long-term process and frequently requires multiple episodes of treatment

☞ Remember!!

As with other chronic illnesses, relapses to drug use can occur during or after successful treatment episodes. Addicted individuals may require prolonged treatment and multiple episodes of treatment to achieve long-term abstinence and fully restored functioning. Participation in self-help support programs during and following treatment often is helpful in maintaining abstinence.

Chapter 45

Myths And Facts About Addiction And Treatment

Myth: Addiction is a bad habit, the result of moral weakness and over-indulgence.

- **Fact:** Addiction is a chronic, life-threatening condition, like hypertension, atherosclerosis, and adult diabetes.
- **Fact:** Addiction has roots in genetic susceptibility, social circumstance, and personal behavior.
- **Fact:** Certain drugs are highly addictive, rapidly causing biochemical and structural changes in the brain. Others can be used for longer periods of time before they begin to cause inescapable cravings and compulsive use.

Myth: If an addict has enough willpower, he or she can stop abusing alcohol and using drugs.

- **Fact:** Few people addicted to alcohol and illicit drugs can simply stop using them, no matter how strong their inner resolve. Most need one or more courses of structured substance abuse treatment to reduce or end their dependence on alcohol and illicit drugs.

About This Chapter: This chapter is from "Myths and Facts about Addiction and Treatment," Connecticut Clearinghouse, a program of Wheeler Clinic, Inc., © September 1997 Connecticut Clearinghouse, 334 Farmington Avenue, Plainville, CT 06062, 800-232-4424, 860-793-9791 (www.ctclearinghouse.org); reprinted with permission.

Myth: Many people relapse, so treatment obviously does not work.

- **Fact:** Like virtually any other medical treatment, addiction treatment cannot guarantee lifelong health. Relapse, often a part of the recovery process, is always possible—and treatable. Even if a person never achieves perfect abstinence, addiction treatment can reduce the number and duration of relapses, minimize related problems such as crime and poor overall health, improve the individual's ability to function in daily life, and strengthen the individual to better cope with the next temptation or craving. These improvements reduce the social and economic costs of addiction.

Myth: We have reached the limits of what we can do to treat addiction.

- **Fact:** The more we learn about addiction, the more effective treatment becomes. Matching clients to the services they most need, while supporting continuous and focused engagement in treatment, is imperative. Today's treatment providers are better able to do this than ever before.

Myth: People with alcohol and illicit drug problems get sent to 28-day treatment programs, where they dry out and emerge new individuals, cured of their problems.

- **Fact:** Treatment is provided in many different settings, in many different ways, for different lengths of time. It is important to provide the most appropriate mix of services and settings for each client based on an assessment of individual needs and cultural relevance.

- **Fact:** Treatment is provided in both outpatient and inpatient settings, with different levels of intensity. Residential treatment is provided in the form of short-term treatment and therapeutic communities. Outpatient treatment is available in three general formats: 1) intensive day treatment; 2) intensive outpatient treatment; and 3) traditional outpatient treatment. General phases of treatment include: 1) detoxification; 2) rehabilitation; 3) continuing care; and 4) relapse prevention.

Chapter 46

If Someone You Care About Has A Drug Problem

This text was developed to assist you in helping a friend who has a problem with alcohol or other drugs. Sometimes, being a good friend means you have to intervene, but before you get involved it is important to understand what is really going on with your friend.

No matter what, in order to get better, your friend eventually has to admit that he or she has a problem and make an effort to get help. You can be the one that encourages and guides your friend to seek this help.

How can I tell if my friend has a drinking or other drug problem?

Sometimes it's tough to tell. Most kids won't walk up to someone they're close to and ask for help. In fact, your friend will probably do everything possible to deny or hide the problem. But, there are signs you can look for.

About This Chapter: This text is excerpted from *A Guide for Teens: Does Your Friend Have an Alcohol or Other Drug Problem? What Can You Do to Help?* produced and published by the Center for Health Communication of the Harvard School of Public Health. Copies of this publication may be downloaded free of charge from the website of the National Clearinghouse for Alcohol and Drug Information at http://www.health.org/govpubs/phd688/. Additional information is excerpted from "If Someone Close...Has a Problem with Alcohol or Other Drugs," an undated fact sheet available from the National Clearinghouse for Alcohol and Drug Information (NCADI) at www.health.org/; accessed November 2001.

People with serious substance abuse problems say things like," I can stop drinking or using other drugs any time I want to" —but they don't. They may be o.k. to hang around with, until they get high—then they often act like jerks or get into fights. No one is sure why some people get into trouble with alcohol or other drugs. There are signs, however, when substances are taking control of someone's life. Some of these signs are easy to see, others aren't, but if you see them happening over and over again, chances are your friend needs help.

If your friend has one or more of the following warning signs, he or she may have a problem with alcohol or other drugs:

- getting drunk or high on drugs on a regular basis
- lying about things, or about how much alcohol or other drugs he or she is using
- avoiding you in order to get drunk or high
- giving up activities he or she used to do, such as sports, homework, or hanging out with friends who don't drink or use other drugs
- planning drinking in advance, hiding alcohol, drinking or using other drugs alone
- having to drink more to get the same high
- believing that in order to have fun you need to drink or use other drugs
- frequent hangovers
- pressuring others to drink or use other drugs
- taking risks, including sexual risks

✤ It's A Fact!!

There are millions of people with alcohol and other drug problems in this country. A recent study reported that 28 million people age 12 and older used illicit drugs during the past year. By current estimates, more than 76 million people have been exposed to alcoholism in the family. Experience shows that for every person with an alcohol or other drug problem, at least four others are affected by their behavior.

- having "blackouts" —forgetting what he or she did the night before while drinking (if you tell your friend what happened, he or she might pretend to remember, or laugh it off as no big deal)
- feeling run-down, hopeless, depressed, or even suicidal
- sounding selfish and not caring about others
- constantly talking about drinking or using other drugs
- getting in trouble with the law
- drinking and driving
- suspension from school for an alcohol- or other drug-related incident

How serious can my friend's drinking or other drug problem be? What can it lead to?

Not all people who drink or use other drugs develop the same symptoms or consequences, but one thing is for sure: If your friend has a drinking or other drug problem and doesn't get help, things can get much worse. People with serious drinking or other drug problems don't like to admit it, even to themselves. In the beginning, they often say they feel great, that drinking or smoking pot or doing a few lines of cocaine is the best thing that ever happened to them. But then things change for the worse. Eventually, if they don't get help, they can develop serious psychological problems such as suicidal depression, and serious physical problems such as liver damage and brain damage; and some will die from an overdose. Getting drunk or high impairs judgment, and may lead to behaviors that people wouldn't do ordinarily if they weren't under the influence of these substances—such as having unsafe sex which could result in pregnancy, AIDS, or other sexually transmitted diseases. Substance abuse is dangerous; it can ruin your friend's health, cause your friend to drop out of school, lose friends, lose values, and even lose his or her self-respect.

Alcohol and other drugs don't care who you are, what color you are, if you're rich or poor, how old you are, your sex, or where you're from. They don't care if you're a jock, a cheerleader, or a genius.

✤ **It's A Fact!!**

If there is one thing true about alcohol and other drug abusers, it is that, as with all people, each one is different—different in human needs and responses, as well as in their reasons for drinking and taking other drugs, their reactions to these drugs, and their readiness for treatment.

You are in a good position to help your relative or friend, because you know a good deal about their unique qualities and their way of life. And having made the effort to gain some understanding of the signs and effects of problem drinking or other drug abuse, you should be in a better position to consider a strategy for helping.

What would cause my friend to have a serious drinking or other drug problem?

Lots of things lead to these problems. For one thing, these difficulties often run in families, just like heart disease and cancer. If your friend's parents are alcoholic, or there is a family history of alcoholism or other drug addiction, your friend is more likely to become alcoholic or drug dependent.

People often drink or use other drugs to avoid things that bother them—pressure from friends, stress in the family, hassles, the feeling that adults are on their case, the lousy feeling that they're different from everyone else in the world. They use these substances just to feel better. The problem is, drinking or using other drugs eventually makes things worse because all you care about is getting high, and once you start it's hard to stop; you need to use more just to feel normal. Alcohol and other substances change the way you think, and you start to believe things are better or worse than they really are. Alcohol and other drugs may make you feel good when you're high, but when they wear off, depression sets in.

Why is it so hard for individuals to get help for themselves?

It's tough for most people to admit that they have a serious substance abuse problem. It's especially hard to admit it when you're young because you think that kind of thing could never happen to you. Many people believe that alcoholics and other drug addicts are old people, or are street people, when, in reality, they can be anyone. People who have a serious problem with drinking or using other drugs might say that they are not using that much and that they won't get addicted. Denying that there's a problem is very common. In fact, this denial, along with hiding the substance abuse from friends, becomes almost as big a problem as the drinking or other drug use itself. Becoming dependent on alcohol or other drugs makes you want to cut off the people who care about you, and you can end up feeling lonely and afraid.

To avoid being found out, serious problem drinkers and other drug users often spend more and more time alone, and think they can solve their problem all by themselves, or that a boyfriend or girlfriend can solve it for them. Getting better doesn't work that way. What has to happen is that your friend has to admit that alcohol and/or other drugs are messing up his or her life. However, you can help even if your friend does not admit to having a problem.

What can I do to help my friend?

It is possible for you to help a friend who is in serious trouble with alcohol or other drugs. Whether or not your friend takes your advice and gets help is really your friend's decision and responsibility. Sometimes, approaching the friend in trouble with another mutual friend can make our intervention easier since there is safety and support in numbers.

The first step in getting help is for your friend to talk to someone about his or her alcohol and drug use. Eventually, your friend will need to admit that there is a problem, and to agree to stop drinking and/or using other drugs completely. Your friend needs support and understanding, and someone he or she can trust to talk to about the problem. You can't force a friend to get help, but you can encourage and support your friend to seek and find professional help.

If you are worried about a friend, it is important for you to speak to someone in private who is knowledgeable and reassuring. Telling someone isn't being disloyal to your friend. It's important to know the facts about

✔ Quick Tip

What Not To Do

- Don't attempt to punish, threaten, bribe, or preach.
- Don't try to be a martyr. Avoid emotional appeals that may only increase feelings of guilt and the compulsion to drink or use other drugs.
- Don't allow yourself to cover up or make excuses for the alcoholic or drug addict or shield them from the realistic consequences of their behavior.
- Don't take over their responsibilities, leaving them with no sense of importance or dignity.
- Don't hide or dump bottles, throw out drugs, or shelter them from situations where alcohol is present.
- Don't argue with the person when they are impaired or high.
- Don't try to drink along with the problem drinker or take drugs with the drug abuser.
- Above all, don't feel guilty or responsible for another's behavior.

What To Do

- Try to remain calm, unemotional, and factually honest in speaking about their behavior and its day-to-day consequences.
- Let the person with the problem know that you are reading and learning about alcohol and other drug abuse, attending Al-Anon, Nar-Anon, Alateen, and other support groups.
- Discuss the situation with someone you trust—someone from the clergy, a social worker, a counselor, a friend, or some individual who has experienced alcohol or other drug abuse personally or as a family member.
- Encourage new interests and participate in leisure time activities that the person enjoys. Encourage them to see old friends.
- Be patient and live one day at a time. Alcoholism and other drug addiction generally takes a long time to develop, and recovery does not occur overnight. Try to accept setbacks and relapses with calmness and understanding.
- Refuse to ride with anyone who's been drinking heavily or using other drugs.

what's happening to your friend if you plan to help. Don't try to help your friend on your own until you have talked to someone you can trust—a counselor, teacher, doctor, nurse, parent, or someone at your church or synagogue. Ask this person to keep the conversation confidential. You don't have to mention your friend by name; you can just talk generally about the problem. Talking to a professional will help you figure out what the best steps are for you to take.

If you decide to speak to your friend, here are some guidelines that you and your advisor should consider in planning how and what you could do to help:

- Make sure the timing is right. Talk to your friend when he or she is sober of straight—before school is a good time.
- Never accuse your friend of being an alcoholic or a drug addict, but do express your concern. Try not to blame your friend for the problem; if you do, he or she might be turned off right away.
- Talk about your feelings. Tell your friend you're worried, and how it feels for you to see him or her drunk or high on other drugs.
- Tell your friend what you've seen him or her do when drinking or using other drugs. Give specific examples. Tell your friend you want to help.
- Speak in a caring and understanding tone of voice, not with pity but with friendship.
- Be prepared for denial and anger. Your friend may say there is nothing wrong and may get mad at you. Many people with alcohol and other drug problems react this way. When confronted, many users will defend their use, blame others for the problem, or give excuses for why they drink or use other drugs.
- Find out where help is available. You could offer to go with your friend to get help, but be prepared to follow through. This gesture will show your friend that you really care.
- You need to tell your friend that you are worried about him or her, and that someone who can help needs to be told. Your friend might get

really mad at you, but if you say nothing, things may get worse and your friend may be in more danger.

- Your friend's problem is probably hard on you, too. The situation may have left you feeling lonely and afraid. Maybe you've thought, "What if I get my friend in trouble? What if I lose my friend over this? What if I don't do anything and something awful happens?" It's hard to keep all of these questions and feelings to yourself. It's important that you talk about them. You can share these feelings with the person that you go to for help about your friend's problem. There are also support groups for people like you who are trying to help a friend, such as Al-Anon or Alateen, where you can learn more about people's alcohol and other drug use problems. Your school may have a substance abuse prevention counselor as well.

What does my friend have to do to get help?

Probably the hardest decision your friend will be faced with is admitting that he or she has a problem. To get better and recover, your friend has to get some help to stop drinking or using other drugs.

Facing such a problem and asking for help can be a scary thing to do. Your friend will have to take an honest look at where drinking or other drug use has brought him or her, and admit that it has caused emotional and maybe physical pain. Your friend will have to see that it has robbed him or her of real friends, creativity, happiness, spirit, the respect of others, and even self-respect, and that it keeps your friend from growing up.

Your friend will not be able to solve this problem alone. He or she will need experienced help. A good counselor will support your friend and direct him or her to the kind of treatment and/or support groups that are most helpful.

Encourage your friend to talk to other people with drinking and other drug problems who are now in recovery, such as members of Alcoholics Anonymous (AA) and Narcotics Anonymous (NA). These groups are confidential, self-help organizations that offer assistance to anyone who has a drinking or other drug problem and wants to do something about it. AA and

NA members are recovering alcoholics and addicts, so they have a special understanding of each other. Talking with others who have experienced similar problems is an important part of recovery. New members are encouraged to stay away from alcohol or other drugs "one day at a time." There is no fee for membership in these organizations. If your friend is afraid to go to a meeting alone, you can go along with him or her to an "open" meeting. Friends and family members are welcome to attend this type of meeting, and there are special meetings in most neighborhoods or communities. Local branches of AA and NA are listed in your phone directory.

If your friend has a drinking or other drug problem, you may be the only one willing to reach out and help. Your friend may not appreciate your help right away, or he or she may realize it means you really care. Ultimately, it's up to your friend to get help. It is not your responsibility to make that happen. In fact, you can't make that happen. All you can do is talk to your friend, show how much you care, and encourage him or her to get help. Your concern and support might be just what is needed to help your friend turn his or her life around.

However, if your friend is in serious trouble with alcohol or other drugs, and you have been unable to get your friend to get help on his or her own, you should consider speaking with your friend's parents or guardian. The potential consequences to your friend's life can be too severe to do nothing.

—by Betsy O'Connor, M.A./L.R.C., Visiting Fellow at the Center for Health Communication of the Harvard School of Public Health and, Director of Interventions at the Gosnold Treatment Center in Falmouth, Massachusetts.

Part 7

Drug Statistics and Policy Controversies

Chapter 47

High School And Youth Trends

2000 Monitoring The Future Study

Since 1975, the Monitoring the Future (MTF) survey has annually studied the extent of drug abuse among high school 12th graders. The survey was expanded in 1991 to include 8th and 10th graders. It is funded by the National Institute on Drug Abuse (NIDA) and is conducted by the University of Michigan's Institute for Social Research. The goal of the survey is to collect data on past month, past year, and lifetime drug use among students in these grade levels. ("Lifetime" refers to use at least once during a respondent's lifetime. "Past year" refers to an individual's drug use at least once during the year preceding their response to the survey. "Past month" refers to an individual's drug use at least once during the month preceding their response to the survey.) This, the 26th annual study, was conducted during spring 2000.

The 2000 MTF marks the fourth year in a row that illicit drug use among 8th, 10th, and 12th graders remained stable or decreased in some cases. Since the 1999 MTF, reductions in cigarette smoking occurred in all three grades, with statistically significant decreases in 2000. Other reductions occurred in cocaine and crack use for 12th graders; hallucinogens and LSD for 10th and

About This Chapter: This chapter includes excerpts from "High School and Youth Trends," National Institute on Drug Abuse (NIDA), Infofax No. 13565, November 2001; and "Youth and Underage Drinking: An Overview," Substance Abuse and Mental Health Services Administration (SAMHSA), 1999.

12th graders; heroin and inhalants for 8th graders; and methaqualone (a sedative) for 12th graders.

The few statistically significant increases from the 1999 MTF to the 2000 MTF were in the use of Ecstasy among all three grade levels, anabolic-androgenic steroids among 10th graders, and heroin use among 12th graders.

✔ **Quick Tip**

You can check out the latest Monitoring the Future results at www.monitoringthefuture.org.

Perceived Risk Of Harm, Disapproval, And Perceived Availability

In addition to surveying for use of drugs among 8th, 10th, and 12th graders, MTF surveys for three indicators of attitudes related to drug use. These are perceived risk of harm in taking a drug, disapproval of others who take drugs, and perceived availability of drugs.

Perceived Risk Of Harm

From 1999 to 2000, perceived risk of harm in smoking one or more packs of cigarettes per day increased among 8th graders, from 54.8 percent in 1999 to 58.8 percent in 2000; and among 10th graders, from 62.7 percent to 65.9 percent.

Perceived risk of harm in regularly using smokeless tobacco increased among 10th graders, from 44.2 percent in 1999 to 46.7 percent in 2000.

However, perceived harm in taking crack occasionally decreased among 10th graders, from 79.1 percent in 1999 to 76.9 percent in 2000. Tenth graders' perceived harm in trying cocaine powder once or twice decreased from 51.6 percent in 1999 to 48.8 percent in 2000; and their perceived harm in trying it occasionally decreased from 73.6 percent to 70.9 percent.

For 12th graders, the perceived risk of harm in taking anabolic steroids decreased, from 62.1 percent in 1999 to 57.9 percent in 2000. Also, 12th graders' perceived harm in taking one or two drinks of alcohol decreased, from 8.3 percent to 6.4 percent.

Disapproval Of Others Who Take Drugs

Disapproving of people who try marijuana once or twice increased among 8th graders, from 70.7 percent in 1999 to 72.5 percent in 2000; and among 12th graders, from 48.8 percent o 52.5 percent. Disapproval of those who take LSD regularly, however, decreased among 8th graders, from 72.5 percent in 1999 to 69.3 percent in 2000.

Perceived Availability

The perceived availability of Ecstasy increased among 12th graders, from 40.1 percent in 1999 to 51.4 percent in 2000. The proportion of 12th graders perceiving increased availability of hallucinogens other than LSD also increased, from 29.5 percent to 34.5 percent. Decreases in perceived availability occurred among 8th graders for alcohol, dropping from 72.3 percent in 1999 to 70.6 percent in 2000; and for cigarettes, dropping from 71.5 percent to 68.7 percent. Among 10th graders, perceived availability decreased for crack, from 36.5 percent in 1999 to 34.0 percent in 2000; for cocaine powder, from 36.7 percent to 34.5; and for cigarettes, from 88.3 percent to 86.8 percent.

Cigarette Use

The 2000 MTF found that cigarette use among teens dropped significantly, with past month smoking down from 17.5 percent in 1999 to 14.6 percent in 2000 among 8th graders, and from 34.6 percent to 31.4 percent among 12th graders. Daily smoking in the past month declined from 15.9 percent in 1999 to 14.0 percent in 2000 among 10th graders, and from 23.1 percent to 20.6 percent among 12th graders.

At the same time, perceived risk of harm from smoking a pack or more of cigarettes per day increased among 8th and 10th graders, from 54.8 percent in 1999 to 58.8 percent in 2000 among 8th graders, and from 62.7 percent to 65.9 percent among 10th graders. Also, the perceived availability of cigarettes declined among 8th and 10th graders (it is not a measure for 12th graders). For example, 71.5 percent of 8th graders in 1999 felt it would be "fairly easy" or "very easy" to get cigarettes, and this percentage dropped to 68.7 percent in 2000.

The use of smokeless tobacco remained stable from 1999 to 2000 among the three grade levels. Its use has decreased since a peak in 1994/1995. Among 12th graders, past month smokeless tobacco use has decreased from 12.2 percent in 1995 to 7.6 percent in 2000. The decrease among 10th graders is from 10.5 percent in 1994 to 6.1 percent in 2000. Among 8th graders, it has decreased from 7.7 percent in 1994 to 4.2 percent in 2000.

> **✤ It's A Fact!!**
>
> Young people begin to take risks and experiment as they transition from childhood to adulthood. Without support and guidance, some young people may engage in behaviors that place them and others at risk—including using alcohol and other drugs.

Ecstasy

From 1999 to 2000, the use of Ecstasy (or "MDMA") increased among all three grade levels. For 10th and 12th graders, this is the second consecutive year MDMA use has increased. Past year use of Ecstasy increased among 8th graders from 1.7 percent in 1999 to 3.1 percent in 2000; from 4.4 percent to 5.4 percent among 10th graders; and from 5.6 percent to 8.2 percent among 12th graders. Also among 12th graders, the perceived availability of Ecstasy rose from 40.1 percent in 1999 to 51.4 percent in 2000 (not measured for 8th and 10th graders).

African American students show considerably lower rates of Ecstasy use than white or Hispanic students. For example, past year use among African American 12th graders is 1.3 percent, compared to 7.6 percent for white 12th graders and 10.6 percent for Hispanic 12th graders.

Steroids (anabolic-androgenic)

Use of steroids remained unchanged among 8th and 12th graders from 1999 to 2000. Among 10th graders, however, the past year use of steroids increased from 1.7 percent in 1999 to 2.2 percent in 2000. Most steroids users are male and, among male students, past year use of these substances was reported by 2.2 percent of 8th graders, 3.6 percent of 10th graders, and 2.5 percent of 12th graders. In addition, the 2000 MTF noted a decrease among 12th graders in the perceived risk of harm from using steroids.

Marijuana

Since 1999, marijuana use has remained stable in all three grades and for all three use categories. The increases in use seen during the mid-1990s have leveled off or decreased and, among 8th graders, have decreased significantly. Among 10th graders, past year use decreased from a peak of 34.8 percent in 1997 to 32.2 percent in 2000. Past year marijuana use among 8th graders decreased from 18.3 percent in 1996 to 15.6 percent in 2000.

Cocaine And Crack

Past year use of cocaine decreased significantly among 12th graders, from 6.2 percent in 1999 to 5.0 percent in 2000; crack use in the past year decreased from 2.7 percent to 2.2 percent for 12th graders. This was the first decrease in cocaine and crack use among 12th graders since the early 1990s. Modest declines have appeared in all other categories and grade levels since 1998. Of note is the past year use of crack by 8th graders, decreased from a 10-year high of 2.1 percent in 1998 to 1.8 percent in 1999, where it remained in 2000.

Although the perceived availability of crack and cocaine decreased among 10th graders from 1999 to 2000, there was also a decrease in their perceived risk of harm from these drugs. The proportion of 10th graders who perceived risk of harm in taking cocaine powder occasionally decreased from 73.6 percent in 1999 to 70.9 percent in 2000; from 51.6 percent to 48.8 percent for trying cocaine once or twice; and from 79.6 percent to 76.9 percent in taking crack occasionally.

Heroin And Other Opiates

Among 8th graders, past year heroin use declined from 1.4 percent in 1999 to 1.1 percent in 2000. This decline in heroin use among 8th graders is the first since 1997 (1.3 percent).

Among 12th graders, however, past year heroin use rose from 1.1 percent in 1999 to 1.5 percent in 2000, resulting in the highest rate of heroin use among 12th graders since the MTF began. This trend may reflect the increasing availability of high-purity heroin in smokable and snortable form.

Use of opiates other than heroin remained stable from 1999 to 2000, but use of opiate drugs is at its highest level since the MTF began, with 10.6 percent of 12th graders reporting lifetime use, 7.0 percent past year, and 2.9 percent past month.

Inhalants

Inhalant use continues to be more prevalent among 8th graders than students in the other two grades. Lifetime use of inhalants among 8th graders decreased from 19.7 percent in 1999 to 17.9 percent in 2000. During the 10 years that data have been collected for 8th graders, inhalant use was highest in 1995, with percentages of 21.6 for lifetime use, 12.8 for past year use, and 6.1 for past month use.

Methamphetamine

This was added to the MTF as a drug category in 1999. Rates of methamphetamine use remained stable from 1999 to 2000 in all three grades, for all three categories. Past year use was reported by 4.3 percent of 12th graders, 4.0 percent of 10th graders, and 2.5 percent of 8th graders.

Alcohol

Alcohol use has generally remained stable in the past few years among 8th and 10th graders and, more recently, among 12th graders. Among 8th graders, daily drinking in the past month decreased significantly from 1.0 percent in 1999 to 0.8 percent in 2000. Among 12th graders, however, the perceived risk of harm in trying one or two alcoholic drinks decreased, from 8.3 percent in 1999 to 6.4 percent in 2000.

In 2000, 30.0 percent of 12th graders, 26.2 percent of 10th graders, and 14.1 percent of 8th graders reported binge drinking (5+ drinks in a row) in the 2 weeks prior to the survey. Nearly one-third (32.3 percent) of 12th graders, 23.5 percent of 10th graders, and 8.3 percent of 8th graders reported having "been drunk" in the month prior to the survey. This is the highest percentage of 10th graders in this category since the MTF began including them, in 1991.

More than 70 percent of 8th graders perceive alcoholic beverages as "fairly easy" or "very easy" to get, although this percentage has decreased, from 72.3 percent in 1999 to 70.6 percent in 2000.

Adolescents' Beliefs About Alcohol

- Very young children—even preschoolers—can tell that alcohol has an effect on people that other beverages do not. In fact, children begin forming opinions about alcohol at an early age, and they tend to view it negatively.
- Boys' beliefs tend to be more favorable toward drinking than those of girls. Boys also tend to associate drinking with being more grown up.
- Adolescents ages 12 to 14 believe that the positive benefits of drinking (feeling good, fitting in with peers) are more likely to occur than the negative effects of drinking (feeling sick, causing serious health problems).
- Youth ages 12 to 14 who expect to gain greater social acceptance from drinking are more likely to begin to drink as well as to consume alcohol at faster rates.
- Fifty-six percent of students in grades 5 through 12 say that alcohol advertising encourages them to drink.
- Eighty percent of 12- to 17-year-olds surveyed think that alcohol negatively affects school performance, and 81 percent believe it increases the likelihood of getting into trouble.

♣ It's A Fact!!

- Peer pressure begins early. One-third of 4th graders and more than half of 6th graders say they have been pressured by friends to drink alcohol.
- On average, young people begin drinking at about age 13, but some start even younger. By the time they are high school seniors, more than 80 percent have used alcohol and approximately 64 percent have been drunk. When adolescents move on to college, they bring their drinking habits with them: more than 40 percent of college students are binge drinkers.
- In 1998, 10.4 million current drinkers were under legal age (age 12-20). Of these, 5.1 million were binge drinkers, including 2.3 million heavy drinkers.

Risk Factors For Adolescent Alcohol Use

The reasons why adolescents use alcohol are complex but include curiosity, a need to fit in with friends, and a desire to relax and escape problems. For some, additional factors may be involved.

- *Genetic Factors:* Children of alcoholic parents are significantly more likely to begin drinking during adolescence and to develop alcohol use disorders, but the relative influences of environment and genetics have not been determined and vary among young people.
- *Childhood Behavior:* Research has shown that children who are very restless and impulsive at age 3 are twice as likely to be diagnosed with alcohol dependency at age 21. Aggressiveness in children as young as ages 5 to 10 has been found to predict alcohol and other drug use in adolescence.
- *Psychiatric Disorders:* Among 12- to 16-year-olds, regular alcohol use has been significantly associated with conduct disorder; in one study, adolescents who reported higher levels of drinking were more likely to have conduct disorder. Whether anxiety and depression lead to or are consequences of alcohol abuse is unresolved.
- *Suicidal Behavior:* Alcohol use among adolescents has been associated with considering, planning, attempting, and completing suicide. Research does not indicate whether drinking causes suicidal behavior, only that the two behaviors are correlated.
- *Parental and Peer Influences:* Parents' drinking behavior and favorable attitudes about drinking have been associated with adolescents' beginning and continuing drinking. Early initiating of drinking has been identified as an important risk factor for later alcohol-related problems. Lack of parental support, monitoring, and communication also has been significantly related to frequency of drinking, heavy drinking, and drunkenness among adolescents. Peer drinking and acceptance also influences adolescent drinking behaviors.
- *Expectancies:* Positive expectations from alcohol use have been found to increase with age and to predict the onset of drinking among adolescents.

Chapter 48

Teen Survey

According to the National Center on Addiction and Substance Abuse (CASA)'s 1999 survey of 2,000 teens and 1,000 parents, some 14 million teens age 12 to 17 (60%) are at moderate or high risk of substance abuse, meaning they have friends who use marijuana, friends who drink regularly, have a classmate or friend who used acid, cocaine, or heroin, can buy marijuana quickly, and expect to use an illegal drug in the future.

Obtaining Drugs

Marijuana is easier to buy than beer, according to our nation's teenagers, while cigarettes are the easiest to buy. Forty-seven percent of all teens say cigarettes are easiest to buy, 27% say marijuana and 12% say beer. The older the teen gets, the easier marijuana is to buy compared to beer.

After marijuana, high school teens cite LSD/acid (23%) as the most popular drug and cocaine (10%) the second most popular. Middle school students rank cocaine higher (11%) compared with 7% for LSD/acid. Among high school students, ecstasy ranks next (4%), heroin, methamphetamine and inhalants tie for 2%, according to the CASA survey. Most teens agree that marijuana leads to use of harder drugs like cocaine, heroin, and acid.

About This Chapter: This chapter contains text from "CASA's Teen Survey," The National Center on Addiction and Substance Abuse at Columbia University (CASA), © 1999 CASA; reprinted with permission. The full text of this report, including references and notes, can be found on CASA's website at http://www.casacolumbia.org.

Attitudes About Drugs

CASA also measured attitudes towards smoking, drinking and using illegal drugs. Drinking beer, by far, was considered the most acceptable with 35% of boys and 30% of girls saying drinking by the opposite sex is "no big deal." Regarding cigarettes, 21% of boys and 17% of girls say smoking cigarettes is "no big deal" while only 18% of boys and 14% of girls say smoking pot is "no big deal."

✤ It's A Fact!!

Teen attitudes are difficult to measure, but CASA's survey did find some lights in the tunnel: The largest proportion of teens still cite drugs as their biggest problem but 23% of teens did so this year, down from 29% in 1998 and 35% in 1997. 60% of teens say they don't expect to use a drug in the future compared to 51% in 1998. 44% of teens say they attend a drug-free school compared to 31% in 1998. 40% say the drug situation in school is getting worse compared to 55% in 1998. 36% of teens say their parents never had a serious discussion with them about the risks of using illegal drugs, down from 43% last year.

Tobacco

More than 4 million kids age 12-17 are current smokers, according to the 1998 National Household Survey on Drug Abuse. Three thousand kids start to smoke every day and more than 5 million children under age 18 alive today will eventually die from smoking-related disease, unless current rates are reversed, according to the U.S. Centers for Disease Control and Prevention. Starting to smoke when you are a teen means trouble in the future. Early smoking can trigger genetic changes in your body that put young smokers at higher risk for cancer even if they quite later on.

According to CASA's survey, boys are five times as likely to get their first cigarette from a boy as from a girl; girls are four times as likely to get their first cigarette from a girl as from a boy. Both boys and girls are more likely to get their first marijuana cigarette from a boy: 28% of boys were offered pot by a boy compared with 2% by a girl, 14% of girls were offered pot by a boy compared with 7% by a girl. Boys and girls are also likely to consume more alcohol when they are with boys than with girls.

CASA also asked teens why they smoke, drink and use marijuana. Teens are most likely to smoke cigarettes or marijuana to "fit in with the crowd" and to drink to "have fun."

Chapter 49

The Controlled Substances Act

Controlling Drugs Or Other Substances

The Controlled Substances Act (CSA), Title II of the Comprehensive Drug Abuse Prevention and Control Act of 1970, is the legal foundation of the government's fight against abuse of drugs and other substances. This law is a consolidation of numerous laws regulating the manufacture and distribution of narcotics, stimulants, depressants, hallucinogens, anabolic steroids, and chemicals used in the illicit production of controlled substances.

Formal Scheduling

The CSA places all substances which were in some manner regulated under existing federal law into one of five schedules. This placement is based upon the substance's medical use, potential for abuse, and safety or dependence liability. The Act also provides a mechanism for substances to be controlled, or added to a schedule; decontrolled, or removed from control; and rescheduled or transferred from one schedule to another.

Proceedings to add, delete, or change the schedule of a drug or other substance may be initiated by the Drug Enforcement Administration (DEA), the Department of Health and Human Services (HHS), or by petition from

About This Chapter: Text in this chapter is excerpted from *Drugs of Abuse*, Drug Enforcement Administration, U.S. Department of Justice. The full text of this book is available online at www.dea.gov; cited November 2001.

any interested party (for example, the manufacturer of a drug, a medical society or association, a pharmacy association, a public interest group concerned with drug abuse, a state or local government agency, or an individual citizen). When a petition is received by the DEA, the agency begins its own investigation of the drug.

The agency also may begin an investigation of a drug at any time based upon information received from law enforcement laboratories, state and local law enforcement and regulatory agencies, or other sources of information.

The threshold issue is whether the drug or other substance has potential for abuse. If a drug does not have a potential for abuse, it cannot be controlled. Although the term "potential for abuse" is not defined in CSA, there is much discussion of the term in the legislative history of the Act. The following items are indicators that a drug or other substance has a potential for abuse:

1. There is evidence that individuals are taking the drug or other substance in amounts sufficient to create a hazard to their health or to the safety of other individuals or to the community; or

2. There is significant diversion of the drug or other substance from legitimate drug channels; or

3. Individuals are taking the drug or other substance on their own initiative rather than on the basis of medical advice from a practitioner licensed by law to administer such drugs; or

4. The drug is a new drug so related in its action to a drug or other substance already listed as having a potential for abuse to make it likely that the drug will have the same potential for abuse. Of course, evidence of actual abuse of a substance is indicative that a drug has a potential for abuse.

In determining into which schedule a drug or other substance should be placed, or whether a substance should be decontrolled or rescheduled, certain factors are required to be considered. Specific findings are not required for each factor. These factors are as follows:

1. The drug's actual or relative potential for abuse.

2. Scientific evidence of the drug's pharmacological effects. For example, it is vital to know whether or not a drug has a hallucinogenic effect if it is to be controlled because of that.

3. The state of current scientific knowledge regarding the substance. Criteria (2) and (3) are closely related. However, (2) is primarily concerned with pharmacological effects and (3) deals with all scientific knowledge with respect to the substance.

4. Its history and current pattern of abuse. To determine whether or not a drug should be controlled, it is important to know the pattern of abuse of that substance.

5. The scope, duration, and significance of abuse.

6. What, if any, risk there is to the public health. If a drug creates dangers to the public health, in addition to or because of its abuse potential, then these dangers must also be considered.

7. The drug's psychic or physiological dependence liability. There must be an assessment of the extent to which a drug is physically addictive or psychologically habit-forming, if such information is known.

✎ Weird Words

Analog: A compound that resembles another in structure

Controlled Substance: A substance subject to the Controlled Substances Act (1970), which regulates the prescribing and dispensing, as well as the manufacturing, storage, sale, or distribution of substances assigned to five schedules according to their 1) potential for or evidence of abuse, 2) potential for psychic or physiologic dependence, 3) contribution to a public health risk, 4) harmful pharmacologic effect, or 5) role as a precursor of other controlled substances.

Precursor: That which precedes another or from which another is derived, applied especially to an inactive substance that is converted to an active substance.

✤ It's A Fact!!

Here are some examples of drugs and the Schedules under which they are classified:

- *Schedule I:* heroin, LSD, marijuana, and methaqualone.
- *Schedule II:* morphine, PCP, cocaine, methadone, and methamphetamine.
- *Schedule III:* anabolic steroids, codeine and hydrocodone with aspirin or Tylenol, and some barbiturates.
- *Schedule IV:* Darvon, Talwin, Equanil, Valium, and Xanax.
- *Schedule V:* Over-the-counter cough medicines with codeine.

8. Whether the substance is an immediate precursor of a substance already controlled. The CSA allows inclusion of immediate precursors on this basis alone into the appropriate schedule and thus safeguards against possibilities of clandestine manufacture.

After considering the above listed factors, the Administrator must make specific findings concerning the drug or other substance. This will determine into which schedule the drug or other substance will be placed. These schedules are established by the CSA.

Schedule I

- The drug or other substance has a high potential for abuse.
- The drug or other substance has no currently accepted medical use in treatment in the United States.
- There is a lack of accepted safety for use of the drug or other substance under medical supervision.

Schedule II

- The drug or other substance has a high potential for abuse.

- The drug or other substance has a currently accepted medical use in treatment in the United States or a currently accepted medical use with severe restrictions.
- Abuse of the drug or other substance may lead to severe psychological or physical dependence.

Schedule III

- The drug or other substance has a potential for abuse less than the drugs or other substances in Schedules I and II.
- The drug or other substance has a currently accepted medical use in treatment in the United States.
- Abuse of the drug or other substance may lead to moderate or low physical dependence or high psychological dependence.

Schedule IV

- The drug or other substance has a low potential for abuse relative to the drugs or other substances in Schedule III.
- The drug or other substance has a currently accepted medical use in treatment in the United States.
- Abuse of the drug or other substance may lead to limited physical dependence or psychological dependence relative to the drugs or other substances in Schedule III.

Schedule V

- The drug or other substance has a low potential for abuse relative to the drugs or other substances in Schedule IV.
- The drug or other substance has a currently accepted medical use in treatment in the United States.
- Abuse of the drug or other substance may lead to limited physical dependence or psychological dependence relative to the drugs or other substances in Schedule IV.

International Treaty Obligations

U.S. treaty obligations may require that a drug or other substance be controlled under the CSA, or rescheduled if existing controls are less stringent than those required by a treaty.

Emergency Or Temporary Scheduling

The CSA was amended by the Comprehensive Crime Control Act of 1984. This Act included a provision which allows the Administrator of DEA to place a substance, on a temporary basis, into Schedule I when necessary to avoid an imminent hazard to the public safety.

This emergency scheduling authority permits the scheduling of a substance which is not currently controlled, is being abused, and is a risk to the public health while the formal rule-making procedures described in the CSA are being conducted. This emergency scheduling applies only to substances with no accepted medical use. A temporary scheduling order may be issued for one year with a possible extension of up to six months if formal scheduling procedures have been initiated.

Controlled Substance Analogues

A new class of substances was created by the Anti-Drug Abuse Act of 1986. Controlled substance analogues are substances which are not controlled substances, but may be found in the illicit traffic. They are structurally or pharmacologically similar to Schedule I or II controlled substances and have no legitimate medical use. A substance which meets the definition of a controlled substance analogue and is intended for human consumption is treated under the CSA as if it were a controlled substance in Schedule I.

☞ Remember!!

The Controlled Substances Act (CSA) provides penalties for the unlawful manufacturing, distribution, and dispensing of controlled substances. The penalties are basically determined by the schedule of the drug or substance. For more information about the CSA, contact:

U.S. Drug Enforcement Administration
Information Services Section
2401 Jefferson Davis Highway
Alexandria, VA 22301
Website: www.dea.gov

Chapter 50

Drug Testing: Questions And Answers

How long do different drugs stay in the body?

The length of time the drug or its metabolites can be detected in the urine is called the "retention time." Retention times differ according to these factors:

- amount of drug consumed
- method of drug use
- whether use is chronic or occasional
- individual rates of metabolism and excretion
- diet
- acidity of the urine
- fluid intake
- time of day

✎ **Weird Words**

Metabolite: Any product or substrate (foodstuff, intermediate, waste product) of metabolism.

Source: From *Stedman's Medical Dictionary, 27th Edition*, Copyright © 2000 Lippincott Williams & Wilkins. All rights reserved.

A list of retention times is given in Table 50.1. Because of all these variables, the values represented in the table should be used as general guidelines only.

About This Chapter: The information in this chapter is from "Q's and A's on Drug Testing," Connecticut Clearinghouse, a program of Wheeler Clinic, Inc., © May 1995 Connecticut Clearinghouse, 334 Farmington Avenue, Plainville, CT 06062, 800-232-4424, 860-793-9791 (www.ctclearinghouse.org); reprinted with permission.

Table 50.1. A Drug's Length Of Stay In The Body

Type of Drug	Retention Time
Amphetamines (crystal, ice, crank, methamphetamines)	1–days
Barbiturates	
short-acting (for example, secobarbital)	1–3 days
long-acting (for example, phenobarbital)	1–3 weeks
Benzodiazepines (Librium, Valium, Serax)	1–14 days
Cannabinoids (marijuana)	
occasional use	1–7 days
chronic use	1–4 weeks
Cocaine	12–48 hours
Methadone	1–3 days
Methaqualone (Quaalude)	1–3 days
Opiates (heroin, morphine, codeine)	1–3 days
Phencyclidine (PCP)	
occasional use	1–8 days
chronic use	up to 30 days
Propoxyphene (Darvon)	1–3 days

How accurate is drug testing?

There are a variety of methods available to test for illegal substances. These methods are accurate and reliable if these two areas of drug testing are adhered to:

1. *Use of confirmation assay.* If a positive result occurs, the specimen is then tested again by a different chemical method to confirm the positive result.

2. *Quality control procedures.* A good laboratory will document how and by whom the sample is handled from the time it is taken from the individual, through the laboratory, until the final assay result is tabulated. This record is referred to as the "chain of custody" for the sample.

Are there any legal substances which can create a "false positive" for illegal drug use?

Here is a list of some of the more often used substances which can affect drug testing:

Over-The-Counter Medications

Some medications contain high concentrations of decongestants that will produce a positive result for amphetamines. Appropriate confirmatory testing will detect when the drug is an decongestant or an amphetamine.

Poppy Seeds

Poppy seeds frequently found on bagels or other baked products do contain sufficient amounts of morphine to produce a detectable test result. This can be resolved by using a test which will detect a substance in the urine which is only found in the illegal substance heroin.

Secondhand Marijuana Smoke

Passive inhalation of marijuana smoke is frequently claimed as a reason for a positive urine test. Yes, passive inhalation of marijuana smoke can be detected, but studies show it is highly unlikely that a nonsmoking individual could unknowingly inhale sufficient smoke by passive inhalation to result in a high enough drug concentration in the urine for detection at the cutoff currently used for urinalysis methods.

Chapter 51

Medical Marijuana

Some of the chemicals in marijuana may be helpful to people with certain illnesses. For example, smoking marijuana is sometimes used as a treatment for weight loss associated with HIV (human immunodeficiency virus). Claims about its effectiveness are based largely on individual experience rather than data from studies and some medical associations, including the American Medical Association, the American Glaucoma Society, and the American Cancer Society, do not support its use. A synthetic form of the most active ingredient in marijuana, called dronabinol (Marinol), is approved by the U.S. Food and Drug Administration. It is available by prescription for treating HIV-related weight loss (anorexia) as well as for treating nausea during chemotherapy treatments.

This chapter describes some of the issues involved in the debate surrounding the use of medical marijuana. Although the text was originally written for people with HIV, much of the information comes from research on people who do not have HIV disease.

Buyers Clubs And The Law

Marijuana is an illegal substance, yet 'buyers clubs' have been established in some areas to provide the drug for people using marijuana for medical purposes. Even though they are illegal under federal law, some cities like San Francisco have local laws permitting them to operate. Some even have programs that provide medical marijuana free or at reduced cost to people with limited incomes.

Legislation was approved on a public vote in California that allows physicians to prescribe marijuana for some medical conditions. HIV-associated wasting is one of four conditions in the legislation. While some healthcare providers have voiced concern over the safety of marijuana smoking, many providers have also been impressed with positive results in weight gain, mood, and quality of life in their HIV-positive patients who use medical marijuana.

Safety Concerns

There are many possibly harmful effects from smoking marijuana, just as there would be from inhaling almost any other form of smoke. Most of the studies citing these effects were conducted many years ago, and conflicting reports can often be found among all of them. Many people question whether political motives may have influenced early studies of marijuana. For people living with HIV, the largest safety concerns when using marijuana are the affects on:

- immune function,
- lung complications (particularly with smoked marijuana),
- hormones, and
- mental state.

Immune Function

Marijuana and/or its psychoactive ingredient THC have been reported to suppress many immune functions. These include the function of cells important in controlling infections commonly seen among people living with HIV. Marijuana may also increase your risk for certain infections, including herpes and a variety of other bacterial, viral, and fungal infections. Some of these infections may result in increased HIV levels. None of this, however, has been clearly documented in HIV-positive people.

Some research suggests that marijuana has no significant effect—good or bad—on the immune system of people living with HIV. Studies from the Multicenter AIDS Cohort Study evaluating outcomes in 1,662 HIV-positive users of psychoactive drugs (marijuana, cocaine, LSD, etc.) found that none of the drugs were linked to a higher rate of HIV disease progression or loss of CD4+ cell counts. Of the men who took part in the study, 89% reported using marijuana in the preceding two years. A recent study, presented in 2000, examined the short-term impact of marijuana, dronabinol, or placebo on HIV levels, CD4+ cell count and HIV levels. After twenty-one days, the use of marijuana did not appear to have harmful affects. Much longer-term studies are needed before concluding that marijuana use is either safe or unsafe for people living with HIV, however.

Lung Complications

Research comparing the effects of tobacco and marijuana smoking on the lungs shows that marijuana smoke can be harmful. Smoking marijuana increases the risks of lung complications, may worsen asthma, and may increase the risk of lung cancer over and above smoking tobacco.

Another possible harmful effect of smoking marijuana is that it may cause lung infections. In particular, a fungus sometimes found in marijuana called aspergillus is thought to be the cause of possible infections. This infection has sometimes been seen in people with advanced HIV disease.

Some recommend putting marijuana in the microwave for ten seconds to kill any fungus that might be growing on it. The exact time needed to kill the fungus will vary depending on the oven settings, the quantity and moisture content of the marijuana, and the wattage of the microwave. There are no standards for this, but in general, smaller microwave ovens put out less power and would therefore require longer "cooking" times to kill a fungus.

Recent studies suggest that smoking marijuana may also decrease the ability of cells in the lung to destroy candida and bacteria. Candida is the fungus responsible for candidiasis, a common condition in people living with HIV. People living with HIV who smoke marijuana may be at higher risk for lung complications.

✤ It's A Fact!!

The use of medical marijuana is controversial.

Pros

- Dronabinol is FDA-approved and legally available by prescription through hospitals and pharmacies.
- People who have tried both dronabinol and medical marijuana contend that they are better able to control drug effects with medical marijuana.
- Some limited studies suggest that marijuana doesn't have negative long-term impact on HIV disease and measures of immune health, like CD4+ cell counts.

Cons

- Dronabinol has absorption problems and individuals' claim difficulty in controlling the drug effect (feeling too "stoned").
- Medical marijuana is not legally available to many people. Third-party payers, like insurance and Federal programs, do not cover its cost.
- Marijuana and its active ingredient THC has been shown in some studies to suppress immune function.
- Smoked marijuana increases the risk of lung infections and complications.
- Marijuana may be contaminated with insecticides, pesticides, fungus and/or bacteria. Ingesting these could have mild-to-severe health consequences.
- Marijuana/THC has short-term impact on mental status. Long-term effects are less clear.
- Some studies suggest that marijuana/THC may decrease testosterone levels.
- It is unknown if marijuana interacts with anti-HIV drug therapies, increases HIV replication or negatively impacts HIV disease progression.

Impact On Hormones

Many men with HIV experience low testosterone levels during the course of HIV infection. Women may also experience lowered testosterone levels and changes in other hormones, both of which may be contributing factors in many menstrual irregularities seen in women living with HIV. Studies in animals and humans show that marijuana may further lower the levels of hormones, including testosterone. This information is important to people with HIV as lowered testosterone levels are associated with AIDS-related wasting. Marijuana could cause or worsen this condition, possibly leading to the necessity of testosterone replacement therapy.

Mental Status

The question of the neurological (change in mental status) effects of marijuana has been addressed by several studies in recent years. Marijuana use has been shown to have short-term impact on a person's ability to think, learn, judge, and perform tasks. Moreover, marijuana use has short-term effects on memory. It's less clear if marijuana has any long-term effects on mental status or mood. It is also less clear whether the effects noted are perceived as "good" or "bad" by those who experience them. Some people feel smoking marijuana offers relief from depression, while others say it increases their anxiety levels.

Marijuana's Impact On Appetite

Extensive research on how smoked marijuana affects appetite has been conducted, although much of it was published 20 to 50 years ago. Anecdotal accounts of increased food intake have always been reported by marijuana smokers—the so-called "munchies." The quality of the food (candy bars and chips vs. vegetables, fruits and protein) and quality of the weight gain (fat vs. muscle) needs to be considered.

Overall, studies suggest that people using marijuana eat more but the food they eat is generally snack food, like cookies and junk food. They also exercise less and sleep more, all of which contributes to weight gain.

It's not at all clear that this kind of weight gain, that consists more of body fat than of lean muscle, will benefit the overall health and longevity of a person with HIV-related wasting. However, if medical marijuana is combined with a comprehensive nutritional and weight maintenance program, as well as exercise, it may prove useful. Because of these concerns, it is important that evaluating the medical effects of marijuana not be limited to measuring weight gain, as this may lead to false conclusions about its value.

Oral THC vs. Marijuana

The oral drug, dronabinol (Marinol), was approved in 1992 for use in treating anorexia in people with HIV-related wasting. The active ingredient in dronabinol is THC, which is one of the main psychoactive agents in marijuana and the chemical that makes someone feel "stoned". For treating HIV-related weight loss, THC probably helps as an appetite stimulant, in the same way people who are "stoned" get the munchies.

People who use dronabinol have mixed experiences. Some report a minimal drug effect while others experience far too much euphoria or feeling "stoned". This is because of the variability in how the oral drug gets into the bloodstream, or perhaps to an individuals' point of view and how they feel about such sensations. Smoking marijuana, or using edible forms of it, may be a more efficient way to get THC throughout the body. People who have tried both forms say that they are better able to control how "stoned" they get by smoking or eating marijuana and thus prefer it over the pill formulation.

Other Possible Uses For Medical Marijuana

For people living with HIV, marijuana may have other uses besides stimulating the appetite. Some research and reports of people's personal experiences support the notion that marijuana/THC can help treat nausea and vomiting. The exact reason why it works is unknown. Dronabinol is approved to ease nausea in people undergoing chemotherapy. Marijuana, therefore, may be a realistic alternative for people who don't benefit from standard anti-nausea medication. This could be an important benefit because so many people report difficulties with nausea when using anti-HIV therapies.

Marijuana has been shown to be an effective treatment for general pain associated with illness or serious injury. As with nausea, how marijuana relieves mild pain is not known. New studies suggest that marijuana may have anti-inflammatory effects.

The Future Of Medical Marijuana

A recent report from the Institute of Medicine (IOM) of the U.S. National Academy of Sciences stated that certain chemicals found in marijuana may help manage certain conditions in some people, but that marijuana smoke, like tobacco smoke, is harmful. Though there is an oral medication (dronabinol) that is supposed to mimic the desired effects of smoking marijuana, many people prefer to smoke or eat marijuana in its natural form.

In an attempt to copy the effects of inhaling marijuana while eliminating the risks involved with smoking, some researchers are looking at the use of a vaporizer (or inhaler) for smokeless inhalation. Though not included in this IOM report, other sources indicate that a vaporizer is now readily available. This device heats marijuana to a certain temperature to release active chemicals without setting the dried plant on fire. Since this has only been around for a short time, it is not known how effective it is in delivering the drug. However, early results seem promising.

Overall, medical marijuana research will likely shift from study of the crude plant material to research and eventually drug development of chemicals derived from marijuana. This has already occurred with isolating THC and the development of dronabinol.

What currently holds back more studies of marijuana (or chemicals associated with marijuana) and its effects on the body is a complex matter. Aside from the obvious political concerns, research scientists are not given much incentive to work on marijuana and its derived chemicals. Namely, funding is scarce from government and private sources, and there is concern that the fruits of research will not be made public because of the controversial nature of the drug. Additionally, many researchers feel their reputations may be affected by working with marijuana because of its status as a street drug and controlled substance.

Nevertheless, more research related to marijuana could benefit many people, especially those living with HIV. There are indications that substances present in marijuana can stimulate appetite, relieve pain and stop nausea. So, research that leads to uncovering the chemicals responsible for these effects and uncovering the best way to deliver them to the body could prove helpful. And though research may not eliminate all the safety concerns associated with medical marijuana, it may make this therapy a more realistic alternative for many people.

☞ Remember!!

- Medical marijuana may be useful in promoting appetite for people with HIV-related anorexia.
- Marijuana may also be useful in managing nausea and may help relieve pain.
- A synthetic form of an active ingredient in marijuana, dronabinol (Marinol) is approved by the FDA for treating HIV-related weight loss and for managing nausea associated with the use of chemotherapy.

Chapter 52

Speaking Out Against Drug Legalization

This text was developed by the Drug Enforcement Administration (DEA) to help people respond to questions about the legalization of drugs. It offers ten assertions, which were developed during an anti-legalization forum, to answer claims made by people and groups who support legalization. DEA believes that legalization is not an alternative, but a surrender that will further reduce our nation's quality of life.

Assertion 1: Crime, Violence, And Drug Use Go Hand-In-Hand

Proponents of legalization contend that if drugs were legalized, crime and violence would decrease. They believe that it is the illegal nature of drug production, trafficking, and use that fuels crime and violence. They state that turf wars, gang activity, and drug-related crimes are the result of the illegal nature of the drug trade. Proponents state that users commit crimes to pay for drugs now because they cannot easily obtain them. If drugs were legal, they say, the enormous profits associated with drugs because of their illegal status would evaporate and, once gone, the black market and criminal activity associated with drugs would also be eliminated.

About This Chapter: Text in this chapter is excerpted from *Speaking Out Against Drug Legalization*, Drug Enforcement Administration, U.S. Department of Justice. The full text is available online at www.usdoj.gov/dea/demand/drugleagl/; cited November 2001.

Sadly, it is the experience of many local police officers that crime is committed not only because people want to buy drugs, but more often because people use drugs. There is no denying the fact that drug use changes behavior and exacerbates criminal activity.

The experts also believe that legalization will lead to greater availability of drugs, which will, in turn, lead to increased use. The use of drugs, especially

✎ Weird Words

Here are some of the terms frequently used by those who support or oppose legalization.

Decriminalization: This term is used to describe the removal of, or reduction in, criminal penalties for particular acts. Used in the context of drug policy, it is a broad term that often encompasses a range of measures such as removal of criminal sanctions for simple possession of drugs or lowering of penalties for possession of small amounts of illegal drugs.

Legalization: Simply put this means making legal what is currently illegal. Used in the context of drug policy, it is a broad term that can mean different things to different people. To some, it means making all illegal drugs legal for anyone to use. To others, it means making certain illegal drugs legal for certain people to use. There is no specific definition of legalization because the parameters of legalization differ among supporters. The term must be further defined by asking: Who will be able to use? Which drugs? At what potency? Where and when? With what regulations? Regulated by whom or by which institutions? Enforced by whom or by which institutions?

Harm Reduction: This term is often used to describe specific programs (for example, needle exchange programs, methadone maintenance clinics, etc.) that attempt to diminish the potential harmful consequences associated with a particular behavior. The term "harm minimization" is also frequently used.

Scheduled Drugs: This term refers to the tiered system at the state and federal levels of regulating psychoactive drugs and access to them. The schedules draw distinctions among drugs with high abuse potential, such as marijuana and heroin, for which the medical and scientific communities have concluded that there are no currently accepted medical or therapeutic uses, and other drugs with abuse potential but accepted medical or therapeutic uses.

cocaine, crack, methamphetamine, and PCP, is often associated with violent criminal behavior. There is ample evidence that demonstrates the links between drugs, violence, and crime. Additionally, links between alcohol, a currently legal substance, and crime are well documented. Police can attest to the fact that alcohol plays a significant role in domestic violence cases. Drug use would only swell the statistics regarding crime, even if the drugs were legally purchased.

Assertion 2: We Have Made Significant Progress In Reducing Drug Use

Legalization advocates claim that the fight against drugs has not been won and is, in fact, unconquerable. They frequently state that people still take drugs, drugs are widely available, and that efforts to change this are futile. Legalization advocates contend that legalization is the alternative.

There have been many positive developments over the past 15 years in reducing drug use, and such positive developments are not afforded adequate publicity. The nation's drug problem did not happen overnight, and it will take a number of years to eliminate. Legalization is not an alternative.

The United States faces a number of challenges today—which like our drug problem are not resolvable through easy solutions—including illegal immigration, the decline of quality education, and public health problems. Should we abdicate ourselves of the need to enforce equitable immigration laws? Should we declare that our education system is an irreparable failure? Should we throw up our hands in frustration about cancer, or AIDS and halt researching for cures? Clearly such suggestions are preposterous. We are a people committed to solving problems, not avoiding them. Why should our commitment to stopping drugs be any different from our approach to other national interests?

Assertion 3: Legalization Of Drugs Will Lead To Increased Use

A cornerstone of the legalization proponents' position is the claim that making illegal drugs legal would not cause more of these substances to be consumed, nor would addiction increase. They claim that many people can use drugs in moderation and that many would choose not to use drugs, just as many abstain from alcohol and tobacco now.

If drugs were more widely available, as they certainly would be if they were legalized, rates of use and addiction would increase. Legalizing drugs sends a message that drug use (like tobacco and alcohol) is acceptable, and encourages drug use among people who currently do not use drugs.

Look to our history. For years, the United States legally refined morphine from opium and hailed it as a miracle drug. Many soldiers on both sides of the Civil War who were given morphine for their wounds became addicted to it.

Early in the 20th century, drugs were plentiful, cheap, and legal in the United States. Some could even be bought from the *Sears Catalog*. But Americans realized that these legalized drugs were harmful to individuals and society, and drug laws were enacted. Legalization proponents would have these statutes repealed and make opium readily available.

The experts believe that legalization of drugs would decrease the perception of risk currently associated with drug use. The government should help protect people from substances and activities that are harmful to them, the community, and society at large.

Assertion 4: Any Revenues Generated By Taxing Legalized Drugs Would Quickly Evaporate In Light Of Increased Social Costs

A favorite argument in support of legalization is that education, health care, road building, and a wide array of other worthwhile causes would benefit from the taxes that could be raised by legalizing drugs and then taxing them. When asked for specifics, the advocates have no answers. Are they taking into account the erosion of the tax base as more and more citizens are unable to work because of drug addiction? Add to this loss the cost of health and welfare benefits for the unemployed.

Health and societal costs of drug legalization would increase. Drug treatment costs, hospitalization for long-term drug-related disease, and

✤ It's A Fact!!

Position Of The Drug Enforcement Administration (DEA)

DEA is unequivocally opposed to the legalization of illicit drugs (including, marijuana, hemp, and hemp seed oil). Legalization of drugs in any form would likely:

1. reduce the perception of the risks and costs of drug use;
2. increase availability of and access to harmful drugs;
3. increase demand, use, abuse, and addiction; and
4. remove the social sanction against drug abuse that is reinforced in legislation.

treatment of the consequences of family violence would further burden our already strapped health care system.

Legalization proponents must realize the increased costs that would be incurred through the damaging effects of drugs. Would the alleged profits from drug legalization offset the acute and chronic effects of increases in fetal defects, loss of workforce productivity, traffic fatalities, industrial accidents, domestic violence, and other problems? The increased financial costs of drug legalization pale in comparison, however, to the increased social and emotional costs that American families would suffer.

Assertion 5: There Are No Compelling Medical Reasons To Prescribe Marijuana Or Heroin

Arguments urging the medical use of marijuana are often used as an entree into the legalization debate. Medical use arguments can garner public support because they seem harmless enough to the well-intended. The experts agreed that these issues are peripheral to the real issue.

Medical professionals best debate the medical pros and cons of prescribing marijuana and heroin to sick people. It should be kept in mind, however, that the American Medical Association, the American Glaucoma Society, the American Academy of Ophthalmology, the International Federation of Multiple Sclerosis Societies, and the American Cancer Society have rejected marijuana as medicine.

Not one American health association accepts marijuana as medicine. Statements issued by these organizations express concern over the harmful effects of the drugs and over the lack of solid research demonstrating that they might do more good than harm.

Assertion 6: Legalization And Decriminalization Of Drugs Have Been A Dismal Failure In Other Nations

The experiences of a number of foreign countries including Great Britain, the Netherlands, and Switzerland are often cited to demonstrate that other nations have successfully controlled drug use by providing areas where drug takers can obtain and use drugs.

Legalization proponents cannot find encouragement in the fact that when drugs were once legal, cheap, and available in the United States, the impact on society was such that laws were enacted to make drugs illegal. They ignore our own history and point to Great Britain, the Netherlands, and Switzerland as free and open societies where drug use is allowed with no adverse effects. It is important to shed light on the foreign experience with increased drug access and liberalized use policies, and explain that this experience has been negative.

England tried prescribing heroin but eventually relented. Until the mid-1960s, British physicians were allowed to prescribe heroin to certain classes of addicts. The British system did not work. Addiction levels rose, especially among teenagers, and many addicts chose to boycott the program and continued to get their heroin from illicit drug distributors. In 1983, English clinics began dispensing methadone instead of heroin, consequently even more addicts departed in search of heroin. According to the late John Kaplan of Stanford University, the number of addicts increased fivefold. James Q. Wilson states that the British Government's experiment with controlled heroin distribution resulted in, at a minimum, a 30-fold increase in the number of addicts in ten years.

The Netherlands, despite its controlled program, is showing signs of failure as well. Under the so-called "expediency principle," Dutch prosecutors have wide discretion in prosecuting, or ignoring, persons in possession of small quantities of drugs for personal use. In practice, marijuana and hashish, for instance, are openly sold and consumed in coffeehouses. The Amsterdam Municipal Health Service showed a rise in hard-core addicts in 1992, attributable to a significant rise in the local heroin supply which led to a price drop of as much as 75 percent.

Switzerland has become a magnet for drug users the world over. Small European nations have discovered firsthand that a modicum of tolerance relative to drugs is capable of attracting innumerable unwelcome visitors. In 1987, Zurich permitted drug use and sales in a part of the city called the Platzspitz, dubbed "Needle Park." Five years later the experiment was curtailed after an influx of addicts, and increased violence and drug-related deaths.

Assertion 7: Alcohol Has Caused Significant Health, Social and Crime Problems In This Country, And Legalized Drugs Would Only Make The Situation Worse

Many legalization advocates are fond of comparing the use of alcohol with the use of drugs, yet draw faulty conclusions from the comparison. People often consume small amounts of wine or beer as a beverage and do not necessarily drink to the point of mental impairment. This is not true of drug use, where the whole point of use is intoxication. A more accurate analogy would be to compare drug use to drunkenness. Yet even that analogy is weak, because drugs are far more addictive than alcohol. Dr. Mitchell Rosenthal points out, for example, that only 10 percent of drinkers become alcoholics, while up to 75 percent of regular illicit drug users become addicted.

Proponents of legalization note correctly that alcohol kills many more Americans than do illegal drugs and currently exact social and financial costs that are higher as well. Advocates point out that many people do not use alcohol, and argue that many Americans may also choose to forego drug use. Additionally, advocates contend that like treatment programs available for alcoholics, treatment programs for other drug addicts should be more widely available.

Health care systems and social service mechanisms are already overburdened and consequently unable to address all the problems associated with alcohol use. The legalization of drugs would compound these problems, adding immeasurably to the burdens on the criminal, health, and social service systems. Alcohol use in this country has taken a tremendous physical toll on Americans, not to mention the social problems that have resulted from its use. Legalization proponents would have us multiply our problems by greatly adding to the class of drug-addicted Americans.

Assertion 8: Compared To The Costs Of Drug Abuse, Drug Control Spending Is Miniscule

Legalization advocates claim that this nation has spent billions of dollars to control drug production, trafficking, and use with few, if any, positive results. They contend that the money spent on drug control should be shifted to other, more productive endeavors.

The truth is, we have made great progress in reducing drug use during the past 15 years. If the relatively modest outlays of Federal dollars had not been made, drug abuse and attendant social costs would have been far greater. The good news is that drug use has continued to decline.

The claim that money allegedly saved from giving up on the drug problem could be better spent on education and social problems is readily disputed. When compared to the amount of funding that is spent on other national priorities, drug control spending is minimal. There has been progress in reducing drug use, and the money spent has been effective and worthwhile.

On the surface, legalization proponents present an appealing, simple argument that by legalizing drugs we can move vast sums of money from drug law enforcement into solving society's ills. They leave unanswered questions about the cost of collecting revenues associated with drug sales, or the cost of regulating drugs. They ignore questions concerning the purity, potency, and quality of legal drugs, the costs of insuring a safe product, and costs associated with increased liability litigation.

Proponents also conveniently fail to mention that unless drugs are made available to children, law enforcement will still be needed to deal with the sale of drugs to minors. But more importantly, in their simplistic arguments, they omit mention of the atrocious social costs that would be incurred with a larger class of drug users. Legalization would also result in lost workforce productivity and a resultant increase in the cost of goods.

Furthermore, it is reasonable to believe that the health and societal costs of drug legalization would also increase. Drug treatment costs, hospitalization for long-term drug-related diseases, and treatment of family violence would place additional demands on our already overburden health-care system. Additionally, there is no guarantee, that criminal justice costs would decline if drugs were legalized. It is possible that law enforcement would be additionally burdened with addressing violations of traffic and family violence laws if more people had access to drugs. Law enforcement is already challenged by significant alcohol-related crimes. More users may result in the commission of additional crimes, causing incarceration costs to increase as well.

Assertion 9: Drug Prohibition Is Working

Legalization advocates claim that drug prohibition is akin to alcohol prohibition earlier this century. Their main premise is that it is impossible to prohibit people from using substances that they want to use.

When the Volstead Act was repealed, arrests for alcohol traffickers disappeared, but arrests in alcohol-related incidents rose, indicating that the prohibition against alcohol had kept people from using it. The same will happen if drugs are legalized. Once the Government sanctions drug use, it is reasonable to suggest that more people will use drugs. It is also important to remember that after Prohibition was repealed, organized crime branched out into other areas, and there is every expectation that current drug organizations would also continue and diversify.

Assertion 10: Legalization Would Have An Adverse Effect On Low-Income Communities

Some proponents of legalization claim that current strict drug control policies have a disproportionately adverse effect on poor communities. The drug laws of the United States, and efforts to stop drug trafficking and abuse, are designed to protect all people from the harm and degradation that illegal drugs cause. If one economic group or another is disproportionately affected by the implementation of current laws, that problem should be dealt with in its proper context, not by legalizing drugs.

Legalization proponents argue that fewer people would be arrested for drug trafficking crime, and the violence associated with the protection of areas of distribution would be reduced if drugs were legalized. That argument assumes that drug-related violence is limited to rival drug gangs disputing areas of distribution, when in fact, most drug violence is committed by people under the influence of drugs.

One can further suggest that the incidence of dysfunctional families, the rate of unemployment, family violence, and ruined lives would increase in low-income communities, just as it would in every other community. Specifically, all communities may experience increased occurrences of child abuse and neglect, family disintegration, fetal damage caused by mothers' drug use, social welfare costs, loss of workforce productivity, increased auto accidents attributable to drug impaired drivers, increased industrial accidents caused by impaired workers, increased absenteeism, and increases in emergency room visits and overdose deaths.

Remember!!

According to DEA, the present social problems in the United States, including crime, health problems, and poverty, are substantial and will only be exacerbated if drugs are legalized. Legalization would increase risks and costs to individuals, families, and communities, indeed, to every part of the nation, without compensating benefits.

Chapter 53

Against Drug Prohibition

More and more ordinary people, elected officials, newspaper columnists, economists, doctors, judges and even the Surgeon General of the United States are concluding that the effects of our drug control policy are at least as harmful as the effects of drugs themselves.

After decades of criminal prohibition and intensive law enforcement efforts to rid the country of illegal drugs, violent traffickers still endanger life in our cities, a steady stream of drug offenders still pours into our jails and prisons, and tons of cocaine, heroin and marijuana still cross our borders unimpeded.

The American Civil Liberties Union (ACLU) opposes criminal prohibition of drugs. Not only is prohibition a proven failure as a drug control strategy, but it subjects otherwise law-abiding citizens to arrest, prosecution, and imprisonment for what they do in private. In trying to enforce the drug laws, the government violates the fundamental rights of privacy and personal autonomy that are guaranteed by our Constitution. The ACLU believes that unless they do harm to others, people should not be punished—even if they do harm to themselves. There are better ways to control drug use, ways that will ultimately lead to a healthier, freer and less crime-ridden society.

About This Chapter: Text in this chapter is from "Against Drug Prohibition," *ACLU Briefing Paper*, Copyright 1996, American Civil Liberties Union. Reprinted with permission of the American Civil Liberties Union (http://www.aclu.org).

Currently Illegal Drugs Have Not Always Been Illegal

During the Civil War, morphine (an opium derivative and cousin of heroin) was found to have pain-killing properties and soon became the main ingredient in several patent medicines. In the late 19th century, marijuana and cocaine were put to various medicinal uses—marijuana to treat migraines, rheumatism and insomnia, and cocaine to treat sinusitis, hay fever, and chronic fatigue. All of these drugs were also used recreationally, and cocaine, in particular, was a common ingredient in wines and soda pop—including the popular Coca Cola.

At the turn of the century, many drugs were made illegal when a mood of temperance swept the nation. In 1914, Congress passed the Harrison Act, banning opiates and cocaine. Alcohol prohibition quickly followed, and by 1918 the U.S. was officially a "dry" nation. That did not mean, however, an end to drug use. It meant that, suddenly, people were arrested and jailed for doing what they had previously done without government interference. Prohibition also meant the emergence of a black market, operated by criminals and marked by violence.

In 1933, because of concern over widespread organized crime, police corruption and violence, the public demanded repeal of alcohol prohibition and the return of regulatory power to the states. Most states immediately replaced criminal bans with laws regulating the quality, potency and commercial sale of alcohol; as a result, the harms associated with alcohol prohibition disappeared. Meanwhile, federal prohibition of heroin and cocaine remained, and with passage of the Marijuana Stamp Act in 1937 marijuana was prohibited as well. Federal drug policy has remained strictly prohibitionist to this day.

Decades Of Drug Prohibition: A History Of Failure

Criminal prohibition, the centerpiece of U.S. drug policy, has failed miserably. Since 1981, tax dollars to the tune of $150 billion have been spent trying to prevent Columbian cocaine, Burmese heroin, and Jamaican marijuana from penetrating our borders. Yet the evidence is that for every ton seized, hundreds more get through. Hundreds of thousands of otherwise law abiding people have been arrested and jailed for drug possession. Between 1968 and 1992, the annual number of drug-related arrests increased from 200,000 to over 1.2 million. One-third of those were marijuana arrests, most for mere possession.

The best evidence of prohibition's failure is the government's current war on drugs. This war, instead of employing a strategy of prevention, research, education and social programs designed to address problems such as permanent poverty, long-term unemployment, and deteriorating living conditions in our inner cities, has employed a strategy of law enforcement. While this military approach continues to devour billions of tax dollars and sends tens of thousands of people to prison, illegal drug trafficking thrives, violence escalates and drug abuse continues to debilitate lives. Compounding these problems is the largely unchecked spread of the AIDS virus among drug-users, their sexual partners and their offspring.

Those who benefit the most from prohibition are organized crime barons, who derive an estimated $10 to $50 billion a year from the illegal drug trade. Indeed, the criminal drug laws protect drug traffickers from taxation, regulation, and quality control. Those laws also support artificially high prices and assure that commercial disputes among drug dealers and their customers will be settled not in courts of law, but with automatic weapons in the streets.

Drug Prohibition Is A Public Health Menace

Drug prohibition promises a healthier society by denying people the opportunity to become drug users and, possibly, addicts. The reality of prohibition belies that promise.

- *No quality control.* When drugs are illegal, the government cannot enact standards of quality, purity, or potency. Consequently, street drugs are often contaminated or extremely potent, causing disease and sometimes death to those who use them.
- *Dirty needles.* Unsterilized needles are known to transmit HIV among intravenous drug users. Yet drug users share needles because laws prohibiting possession of drug paraphernalia have made needles a scarce commodity. These laws, then, actually promote epidemic disease and

death. In New York City, more than 60 percent of intravenous drug users are HIV positive. By contrast, the figure is less than one percent in Liverpool, England, where clean needles are easily available.

- *Scarce treatment resources.* The allocation of vast sums of money to law enforcement diminishes the funds available for drug education, preventive social programs and treatment. As crack use rose during the late 1980s, millions of dollars were spent on street-level drug enforcement and on jailing tens of thousands of low level offenders, while only a handful of public drug treatment slots were created. An especially needy group—low-income pregnant women who abused crack—often had no place to go at all because Medicaid would not reimburse providers. Instead, the government prosecuted and jailed such women without regard to the negative consequences for their children.

Drug Prohibition Creates More Problems Than It Solves

Drug prohibition has not only failed to curb or reduce the harmful effects of drug use, it has created other serious social problems.

- *Caught in the crossfire.* In the same way that alcohol prohibition fueled violent gangsterism in the 1920s, today's drug prohibition has spawned a culture of drive-by shootings and other gun-related crimes. And just as most of the 1920s violence was not committed by people who were drunk, most of the drug-related violence today is not committed by people who are high on drugs. The killings, then and now, are based on rivalries: Al Capone ordered the executions of rival bootleggers, and drug dealers kill their rivals today. A 1989 government study of all 193 "cocaine-related" homicides in New York City found that 87 percent grew out of rivalries and disagreements related to doing business in an illegal market. In only one case was the perpetrator actually under the influence of cocaine.
- *A Nation of Jailers.* The "lock 'em up" mentality of the war on drugs has burdened our criminal justice system to the breaking point. Today, drug-law enforcement consumes more than half of all police resources nationwide, resources that could be better spent fighting violent crimes like rape, assault, and robbery. The recent steep climb in our incarceration rate has made the U.S. the world's leading jailer, with a prison

population that now exceeds one million people, compared to approximately 200,000 in 1970. Nonviolent drug offenders make up 58 percent of the federal prison population, a population that is extremely costly to maintain. In 1990, the states alone paid $12 billion, or $16,000 per prisoner. While drug imprisonments are a leading cause of rising local tax burdens, they have neither stopped the sale and use of drugs nor enhanced public safety.

- *Not Drug Free—Just Less Free.* We now have what some constitutional scholars call "the drug exception to the Bill of Rights." Random drug testing without probable cause, the militarization of drug law enforcement, heightened wiretapping and other surveillance, the enactment of vaguely worded loitering laws and curfews, forfeiture of people's homes and assets, excessive and mandatory prison terms—these practices and more have eroded the constitutional rights of all Americans.

Prohibition Is A Destructive Force In Inner City Communities

Inner city communities suffer most from both the problem of drug abuse and the consequences of drug prohibition.

Although the rates of drug use among white and non-white Americans are similar, African Americans and other racial minorities are arrested and imprisoned at higher rates. For example, according to government estimates only 12 percent of drug users are black, but nearly 40 percent of those arrested for drug offenses are black. Nationwide, one-quarter of all young African American men are under some form of criminal justice supervision, mostly for drug offenses. This phenomenon has had a devastating social impact in minority communities. Moreover, the abuse of drugs, including alcohol, has more dire consequences in impoverished communities where good treatment programs are least available.

Finally, turf battles and commercial disputes among competing drug enterprises, as well as police responses to those conflicts, occur disproportionately in poor communities, making our inner cities war zones and their residents the war's primary casualties.

Drugs Are Here To Stay—Let's Reduce Their Harm

The universality of drug use throughout human history has led some experts to conclude that the desire to alter consciousness, for whatever reasons, is a basic human drive. People in almost all cultures, in every era, have used psychoactive drugs. Native South Americans take coca-breaks the way we, in this country, take coffee-breaks. Native North Americans use peyote and tobacco in their religious ceremonies the way Europeans use wine. Alcohol is the drug of choice in Europe, the U.S. and Canada, while many Muslim countries tolerate the use of opium and marijuana.

A "drug free America" is not a realistic goal, and by criminally banning psychoactive drugs the government has ceded all control of potentially dangerous substances to criminals. Instead of trying to stamp out all drug use, our government should focus on reducing drug abuse and prohibition-generated crime. This requires a fundamental change in public policy: repeal of criminal prohibition and the creation of a reasonable regulatory system.

Ending Prohibition Would Not Necessarily Increase Drug Abuse

While it is impossible to predict exactly how drug use patterns would change under a system of regulated manufacture and distribution, the iron rules of prohibition are that 1) illegal markets are controlled by producers, not consumers, and 2) prohibition fosters the sale and consumption of more potent and dangerous forms of drugs.

During alcohol prohibition in the 1920s, bootleggers marketed small bottles of 100-plus proof liquor because they were easier to conceal than were large, unwieldy kegs of beer. The result: Consumption of beer and wine went down while consumption of hard liquor went up. Similarly, contemporary drug smugglers' preference for powdered cocaine over bulky, pungent coca leaves encourages use of the most potent and dangerous cocaine products. In contrast, under legal conditions, consumers—most of whom do not wish to harm themselves—play a role in determining the potency of marketed products, as indicated by the popularity of today's light beers, wine coolers, and decaffeinated coffees. Once alcohol prohibition was repealed, consumption increased somewhat, but the rate of liver cirrhosis went down because people tended to choose beer and wine over the more potent, distilled spirits previously promoted by bootleggers. So, even though the number of drinkers went up, the health risks of drinking went down. The same dynamic would most likely occur with drug legalization: some increase in drug use, but a decrease in drug abuse.

Another factor to consider is the lure of forbidden fruit. For young people, who are often attracted to taboos, legal drugs might be less tempting than they are now. That has been the experience of The Netherlands: After the Dutch government decriminalized marijuana in 1976, allowing it to be sold and consumed openly in small amounts, usage steadily declined—particularly among teenagers and young adults. Prior to decriminalization, 10 percent of Dutch 17- and 18-year-olds used marijuana. By 1985, that figure had dropped to 6.5 percent.

Would drugs be more available once prohibition is repealed? It is hard to imagine drugs being more available than they are today. Despite efforts to stem their flow, drugs are accessible to anyone who wants them. In a recent government-sponsored survey of high school seniors, 55 percent said it would be "easy" for them to obtain cocaine, and 85 percent said it would be "easy" for them to obtain marijuana. In our inner-cities, access to drugs is especially easy, and the risk of arrest has proven to have a negligible deterrent effect. What would change under decriminalization is not so much drug availability as the conditions under which drugs would be available. Without prohibition, providing help to drug abusers who wanted to kick their habits would be easier because the money now being squandered on law enforcement could be used for preventive social programs and treatment.

What The United States Would Look Like After Repeal

Some people, hearing the words "drug legalization," imagine pushers on street corners passing out cocaine to anyone—even children. But that is what exists today under prohibition. Consider the legal drugs, alcohol and tobacco: Their potency, time and place of sale, and purchasing age limits are set by law. Similarly, warning labels are required on medicinal drugs, and some of these are available by prescription only.

After federal alcohol prohibition was repealed, each state developed its own system for regulating the distribution and sale of alcoholic beverages. The same could occur with currently illegal drugs. For example, states could create different regulations for marijuana, heroin and cocaine.

Remember!!

The American Civil Liberties Union (ACLU) says: Ending prohibition is not a panacea. It will not by itself end drug abuse or eliminate violence. Nor will it bring about the social and economic revitalization of our inner cities. However, ending prohibition would bring one very significant benefit: It would sever the connection between drugs and crime that today blights so many lives and communities. In the long run, ending prohibition could foster the redirection of public resources toward social development, legitimate economic opportunities and effective treatment, thus enhancing the safety, health and well-being of the entire society.

Part 8

Resources For Help And Additional Information

Chapter 54

National Organizations For Drug Information

Federal Agencies

Center for Food Safety and Applied Nutrition

U.S. Food and Drug Administration
5100 Paint Branch Parkway
College Park, MD 20704-3835
Phone: 301-436-1600
Toll Free: 888-723-3366
Web site: http://www.cfsan.fda.gov

Center for Substance Abuse Prevention (CSAP)

Substance Abuse and Mental
Health Services Administration
5600 Fishers Lane
Rockville, MD 20857
Phone: 301-443-0365
Fax: 301-443-5447
Web site: http://www.samhsa.gov/csap

Center for Substance Abuse Treatment (CSAT)

Nicholson Lane Research Center
5516 Nicholson Lane, Suite 615
Kensington, MD 20895
Toll Free: 800-662-HELP
Toll Free: 800-787-8432 (Spanish)
Phone: 301-443-5700
Fax: 301-443-8751
Web site: http://www.samhsa.gov/csat

Centers for Disease Control and Prevention

1600 Clifton Rd.
Atlanta, GA 30333
Toll Free: 800-311-3435
Phone: 404-639-3534 or 639-3311
Web site: http://www.cdc.gov

About This Chapter: Information in this chapter was excerpted from "What You Can Do About Drug Use in America," Office for Substance Abuse Prevention, U.S. Department of Health and Human Services, DHHS Pub. No. ADM 91-1572 and compiled from other sources deemed accurate. All information was updated and verified in May 2002.

Drug Enforcement Administration (DEA)

Information Services Section
2401 Jefferson Davis Highway
Alexandria, VA 22301
Phone: 202-307-1000
Fax: 202-307-8320
Web site: http://www.dea.gov

National Clearinghouse for Alcohol and Drug Information (NCADI)

P.O. Box 2345
Rockville, MD 20847-2345
Toll Free: 800-729-6686
Phone: 301-468-2600
TDD: 800-487-4889
Fax: 301-468-6433
Linea gratis en Español 877-767-8432
Web site: http://www.health.org
E-Mail: info@health.org

National Institute on Alcohol Abuse and Alcoholism

6000 Executive Boulevard
Willco Building
Bethesda, MD 20892-7003
301-443-3860
Web site: http://www.niaaa.nih.gov

National Institute of Drug Abuse (NIDA)

6001 Executive Blvd., Room 5213
Bethesda, MD 20892
Phone: 301-443-1124
Fax: 301-443-9127
Web site: http://www.nida.nih.gov

National Institute of Justice

810 7th Street NW, 7th Floor
Washington, DC 20531
Toll Free: 800-851-3420
Phone: 202-307-2942
Fax: 202-307-6394
Web site: http://www.ojp.usdoj.gov/nij

National Institutes of Health

Bethesda, MD 20892
Toll Free: 800-729-6686
TTY: 888-889-6432
Phone: 301-496-4000
Web site: http://www.nih.gov
E-Mail: NIHInfo@od.nih.gov

Substance Abuse and Mental Health Services Administration (SAMHSA)

5600 Fishers Lane, Parklawn Bldg.
Rockville, MD 20857
Phone: 301-443-8956
Fax: 301-443-9050
Web site: http://www.samhsa.gov
E-Mail: info@samhsa.gov

U.S. Bureau of Alcohol, Tobacco, and Firearms (ATF)

650 Massachusetts Avenue, NW,
Room 8290
Washington, DC 20226
Toll Free: 888-283-2662
Toll Free: 800-ATF-GUNS (To report illegal firearms activity)
Web site: http://www.atf.treas.gov
E-Mail: atfmail@atfhq.atf.treas.gov

U.S. Food and Drug Administration

5600 Fishers Lane
Rockville, MD 20857
Toll Free: 888-463-6332
Web site: http://www.fda.gov

U.S. Indian Health Service

The Reyes Building
801 Thompson Avenue, Suite 400
Rockville, MD 20852-1627
Phone: 301-443-2038
Web site: http://www.ihs.gov

Private Organizations, Civic Groups, and Religious Organizations

Action on Smoking and Health (ASH)

2013 H Street, NW
Washington, DC 20006
Phone: 202-659-4310
Web site: http://www.ash.org

Al-Anon/Alateen Family Groups

1600 Corporate Landing Parkway
Virginia Beach, VA 23454-5617
Toll Free: 888-4AL-ANON
Phone: 757-563-1600
Fax: 757-563-1655
Web site: http://www.al-anon.org
E-Mail: WSO@al-anon.org

Alcoholics Anonymous (AA)

475 Riverside Dr., 11th Floor
New York, NY 10015
Phone: 212-870-3400
Web site: http://www.alcoholics-anonymous.org

American Council for Drug Education

164 W. 74th Street
New York, NY 10023
Toll Free: 800-488-DRUG
Web site: http://www.acde.org

Boys and Girls Clubs of America
1230 West Peachtree Street, NW
Atlanta, GA 30309
Toll Free: 800-854-CLUB
Phone: 404-815-5700
Fax: 404-487-5757
Web site: http://www.bgca.org

CoAnon Family Groups
P.O. Box 12722
Tucson, AZ 85732-2722
Phone: 520-513-5028
Web site: http://www.co-anon.org

Connecticut Clearinghouse
334 Farmington Ave.
Plainville, CT 06062
Toll Free: 800-232-4424
Phone: 860-793-9791
Fax: 860-793-9813
Web site: http://
www.ctclearinghouse.org
E-mail: info@ctclearinghouse.org

Do It Now Foundation
P.O. Box 27568
Tempe, AZ 85285-7568
Phone: 480-736-0599
Fax: 480-736-0771
Web site: http://www.doitnow.org
Feedback@doitnow.org

Families Anonymous, Inc.
P.O. Box 3475
Culver City, CA 90231-3475
Phone: 800-736-9805
Fax: 310-815-9682
Web site: http://www.families
anonymous.org
E-Mail:
famanon@familiesanonymous.org

Focus Adolescent Services
1113 Woodland Road
Salisbury, MD 21801
Toll Free: 877-362-8727
Phone: 410-341-4342
Web site: http://www.focusas.com
E-Mail: help@focusas.com

Hazelden Foundation
P.O. Box 11, CO3
Center City, MN 55012-0011
Toll Free: 800-257-7810
Toll Free: 800-I-DO-CARE
Phone: 651-213-4000
Web site: http://www.hazelden.org
E-Mail: info@hazelden.org

Indiana Prevention Resource Center

Creative Arts Building
2735 E. 10th St., Rm. 110
Bloomington, IN 47408-2606
Toll Free: 800-346-3077 (Indiana only)
Phone: 812-855-1237
Fax: 812-855-4940
Web site: http://www.drugs.indiana.edu
E-Mail: drugprc@Indiana.edu

Institute on Black Chemical Abuse

African American Family Services
2616 Nicollet Avenue
Minneapolis, MN 55408
Phone: 612-871-7878
Fax: 612-871-2567
Web site: http://www.aafs.net
E-Mail: contact@aafs.net

International Institute for Inhalant Abuse

450 West Jefferson Avenue
Englewood, CO 80110-3536
Phone: 303-788-3272
Fax: 303-788-1860

Kickbutt Learning Center

Washington DOC AOC, ANB-1
12401 East Marginal Way South
Tukwila, WA 98168
Phone: 206-988-7832
Web site: http://www.kickbutt.org
E-mail: office@kickbutt.org

Minnesota Drug Information Service

Bio-Medical Library
Diehl Hall
University of Minnesota
Minneapolis, MN 55455-0334
Phone: 612-624-6492
Fax: 612-626-2454
Web site: http://biomed.lib.umn.edu/dis/dismain.html
E-Mail: drugref@tc.umn.edu

Mothers Against Drunk Driving (MADD)

511 E. John Carpenter Fwy., Suite 700
Irving, TX 75062
Toll Free: 800-438-6233
Phone: 214-744-6233
Web site: http://www.madd.org

Nar-Anon Family Groups

P.O. Box 2562
Palos Verdes Peninsula, CA 90274
Phone: 310-547-5800
Web site: http://ww.onlinerecovery.org/co/nfg

The National Alliance for Hispanic Health

1501 16th Street, N.W.
Washington, DC 20036
Phone: 202-387-5000
Fax: 202-797-4353
Web site: http://www.hispanichealth.org

National Asian Pacific American Families Against Drug Abuse

340 East Second Street, Suite 409
Los Angeles, CA 90012
Phone: 213-625-5795
Fax: 213-625-5796
Web site: http://www.napafasa.org
E-Mail: napafasa@apanet.org

National Association of State Alcohol and Drug Abuse Directors (NASADAD)

808 17th Street, NW, Suite 410
Washington, DC 20006
Phone: 202-293-0090
Fax: 202-293-1250
Web site: http://www.nasadad.org
E-Mail: dcoffice@nasadad.org

National Black Alcoholism and Addictions Council (NBAC)

1101 14th Street N.W., Suite 630
Washington, DC 20005
Phone: 202-296-2696
Web site: http://www.borg.com/~nbac
E-Mail: nbac@borg.com

The National Center on Addiction and Substance Abuse at Columbia University (CASA)

633 Third Avenue, 19th Floor
New York, NY 10017-6706
Phone: 212-841-5200
Fax: 212-956-8020
Web site: http://www.casacolumbia.org

National Council on Alcoholism and Drug Dependence, Inc.

20 Exchange Place, Suite 2902
New York, NY 10005
Toll Free: 800-622-2255
Phone: 212-269-7797
Fax: 212-269-7510
Web site: http://www.ncadd.org
E-Mail: national@ncadd.org

National Families in Action

2957 Clairmont Road, Suite 150
Atlanta, GA 30329
Phone: 404-248-9676
Fax: 404-248-1312
Web site: http://www.emory.edu/NFIA
E-Mail: nfia@nationalfamilies.org

National Family Partnership

2490 Coral Way, Suite 501
Miami, Fl 33145
Toll Free: 800-705-8997
Phone: 305-856-4886
Fax: 306-856-4815
Web site: http://www.nfp.org

National Inhalant Prevention Coalition

2904 Kerbey Lane
Austin, TX 78703
Toll Free: 800-269-4237
Phone: 512-480-8953
Fax: 512-477-3932
Web site: http://www.inhalants.org
E-Mail: nipc@io.com

National Latino Council on Alcohol and Tobacco Prevention

1875 Connecticut Avenue NW,
Suite 732
Washington, DC 20009
Phone: 202-265-8054
Fax: 202-265-8056
Web site: http://www.nlcatp.org
E-Mail: lcat@nlcatp.org

National Parents Resource Institute for Drug Education (PRIDE)

PRIDE Youth Program
4684 South Evergreen
Newaygo, MI 49337
Toll Free: 800-668-9277
Phone: 231-652-4400
Web site: http://www.prideusa.org

National Prevention Network

NASADAD
808 17th Street NW, Suite 410
Washington, DC 20006
Phone: 202-293-0090
Fax: 202-293-1250
Web site: http://www.nasadad.org
E-Mail: dcoffice@nasadad.org

Online Drug Policy Library

Web site: http://
www.druglibrary.org

Partnership for a Drug-Free America

405 Lexington Avenue
Suite 1601
New York, NY 10174
Phone: 212-922-1560
Fax: 212-922-1570
Web site: http://
www.drugfreeamerica.org

Phoenix House

164 W. 74th Street
New York, NY 10023
Toll Free: 800-DRUG HELP
Phone: 212-595-5810
Fax: 212-496-6035
Web site: http://
www.phoenixhouse.org

Project Cork Institute

Office of Alcohol and Drug Abuse Programs
Department of Health
108 Cherry Street
Box 70
Burlington, VT, 05402
Phone: 802-651-1573
Web site: http://www.state.vt.us/
adap/Cork/cork1.htm
E-Mail: cork@vdh.state.vt.us

Red Ribbon Works

617 East McBee Avenue
P.O. Box 10203
Greenville, SC 29603
Toll Free: 800-732-4099
Phone: 864-467-4099
Fax: 864-467-4102
Web site: http://
www.redribbonworks.org

Students Against Destructive Decisions (SADD)

SADD National
Box 800
Marlboro, MA 10752
Toll Free: 877-SADD-INC
Fax: 508-481-5759
Web site: http://
www.saddonline.com

Youth Media Network

17872 Moro Road
Prunedale, CA 93907
Toll Free: 800-733-8377
Phone: 831-663-9208
Fax: 831-663-1328
Web site: http://www.ymn.org
E-mail: ymedia@ix.netcom.com

Resources for Children of Alcoholics and Other Drug Users

Children of Alcoholics Foundation

164 West 74th Street
New York, NY 10023
Phone: 646-505-2065
Fax: 212-595-2553
Web site: http://www.coaf.org
E-Mail: coaf@phonenixhouse.org

National Association for Children of Alcoholics

11426 Rockville Pike, #100
Rockville, MD 20852
Toll Free: 888-554-2627
Phone: 301-468-0985
Fax: 301-468-0987
Web site: http://www.nacoa.net
E-mail: nacoa@nacoa.org

Chapter 55

Where Can I Go For Help?

Sometimes the quickest way to find out what help is available in your local area is to join a group such as Alcoholics Anonymous or Al-Anon. People in these groups often know where help is available in the community. Other sources of help and information are listed below.

Hotlines and Helplines

Alcohol Hotline

1-800-ALCOHOL
7 days a week, 24 hours a day

Al-Anon/Alateen

1-800-344-2666
Mon.–Fri.; 8:00 a.m.–6:00 p.m. EST

Boys Town National Hotline

1-800-448-3000

Marijuana Anonymous

1-800-766-6779
7 days a week, 24 hours a day

National Clearinghouse for Alcohol and Drug Information

1-800-729-6686
Mon.–Fri.; 9:00 a.m.–7:00 p.m. EST

National Council on Alcoholism and Drug Dependence

1-800-622-2255
7 days a week, 24 hours a day

National Drug and Alcohol Treatment Referral Service

1-800-662-HELP
Mon.– Fri.; 9:00 a.m.–3:00 a.m.

About This Chapter: Information in this chapter was excerpted from "What You Can Do About Drug Use in America," Office for Substance Abuse Prevention, U.S. Department of Health and Human Services, DHHS Pub. No. ADM 91-1572 and compiled from other sources deemed accurate. All information was updated and verified in May 2002.

National Hopeline Network
1-800-SUICIDE
7 days a week, 24 hours a day

National Mental Health Association Help Line
1-800-950-6264
Mon.–Fri.; 10:00 a.m.–5:00 p.m. EST

National Runaway Hotline
1-800-231-6946
7 days a week, 24 hours a day

Steroids Hotline
1-800-STEROIDS

Victims of Crime Help Line
1-800-FYI-CALL
Mon.—Fri.: 8:30 a.m.–8:30 p.m. EST

Finding Treatment Resources And Support Groups

For information on where to find treatment for alcohol and other drug problems, the best place to look is in the telephone book's Yellow Pages under "Alcoholism Information" or "Drug Abuse and Addiction Information." Usually there is a listing of the nearest Council on Alcoholism (or Council on Alcohol and Drug Abuse). These Councils provide information over the phone on the availability of the nearest alcohol treatment programs. Alcoholics Anonymous (AA) or Narcotics Anonymous (NA) may also be listed. Both offer immeasurable help in enabling people to cope with problems with alcohol and other drugs.

Alcoholics Anonymous (AA)
475 Riverside Drive
New York, NY 10015
Phone: 212-870-3400
Fax: 212-870-3003
Web site: http://www.alcoholics-anonymous.org

Alcoholics Victorious
1045 Swift Street
Kansas City, MO 64116-4127
Phone: 816-471-8020
24-Hour Hotline: 503-245-9629
Fax: 816-471-3718
Web site: http://av.iugm.org

American Council for Drug Education
164 W. 74th Street
New York, NY 10023
Toll Free: 800-488-DRUG
Web site: http://www.acde.org
E-Mail: acde@phoenixhouse.org

Chemically Dependent Anonymous
CDA Communications, Inc.
P.O. Box 423
Severna Park, MD 21146-0423
Toll Free: 888-CDA-HOPE
Web site: http://www.cdaweb.org

Christian Recovery International
P.O. Box 215
Brea, CA 92822
Phone: 714-529-6227
Fax: 714-529-1120
Web site: http://www.christianrecovery.com

Co-Anon Family Groups World Services
P.O. Box 12722
Tucson, AZ 85732-2722
Phone: 520-513-5028
Web site: http://www.co-anon.org

Cocaine Anonymous (CA)
3740 Overland Avenue, Suite C
Los Angeles, CA 90034
Phone: 310-559-5833
Toll Free: 800-347-8998
Web site: http://www.ca.org
E-Mail: cawso@ca.org

Crystal Meth Anonymous
8205 Santa Monica Blvd.
PMB 1-114
West Hollywood, CA 90046-5977
Phone: 213-488-4455 (24 hour information line)
Web site: http://www.crystalmeth.org
E-Mail: generalservice@crystalmeth.org

Dual Recovery Anonymous
World Service Central Office
P.O. Box 218232
Nashville, TN 37221-8232
Toll Free: 877-883-2332
Web site: http://draonline.org

JACS (Jewish Alcoholics, Chemically Dependent Persons, and Significant Others)
850 Seventh Avenue
New York, NY 10019
Phone: 212-397-4197
Fax: 212-399-3525
Web site: http://www.jacsweb.org
E-mail: jacs@jacsweb.org

Marijuana Anonymous World Services
P.O. Box 2912
Van Nuys, CA 91404
Toll Free: 800-766-6779
Web site: http://www.marijuana-anonymous.org
E-mail: office@marijuana-anonymous.org

Narcotics Anonymous (NA)
P.O. Box 9999
Van Nuys, CA 91409
Phone: 818-733-9999
Fax: 818-700-0700
Web site: http://www.na.org

National Association of State Alcohol and Drug Abuse Directors (NASADAD)
808 17th Street NW, Suite 410
Washington, DC 20006
Phone: 202-293-0090
Fax: 202-293-1250
Web site: http://www.nasadad.org
E-Mail: dcoffice@nasadad.org

National Council on Alcoholism and Drug Dependence, Inc.
20 Exchange Place, Suite 2902
New York, NY 10005
Phone: 212-269-7797
Toll Free: 800-NCA-CALL
Fax: 212-269-7510
Web site: http://www.ncadd.org
E-Mail: national@ncadd.org

Nicotine Anonymous World Services
419 Main Street, PMB #370
Huntington Beach, CA 92648
Phone: 415-750-0328
Web site: http://nicotine-anonymous.org
E-mail: info@nicotine-anonymous.org

Overcomers Outreach
P.O. Box 2208
Oakhurst, CA 96344
Toll Free: 800-310-3001
Web site: http://www.overcomersoutreach.org
E-mail: info@overcomersoutreach.org

Prescription Anonymous
P.O. Box 1297
Powder Springs, GA 30127-1287
Phone: 770-428-1220
Web site: http://www.prescription anyonymous.org

SMART Recovery
7537 Mentor Avenue, Suite #306
Mentor, OH 44060
Phone: 440-951-5357
Fax: 440-951-5358
Web site: http://www.smartrecovery.org
E-mail: SRMail1@aol.com

Women for Sobriety
P.O. Box 618
Quakertown, PA 18951-0618
Phone: 215-536-8026
Fax: 215-538-9026
Web site: http://wwwwomenforsobriety.org
E-Mail: newlife@nni.com

Chapter 56

State-By-State List Of Alcohol And Drug Referral Phone Numbers

National Information

National Association of State Alcohol and Drug Abuse Directors

808 17th Street NW, Suite 410
Washington, DC 20006
Phone: 202-293-0090; Fax: 202-293-1250
Website: http://www.nasadad.org
E-Mail: dcoffice@nasadad.org

States

Alabama

Div. of Mental Health, Illness, and Substance Abuse Community Programs
Department of Mental Health
100 N. Union Street
Montgomery, AL 36130
Phone: 334-242-3174
Website: http://www.mh.state.al.us

Alaska

Office of Alcoholism and Drug Abuse
Dept. of Health and Social Services
249 Main Street
P.O. Box 110608
Juneau, AK 99811-0608
Toll Free: 888-464-8920
Phone: 907-465-8920
Fax: 907-465-4410
Website: http://www.abda.com

About This Chapter: Information in this chapter was excerpted from "What You Can Do About Drug Use in America," Office for Substance Abuse Prevention, U.S. Department of Health and Human Services, DHHS Pub. No. ADM 91-1572. All information was updated and verified in May 2002.

Arizona

Alcoholism and Drug Abuse
Office of Community Behavior Health
Department of Health Services
2122 East Highland Avenue
Phoenix, AZ 85016
Phone: 602-381-8999
Fax: 602-553-9140
Website: http://www.hs.state.az.us

Arkansas

Office on Alcohol and Drug Abuse Prevention
Donaghey Plaza, North
Suite 400
P.O. Box 1437
Little Rock, AR 72203-1437
Phone: 501-280-4500
Fax: 510-280-4519
Website: http://www.healthyarkansas.com

California

Department of Alcohol and Drug Programs
1700 K Street
Sacramento, CA 95814
Toll Free: 800-879-2772
Phone: 916-445-0834
Website: http://www.dhs.cahwnet.gov/ps/index.htm

Colorado

Alcohol and Drug Abuse Division
Department of Health
4055 S. Lowell Blvd.
Denver, CO 80236
Phone: 303-866-7480
Fax: 303-866-7481
Website: http://www.cdhs.state.co.us/ohr/adad/index.html

Connecticut

Department of Mental Health and Addiction Services
410 Capitol Avenue
P.O. Box 341431
Hartford, CT 06134
Toll Free: 800-446-7348
Phone: 860-418-7000
TDD: 860-418-6707 or 888-621-3551
Website: http://ww.dmhas.state.ct.us

Delaware

Delaware Division of Substance Abuse and Mental Health
1901 North DuPont Highway
Newcastle, DE 19720
Toll Free Helpline: 800-464-HELP
Phone: 302-577-4460
Fax: 302-577-4000
Website: http://www.state.de.us/dhss/dsamh/about.htm
E-Mail: dhssinfo@state.de.us

District of Columbia

Addiction Prevention and Recovery Administration
1300 First Street, NE
Washington, DC 20002
Phone: 202-727-9393 or 202-727-0672
Fax: 202-727-0092
Website: http://dchealth.dc.gov

Florida

Alcohol and Drug Abuse Program
Department of Health and Rehabilitative Services
2639 North Monroe Street
Suite A-118
Tallahassee, FL 32303
Phone: 850-488-2419
Fax: 850-487-9469
Website: http://www.doh.state.fl.us

Georgia

Alcohol and Drug Services
878 Peachtree Street, NE
Suite 319
Atlanta, GA 30309
Toll Free Helpline: 800-338-6745
Phone: 404-657-2272
Website: http://www.legis.state.ga.us/departments/dhr/mhmrsa.html

Hawaii

Alcohol and Drug Abuse Division
Department of Health
601 Kamokila Blvd.
Kapolei, HI 96707
Phone: 808-692-7506
Website: http://tako.icsd.hawaii.gov/doh/resource/drug_abuse.html

Idaho

Department of Health and Welfare
Family and Children's Services
Drug and Alcohol Abuse Division
450 West State Street, 5th Floor
Boise, ID 83720
Toll Free Idaho CareLine: 800-926-2588
Phone: 208-334-5700
TDD: 208-332-7205
Fax: 208-334-6558
Website: http://www2.state.id.us/dhw/mentalhealth/index.htm

Illinois

Department of Alcoholism and Substance Abuse
100 West Randolph St., Suite 5-600
Chicago, IL 60601
Toll Free: 800-444-9999 (Alcohol)
Toll Free: 800-272-2544 (Other Drugs)
Phone: 312-814-1737
Fax 312-814-2419
Website: http://www.state.il.us/agency/dhs/indexasanp.html

Indiana

Division of Addiction Services
Department of Mental Health
Indiana Government Center
3rd Floor South, Room W353
Indianapolis, IN 46204
Phone: 317-232-7800
Fax: 317-233-3472
Website: http://www.in.gov/fssa/serviceaddict

Iowa

Department of Public Health
Division of Substance Abuse and Health Promotion
Lucas State Office Building
321 East 12th Street, 3rd Floor
Des Moines, IA 50319-0075
Phone: 515-281-4404

Kansas

Alcohol and Drug Abuse Prevention, Treatment, and Recovery
Docking State Office Building
915 SW Harrison, 10th Floor
Topeka, KS 66612-1570
Phone: 785-296-6807
Fax: 785-296-7275

Kentucky

Division of Substance Abuse
Department for Mental Health and Mental Retardation Services
100 Farrow, 4th Floor
Frankfort, KY 40601
Phone: 502-564-2880
Fax: 502-564-7152
Website: http://dmhmrs.chr.state.ky.us/preventatodky

Louisiana

Office of Human Services
Office for Addictive Disorders
1201 Capitol Access Road
P.O. Box 2790, Bin 18
Baton Rouge, LA 70821-2790
Phone: 225-342-6717
Fax: 225-342-3875
Website: http://www.dhh.state.la.us/oada/prevention_services.htm

Maine

Office of Substance Abuse
A.M.H.I. Complex, Marquardt Bldg.
#159 State House Station
Augusta, ME 04333-0159
Toll Free: 800-499-0027 (Maine only)
Phone: 207-287-2595
TTY: 207-287-4475
Fax: 207-287-4334
Website: http://www.state.me.us/bds/osa/homepage.htm

Maryland

Maryland State Alcohol and Drug Abuse Administration
55 Wade Avenue
Cantonsville, MD 21228
Phone: 410-402-8600
Fax: 410-402-8601
TTY: 410-528-2258
Website: http://www.dhmh.state.md.us/adda
E-Mail: addainfo@dhmh.state.md.us

Massachusetts

Division of Substance Abuse Services
250 Washington Street, 3rd Floor
Boston, MA 02108
Toll Free: 800-327-5050 (Massachusetts only)
Phone: 617-624-5300
Fax: 617-624-5399
Website: http://www.state.ma.us/dph/dphhome.htm

Michigan

Office of Substance Abuse Services
Department of Public Health
2150 Apollo Drive
P.O. Box 30206
Lansing, MI 48909
Phone: 517-335-8831

Minnesota

Chemical Dependency Program Division
Department of Human Services
444 Lafayette Road
St. Paul, MN 55155-3823
Phone: 651-582-1900
Fax: 651-582-1865

Mississippi

Division of Alcohol and Drug Abuse
Department of Mental Health
Robert E. Lee State Office Bldg.
9th Floor
239 North Lamar Street
Jackson, MS 39201
Phone: 601-359-6220
Fax: 601-576-4040

Missouri

Division of Alcohol and Drug Abuse
Department of Mental Health
1706 East Elm Street
P.O. Box 687
Jefferson City, MO 65102
Phone: 573-751-4942
Fax: 573-751-7814
Website: http://www.modmh.state.mo.us/ada
E-Mail: dmhmail@mail.dmh.state.mo.us

Montana

Addictive and Mental Disorders Division
Department of Institutions
555 Fuller
Helena, MT 59620
Phone: 406-444-3964
Fax: 406-444-4435
Website: http://www.dphhs.state.mt.us/divisions/amd/amd.htm

Nebraska

Division of Alcoholism and Drug Abuse
Department of Public Institution
P.O. Box 94728
Lincoln, NE 68509
Phone: 402-479-5583
Fax: 402-479-5162
Website: http://www.hhs.state.ne.us/beh/mhsa.htm

Nevada

Alcohol & Drug Abuse Bureau
Department of Human Resources
505 East King Street, Room 500
Carson City, NV 89710
Phone: 775-684-4190 or 702-486-8250 (Las Vegas)
Fax: 775-684-4185
Website: http://health2k.state.nv.us/bada

New Hampshire

Office of Alcohol and Drug Abuse Prevention
State Office Park South
105 Pleasant Street
Concord, NH 03301
Toll Free: 800-804-0909
Phone: 603-271-6100
Fax: 603-271-6116
Website: http://www.dhhs.state.nh.us

New Jersey

Department of Health
Addiction Services
120 South Sockton Street
PO Box 362
Trenton, NJ 08625-0362
Toll Free: 800-322-5525 (New Jersey only)
Phone: 609-292-7232
Website: http://www.state.nj.us/health/as/abuse.htm

New Mexico

Behavioral Health Services Division
1190 St. Francis Drive
Room 3300 North
P.O. Box 26110
Santa Fe, NM 87502
Toll Free: 800-962-8936 (outside Albuquerque)
Phone: 505-827-2658
Fax: 505-827-0097

New York

Division of Alcoholism and Substance Abuse Services
1450 Western Avenue
Albany, NY 12203
Phone: 518-485-2156
Fax: 518-485-2142
Website: http://oasas.state.ny.us/pio/prevent.htm

North Carolina

Alcohol and Drug Abuse Section
Division of Mental Health and Mental Retardation Services
325 North Salisbury Street
Raleigh, NC 27699
Phone: 919-733-4670
Fax: 919-733-9455
Website: http://www.dhhs.state.nc.us/mhddsas/sas

North Dakota

Division of Alcoholism and Drug Abuse
600 South 2nd Street, Suite 1E
Bismark, ND 58504
Phone: 701-328-8920
Fax: 701-328-8969
E-Mail: dhsmed@state.nd.us

Ohio

Bureau on Alcohol Abuse and Recovery
Ohio Department of Health
Two Nationwide Plaza
280 North High Street, 12th Floor
Columbus, OH 43215
Phone: 614-466-3445
Fax: 614-752-8645
Website: http://www.drc.state.oh.us/web/recovery.htm

Oklahoma

Oklahoma Dept. of Mental Health and Substance Abuse Services
1200 NE 13th Street
P.O. Box 53277
Capitol Station
Oklahoma City, OK 73152-3277
Toll Free: 800-522-9054 (Oklahoma only)
Phone: 405-522-3908
Fax: 405-522-3650
Website: http://www.odmhsas.org

Oregon

Office of Mental Health and Addiction
500 Summer St., NE, E86
Salem, OR 97301-1118
Phone: 503-945-5763
Fax: 503-378-8467
TDD: 503-945-5893
Website: http://www.oadap.hr.state.or.us

Pennsylvania

Drug and Alcohol Programs
Department of Health
P.O. Box 90
Harrisburg, PA 17108
Toll Free: 800-582-7746
Phone: 717-787-2712
Fax: 717-787-6285

Rhode Island

Council on Alcoholism
Department of Mental Health, Retardation and Hospitals
500 Prospect St.
Pawtucket, RI 02860
Toll Free: 866-252-3784
Phone: 401-725-0410
Fax: 401-725-0768
Website: http://www.mhrh.state.ri.us

South Carolina

South Carolina Commission on Alcohol and Drug Abuse
101 Business Park Boulevard
Columbia, SC 29203-9498
Phone: 803-896-5555
Fax: 803-896-5557
Website: http://www.daodas.state.sc.us/web

South Dakota

Division of Alcohol and Drug Abuse
E. Hwy. 34, Hillsview Plaza
c/o 500 E. Capital Avenue
Pierre, SD 57501
Phone: 605-773-3123
Fax: 605-773-7076
Website: http://www.state.sd.us/dhs/ADA

Tennessee

Alcohol and Drug Abuse Services
Department of Mental Health and Mental Retardation
Cordell Hull Building, 3rd Floor
425 5th Avenue North
Nashville, TN 37247-4401
Phone: 615-741-1921
Fax: 615-532-2419
Website: http://www.state.tn.us/health/A&D

Texas

Texas Commission on Alcohol and Drug Abuse
9001 N. IH 35, Suite 105
P.O. Box 80529
Austin, TX 78708
Toll Free: 800-832-9623
Fax: 512-821-4419
Website: http://www.tcada.state.tx.us

Utah

Division of Substance Abuse
Department of Social Services
120 North 200 West, 2nd Floor
P.O. Box 45500
Salt Lake City, UT 84103
Toll Free Hotline: 888-633-4673
Phone: 801-538-3939
Website: http://
www.hsdsa.utah.gov

Vermont

Office of Alcohol and Drug Abuse
Programs
108 Cherry Street
Burlington, VT 05401
Phone: 802-651-1550
Fax: 802-651-1573
Website: http://www.state.vt.us/adap

Virginia

Office of Substance Abuse Services
Dept. of Mental Health, Mental
Retardation and Substance Abuse
Ninth Street Office Building
202 North Ninth Street
Sixth Floor
Richmond, VA 23219
Toll Free: 800-451-5544 (Virginia
only)
Phone: 804-786-9072
Fax: 804-786-1807
Website: http://
www.gosap.state.va.us
E-Mail: gosap@gov.state.va.us

Washington

Bureau of Alcoholism and
Substance Abuse
P.O. Box 45330
Olympia, WA 98504-5330
Toll Free: 877-301-4557
Phone: 360-438-8200
Fax: 360-438-8057

West Virginia

Office of Behavioral Health Services
350 Capitol Street
Room 350
Charleston, WV 25301-3702
Phone: 304-558-0627
Fax: 304-558-1008
Website: http://www.wvdhhr.org/
obhs/preventing.htm

Wisconsin

Office of Alcohol and Other
Drug Abuse
1 West Wilson Street
Room 434
P.O. Box 7851
Madison, WI 53707
Phone: 608-266-2717
Fax: 608-266-1533

Wyoming

Alcohol and Drug Abuse Programs
2424 Pioneer Avenue, Suite 306
Cheyenne, WY 82002
Toll Free: 800-535-4006
Phone: 307-777-6840
Fax: 307-777-7006
Website: http://substanceabuse.state.wy.us/index.html
E-Mail: info@state.wy.us

Territories

Guam

Department of Mental Health and Substance Abuse
790 Gov. Carlos G. Camacho Way
Tamuning, GU 96911
Phone: 671-647-5445
Fax: 671-649-6948

Puerto Rico

Departmento de Servicios Contra la Adiccion
Box 70184
San Juan, Puerto Rico 00936
Phone: 787-274-5634
Fax: 787-274-5523

Virgin Islands

Division of Mental Health Alcoholism and Drug Dependency Services
P.O. Box 520
St. Croix, VI 00820
Phone: 340-773-2323

American Samoa

Social Services Division
Alcohol and Drug Program
Government of America Samoa
Pago Pago 96799
Phone: 684-633-5139

Chapter 57

Additional Reading

Books

Bichler, Christine. *Teen Drinking*. New York: Rosen Publishing Group, Incorporated, 1999. ISBN: 0823928306.

Gorski, Terence T. *Adolescent Relapse Prevention Workbook : A Brief Strategic Approach*. Independence: Herald Publishing Company, August 1996. ISBN: 0830907696.

Leite, Evelyn and Pamela Espeland. *Different like Me: A Book for Teens Who Worry about Their Parent's Use of Alcohol/Drugs*. Center City, MN: Hazelden Information & Educational Services, March 1989. ISBN: 093590834X.

Masline, Shelagh Ryan. *Drug Abuse and Teens*, Berkley Heights: Enslow Publishers, Inc., October 2000. ISBN: 0766013723.

Mass, Wendy. *Teen Drug Abuse (Lucent Overview Series)*. Farmington Hills, MI: Lucent Books, January 1998. ISBN: 1560061960.

Miller, Michelle A., Michael L. Hecht, Jess Alberts, Melanie Trost, and Robert Krizek. *Adolescent Relationships and Drug Use*. Mahwah, NJ: Lawrence Erlbaum Associates, Inc., May 2000. ISBN: 0805834362.

About This Chapter: There is a vast amount of material about alcohol and drug use. The resources listed in this chapter are intended to serve as a starting point for further research. They represent a sampling of available material; this list is not complete. Inclusion does not constitute endorsement.

Mitchell, Hayley R. *Teen Alcoholism*. Farmington Hills, MI: Gale Group, January 1997. ISBN: 1560065141

Moe, Barbara A. *Drug Abuse Relapse: Helping Teens to Get Clean Again*. New York: Rosen Publishing Group, Inc., 2000. ISBN: 0823931579.

Stewart, Gail Stewart and Carl Franzen (Illustrator). *Teen Addicts*. Farmington Hills, MI: Lucent Books, January 2000. ISBN: 1560065745

Winters, Paul A. (Ed.) *Teen Addiction (Current Controversies Series)*. Farmington Hills, MI: Greenhaven Press, March 1997. ISBN: 1565105354.

Magazine/Journal Articles

Brener, N.D., S.S. Hassan, and L.C. Barrios. "Suicidal Ideation among College Students in the United States," *Journal of Consulting and Clinical Psychology*, vol. 67, no. 6, 1999, p. 1004(5).

Califano, Joseph A., "It's All in the Family," *America*, January 15, 2000, p. 6(3).

Centers for Disease Control and Prevention, "Cigarette Smoking among High School Students—11 States, 1991-1997," *Morbidity and Mortality Weekly Report*, August 13, 1999, p. 686(8).

Centers for Disease Control and Prevention, "Effectiveness of School-Based Programs as a Component of a Statewide Tobacco Control Initiative—Oregon, 1999-2000," *Morbidity and Mortality Weekly Report*, August 10, 2001, p. 663(4).

Centers for Disease Control and Prevention, "Guidelines for School Health Programs to Prevent Tobacco Use and Addiction," *Morbidity and Mortality Weekly Report*, February 25, 1994, p. 1(18).

Centers for Disease Control and Prevention, "Tobacco Use among High School Students—United States, 1997," *Morbidity and Mortality Weekly Report*, April 3, 1998, p. 229(4).

Centers for Disease Control and Prevention, "Trends in Cigarette Smoking among High School Students—United States, 1991-1999," *Morbidity and Mortality Weekly Report*, August 25, 2000, p. 755(4).

Centers for Disease Control and Prevention, "Youth Tobacco Surveillance—United States, 2000," *Morbidity and Mortality Weekly Report*, November 2, 2001, p. 1(84).

Crossett L.S., C. Husten, A. Malarcher, J. Moskowitz, and J. Ockene (eds.), "Tobacco Cessation and Youth," *Preventive Medicine*, supplemental issue, 1998, p. 27(5).

Crossett L.S., S.A. Everett, N.D. Brener, J.A. Fishman, and T.F. Pechacek. "Measuring Adherence to the CDC Guidelines for School Health Programs to Prevent Tobacco Use and Addiction," *Journal of Health Education*, vol. 30, no. 5, p. S4(8).

Etheridge, Rose M., et al. "Drug Abuse Treatment and Comprehensive Services for Adolescents," *Sage Family Studies Abstracts*, vol. 24, no. 2, 2002, pp. 143(134).

Etheridge, Rose M., Jeff C. Smith, Jennifer L. Rounds-Bryant, and Robert L. Hubbard, "Drug Abuse Treatment and Comprehensive Services for Adolescents, *Journal of Adolescent Research*, vol. 16, no. 6, 2001, p. 563(27).

Everett S.A., A.M. Malarcher, D.J. Sharp, C.G. Husten, and G.A. Giovino, "Relationship between Cigarette, Smokeless Tobacco, and Cigar Use, and Other Health Risk Behaviors among U.S. High School Students," *Journal of School Health*, vol. 70, no. 6, 2000, p. 234(7).

Everett S.A., C.W. Warren, D. Sharp, L. Kann, C.G. Husten, and L.S. Crossett L.S., "Initiation of Cigarette Smoking and Subsequent Smoking Behavior among U.S. High School Students," *Preventive Medicine*, vol. 29, no. 5, 1999 p. 327(7).

Everett, S.A., G.A. Giovino, C.W. Warren, L. Crossett, and L. Kann, "Other Substance Use among High School Students Who Use Tobacco," *Journal of Adolescent Health*, vol. 23, 1998, p. 289(8).

Everett, S.A., R. Lowry, L.R. Cohen, and A.M. Dellinger, "Unsafe Motor Vehicle Practices among Substance-Using College Students," *Accident Analysis and Prevention*, vol. 31, 1999 p. 667(7).

Jeynes, William H. "The Relationship between the Consumption of Various Drugs by Adolescents and Their Academic Achievement," *American Journal of Drug and Alcohol Abuse*, vol. 28, no. 1, 2002, p. 15.

Lowry R., L.R. Cohen, W. Modzeleski, L. Kann, J.L. Collins, and L.J. Kolbe, "School Violence, Substance Use, and Availability of Illegal Drugs on School Property among U.S. High School Students," *Journal of School Health*, vol. 69, no. 9, 1999 p. 347(9).

Marsa, Linda, "Special Report: Teens and Party Drugs: The Dangerous Search for a Good Time," *Family Circle*, June 1999, p. 90(3).

Meadows, Michelle, "Prescription Drug Use and Abuse," *FDA Consumer*, September/October 2001), p.18(6).

Modzeleski W., M.L. Small, and L.K. Kann, "Alcohol and Other Drug Prevention Policies and Education in the United States," *Journal of Health Education*, vol. 30, no. 5, 1999, p. S42(8).

Nordenberg, Tamar, "The Death of the Party: All the Rave, GHB's Hazards Go Unheeded," *FDA Consumer*, March/April 2000, p.14(5).

"Substance Abuse: The Moment of Truth," *Scholastic Choices*, January 1, 1999, p. 20.

Vilbig, Peter, New Highs, New Risks," *New York Times*, Upfront, May 8 2000, p. 10(6).

Web Page Documents

Alcohol Alert (series)

National Institute on Alcohol Abuse and Alcoholism
http://www.niaaa.nih.gov/publications/alalerts.htm

Alcohol and Teen Drinking

Focus Adolescent Services
http://www.focusas.com/Alcohol.html

Alcohol Research and Health

National Institute on Alcohol Abuse and Alcoholism
http://www.niaaa.nih.gov/publications/aharw.htm

Alcohol Use among Girls
Substance Abuse and Mental Health Services Administration
http://www.health.org/govpubs/rpo993/

Alcoholism Shows Its Youthful Side, by B. Bower
Science News Online
http://www.sciencenews.org/sn_arc98/1_24_98/fob1.htm

Alive and Free (newsletter)
Hazelden Foundation
http://www.hazelden.org/newsletter_detail.dbm?id=460

Articles and Directories (links)
NI-COR (Network International—Coalition for On-line Resources)
http://www.ni-cor.com

Assessing Health Risk: Behaviors among Young People
National Center for Chronic Disease Prevention and Health Promotion
http://www.cdc.gov/nccdphp/dash/yrbs/yrbsaag.htm

Does My Parent Really Have an Alcohol or Drug Problem?
Children of Alcoholics Foundation
http://www.coaf.org/Coas/kdparadd.htm

Drug Use and Alcohol Dependence
American Psychological Association
http://www.apa.org/divisions/div12/rev_est/drugs.shtml

Inhalant Abuse: It's Deadly
Focus Adolescent Services
http://www.focusas.com/Inhalants.html

Keep Kids Alcohol Free: Strategies for Action
Leadership to Keep Children Alcohol Free
http://www.alcoholfreechildren.org/gs/pubs/html/Prev.htm

Mind Over Matter
National Institute on Drug Abuse
http://www.drugabuse.gov/MOM/MOMIndex.html

Monitoring the Future: Overview of Key Findings
The University of Michigan Institute for Social Research and National Institute on Drug Abuse
http://www.monitoringthefuture.org/pubs/monographs/overview2001.pdf

NIDA Research Report (journal)
National Institute on Drug Abuse
http://www.drugabuse.gov/ResearchReports/ResearchIndex.html

The Phoenix Newspaper
National Counseling Intervention Services, Inc.
http://www.phoenixrecovery.org

Straight Talk (series of publications)
Do-It-Now Foundation
http://www.doitnow.org/pages/straighttalk.html

Substance Abuse and Addiction
American Psychiatric Association
http://www.psych.org/public_info/substance.cfm

When Your Teen Is in Trouble with the Law
Focus Adolescent Services
http://www.focusas.com/JuvenileJustice.html

Why Adolescents Should Not Use Alcohol At All
Connecticut Clearinghouse
http://www.ctclearinghouse.org/fadol.pdf

Index

Index

Page numbers that appear in *Italics* refer to illustrations. Page numbers that have a small 'n' after the page number refer to information shown as Notes at the beginning of each chapter. Page numbers that appear in **Bold** refer to information contained in boxes on that page (except Notes information at the beginning of each chapter).

A

C

D

G

H

I

J

K

L

M

N

Q

R

X

Y

Z